£19·05

THE
COMPLETE
REVIEW OF
RADIOGRAPHY

THE
COMPLETE
REVIEW OF
RADIOGRAPHY

COAUTHORS

KATHRYN M. MARZANO, AS, RTR
Program Director
Hartford Hospital Radiologic Technology Program
Hartford, Connecticut

PAULINE D. LYONS, AS, RTR
Instructor
Hartford Hospital Radiologic Technology Program
Hartford, Connecticut

Library of Congress Cataloging in Publication Data:

Marzano, Kathryn M.
  The Complete Review of Radiography

  (A Wiley medical publication)
  1. Radiography, Medical—Examinations, questions,
etc. I. Lyons, Pauline D. II. Title. III. Series.
[DNLM: 1. Radiography—examination questions. WN 18 M393c]
RC78.15.M37 1986   616.07'57'076   86–9117
ISBN 0-471-80817-2

Printed in the United States of America

10 9 8 7 6 5 4 3 2 1

To Jerry Hrycyna
Our Mentor and Close Friend
With Love and Appreciation

Both authors wish to acknowledge the constructive suggestions provided by the reviewers of the original manuscript drafts. Our sincere appreciation and thanks to Drs. Arnold Janzen and William Lynch, and Physicists Larry Oresick and Robert Rice. We also extend our appreciation to our typists Ruth Catalano and Julie Kowalsky and a very special thank you to our families for their love and support throughout the writing of this manuscript.

CONTENTS

PREFACE

This book is designed to prepare the radiologic technology student or other registry-eligible individuals to take the National Registry Exam for Radiologic Technologists (A.R.R.T.). When used in conjunction with the references available, this book can help students assess their understanding of the major subject areas in radiologic technology, recognize deficient areas of knowledge, and introduce factual information extracted from its references.

This book may also be valuable to students in radiologic technology programs in preparing for individual course and final examinations and to adjunct allied health students in nuclear medicine, radiation therapy, and ultrasonography programs for self-assessment and individual course examination preparation.

Educators in the field of radiologic technology may find the organization of this question-answer analysis book instrumental in organizing tools for evaluating learning objectives for their students.

Staff Technologists as well as Radiology departmental inservice programs may benefit by this self-assessment model for remedial training and update.

The organization of this text is such that a pretest covering the five major subject areas can be taken first to assess entry-level comprehension of radiography. The body of the text offers a more copious selection of questions with referenced analysis inclusive of Anatomy and Physiology, Medical Terminology, Radiographic Positioning and Procedures, Radiographic Imaging and Equipment, Physics, Processing and Darkroom Chemistry, Radiation Protection and Radiobiology, Special Procedures and Pathology. The final post-test is designed to examine the student's progress and simulate the 200-question test administered by the A.R.R.T. All 600 questions are explained and referenced. It should be noted that the intention of this book is not that of a substitution for basic study in radiologic technology nor is it meant to replicate actual Registry questions.

Unlike many review books in radiography, this book offers thorough explanations and references to ALL multiple choice questions. New modalities in diagnostic imaging are also included such as: computed tomography and magnetic resonance imaging as well as quality assurance. Diagrams and radiographic representations are used in the questioning process accompanied by in-depth interpretations. All required physics and exposure equations are included with step-by-step solutions.

When used systematically with available references, it can enhance one's understanding of major subject areas as well as point out areas of inadequate preparation. The student can then refer to the reference for a more in-depth review.

ABBREVIATIONS AND SYMBOLS

A	ampere
AP	anteroposterior
cm	centimeter
CT	computed tomography
DNA	deoxyribonucleic acid
FFD	focus-film distance
FOD	focus-object distance
HVL	half value layer
Hz	hertz
keV	kilo electron volts
kV	kilovolts
kVp	kilovolts peak
kW	kilowatts
LAO	left anterior oblique
LET	linear energy transfer
LPO	left posterior oblique
μm	micrometer
mA	milliampere
mAs	milliampere seconds
meV	million electron volts
ml	milliliter
mm	millimeter
MPD	maximum permissible dose
mR	milliroentgen
mrad	millirad
mrem	millirem
mSv	milliseivert
nm	nanometer
OFD	object-film distance
OID	object-image distance
PA	posteroanterior
R	roentgen
rad	radiation absorbed dose
RAO	right anterior oblique
RBC	red blood cell
RBE	relative biologic effectiveness
rem	rad equivalent man
rpm	revolutions per minute
RPO	right posterior oblique
s	second
SID	source-image distance
V	volt
W	watt
WBC	white blood cell

PRETEST

ANATOMY AND PHYSIOLOGY
(including Medical Terminology and Pathology)

1. The imaginary plane that divides the body into equal left and right halves is the

    A. coronal or frontal
    B. sagittal
    C. median or midsagittal
    D. transverse or horizontal

2. Which of the following occur(s) during ventricular diastole?

    1. The semilunar valves remain closed
    2. The ventricles of the heart fill with blood
    3. The atrioventricular valves open

    A. 1 only
    B. 2 only
    C. 3 only
    D. 1, 2, and 3

3. Which of the following is NOT part of the functional units of the kidney, called nephrons?

    A. Glomerulus
    B. Trigone
    C. Convoluted tubules
    D. Bowman's capsule

4. The central nervous system comprises the brain and spinal cord. Which of the following statements are true concerning the spinal cord?

    1. It extends from the medulla oblongata to the level of the second lumbar vertebral body
    2. The cord gives rise to 12 pairs of spinal nerves
    3. The pia mater is a protective membrane in contact with the cord

    A. 1 and 2
    B. 1 and 3
    C. 2 and 3
    D. 1, 2, and 3

5. The eustachian tubes extend from the middle ear to the

    A. buccal cavity
    B. nasal cavity
    C. maxillary sinuses
    D. nasopharynx

6. The vital reflex centers that regulate heartbeat, breathing rate, and blood vessel diameter are located in the

    A. cerebellum
    B. cerebrum
    C. medulla
    D. pons

7. Which of the following vessels does NOT usually arise directly off the aortic arch?

    A. Left common carotid artery
    B. Brachiocephalic artery (innominate)
    C. Left subclavian artery
    D. Left vertebral artery

8. Cells are the basic structural units of the body and are responsible for carrying out vital life processes. The cell membrane allows for movement of substances into and out of the cell; these movements may involve passive (nonliving) or active (living) mechanisms. Which of the following processes involves active engulfment and digestion of solid particles?

    A. Dialysis
    B. Pinocytosis
    C. Filtration
    D. Phagocytosis

Questions 9–12 consist of four lettered headings followed by a list of numbered words. For each bony process or surface listed below, select the name of the bone on which it is located. Each lettered heading may be used once, more than once, or not at all.

    A. Tibia
    B. Fibula
    C. Femur
    D. Patella

9. Patellar surface

10. Intercondylar eminence

11. Lateral malleolus

12. Lesser trochanter

13. The most posterior part of the vertebral arch of a typical vertebra is called the

A. lamina
B. spinous process
C. pedicle
D. transverse process

14. The medical term for hives or skin eruption is

A. erythema
B. urticaria
C. petechiae
D. tinea

15. Which of the following statements regarding the function of the thyroid gland are true?

1. Its hormone secretions regulate the metabolism of proteins, fats, and carbohydrates in the body
2. Overactivity of the thyroid gland may produce restlessness, weight loss, exophthalmos, and goiters
3. Dietary deficiency of iodine may cause hypothyroidism

A. 1 and 2
B. 1 and 3
C. 2 and 3
D. 1, 2, and 3

16. All of the following bones form part of the bony orbit EXCEPT the

A. vomer
B. lacrimal
C. sphenoid
D. maxilla

17. In which of the following cranial types is the skull oval in shape, narrower in the front than the back, with the superior border of the petrous pyramids opening medially and forward at an angle of approximately 47° to the midsagittal plane?

A. Brachycephalic
B. Dolichocephalic
C. Mesocephalic
D. Macrocephalic

18. Which of the following are structural components of adult compact bone?

1. Haversian canals
2. Trabecular spaces filled with marrow
3. Lamellae

A. 1 and 2
B. 1 and 3
C. 2 and 3
D. 1, 2, and 3

19. Saliva is conveyed from the parotid glands to the oral cavity by way of which of the following ducts?

    A. Bartholin's
    B. Stensen's
    C. Santorini's
    D. Wharton's

20. All of the following are true statements concerning the large intestine EXCEPT that

    A. its proximal portion is called the cecum
    B. it is arranged in sacculated folds called haustra
    C. it contains numerous villi within its mucosal layer
    D. it absorbs water from remaining chyme

21. The visual receptor cells called rods are correctly described as

    1. much more sensitive to light than cones
    2. allowing color visualization
    3. allowing perception of detail sharpness

    A. 1 only
    B. 2 only
    C. 3 only
    D. 1, 2, and 3

22. The term that is best defined as "reduced blood supply to a body organ or tissues" is

    A. anemia
    B. infarction
    C. ischemia
    D. erythropenia

23. The human heart contains its own electric conduction system consisting of specialized cardiac muscle tissue that is responsible for initiating and conducting impulses that will eventually cause contraction of the heart chambers. All of the following are part of the heart's conduction system EXCEPT the

    A. chordae tendineae
    B. sinoatrial node
    C. Purkinje's fibers
    D. bundle of His

24. Which of the following bones are part of the visceral cranium?

    1. Ethmoid
    2. Zygomatic (malar)
    3. Palatine

    A. 1 and 2
    B. 1 and 3
    C. 2 and 3
    D. 1, 2, and 3

PRETEST—ANATOMY AND PHYSIOLOGY
ANSWERS, EXPLANATIONS, AND REFERENCES

1. The answer is C.   The diagrams in the following figure illustrate the imaginary planes that are used when positioning the body for various radiographic examinations:

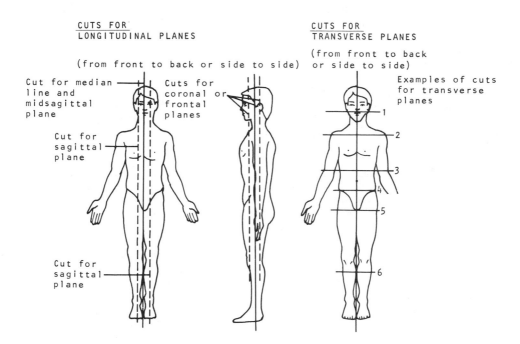

The median, or midsagittal, plane is a longitudinal plane passing down the center of the body from front to back, dividing the body into equal halves. The coronal, or frontal, plane is the imaginary plane that passes down the sides of the body at right angles to the median plane, dividing the body into front and back portions. A sagittal plane is any plane that runs parallel to the median (midsagittal) plane, dividing the body into unequal left and right portions. The transverse plane is a horizontal plane passing at right angles to the coronal and median plane, dividing the body into upper and lower portions. *(Austrin, p 50–51; Hole, p 152–154; Tortora and Anagnostakos, p 13–15)*

2. The answer is D.   During ventricular diastole (ventricles relaxed), the atrioventricular valves open to allow blood to flow through the atria into the ventricles. During this time, the pulmonary and aortic semilunar valves remain closed so that the ventricles can fill with blood. As the pressure in the ventricles builds up and contraction is initiated, ventricular systole occurs. The atrioventricular valves close and the semilunar valves open, allowing blood to flow into the aorta and pulmonary artery. *(Tortora and Anagnostakos, p 470; Hole, p 661–662)*

3. The answer is B.   Each kidney contains about 1 million functional units (nephrons), which are responsible for filtering out various constituents of the blood and urine. Each nephron comprises a tuft of capillaries, called a glomerulus, surrounded by a Bowman's capsule, which is an expansion of a renal tubule. The Bowman's capsules lead into a system of convoluted tubules, which include proximal and distal convoluted tubules and a Henle's loop. Blood from the renal artery is eventually brought to the glomerulus by way of an afferent arteriole and enters the efferent arteriole after passing through the coiled capillary tuft. Various components of the blood, including water and wastes, within the glomerulus are forced out into the Bowman's capsule. This marks the beginning of glomerular filtration. The filtrate passes into the Bowman's capsules and into the convoluted tubules of the nephron, where peritubular capillaries, surrounding the tubules, can reabsorb necessary components back into the bloodstream and secrete certain substances into the tubules. After passing through the tubules, urine enters the collecting ducts of the renal pyramids and then passes through papillae into the minor and major calyces, renal pelvis, and ureter, respectively. The trigone is not part of the nephron of the kidney; however, it is part of the base of the urinary bladder. This smooth triangular region does not contain rugae like the rest of the urinary bladder, and its angles are bounded by the two ureteral orifices and one urethral orifice. *(Hole, p 754–771; Tortora and Anagnostakos, p 661–671, 678)*

4. The answer is B. The spinal cord extends from the lower portion of the brain called the medulla oblongata through the vertebral canal, tapering at about the level of the second lumbar vertebra. The tapered portion of the cord is referred to as the conus medullaris, and the numerous inferior nerve extensions from the end of the cord are collectively called the cauda equina. As the spinal cord passes through the vertebral foramina, it gives rise to 31 pairs of spinal nerves. The spinal cord is surrounded by three protective membranes, called meninges; the innermost meninx is called the pia mater, the middle meninx—the arachnoid, and the outer membrane—the dura mater. The meninges not only surround and protect the cord but cover the brain as well. The spinal cord is extremely important for the maintenance of homeostasis, as it conducts impulses in both directions between the brain and periphery and also serves to coordinate reflexes. *(Hole, p 338–341; Tortora and Anagnostakos, p 288–294)*

5. The answer is D. The eustachian, or auditory, tubes are passageways for air between the middle ear and the nasopharynx. The function of this tube is to equalize pressure on either side of the tympanic membrane. Sudden internal or external pressure changes could cause rupture of the tympanic membrane and hearing impairment in the absence of the eustachian tube, which opens to allow air to pass into or out of the middle ear during swallowing, yawning, or chewing. Abrupt altitude changes demonstrate the pressure-equalizing capabilities of the eustachian tubes: when the forced passage of air equalizes the pressure on either side of the eardrum membrane, the ear "pops" and hearing is improved. *(Hole, p 403; Tortora and Anagnostakos, p 389)*

6. The answer is C. The medulla (oblongata) is the expanded portion of the spinal cord above the foramen magnum, forming the lower brain, or brain stem, which contains the cardiac and vasomotor centers and the medullary rhythmicity region. Besides its function in regulating heartbeat, breathing rate, and blood vessel contraction, the medulla oblongata gives rise to seven pairs of cranial nerves and houses the reticular formation. The medulla also serves to conduct motor and sensory impulses between the spinal cord and brain. The cerebellum controls motor coordination and balance, whereas the cerebrum's numerous functions include memory; behavior; muscular movements; and emotional, intellectual, and sensory interpretation. The pons (varoli), located above the medulla in the brain stem, is a conduction pathway between the cerebrum and cerebellum, the brain and spinal cord, and other parts of the brain with one another. The pons, along with the medulla, controls respiration. *(Hole, p 348–362; Tortora and Anagnostakos, p 315–331)*

7. The answer is D. The left vertebral artery, as well as the right vertebral artery, originates from the subclavian arteries at the base of the neck. The brachiocephalic artery is the first branch off the aortic arch and is located slightly right of the midline; it supplies blood to the right arm and head. The left common carotid is the second (middle) branch of the aortic arch, which supplies blood to the left side of the head and brain. The left subclavian artery is the third branch, which supplies blood to the left shoulder and arm. *(Hole, p 691; Tortora and Anagnostakos, p 496)*

8. The answer is D. Phagocytosis involves the active process of cell eating; it is through this process that the WBCs of the body engulf and destroy bacteria and other foreign substances, constituting a vital defense mechanism. Pinocytosis is an active process similar to phagocytosis but involves cell drinking and engulfment of liquids rather than solids. Filtration is a passive process involving movement of materials into and out of cells as a result of a pressure gradient, with flow occurring from areas of high concentration to low. Dialysis is another passive process of diffusion, involving the separation of small from large molecules by a semipermeable membrane, as occurs in hemodialysis for treatment of kidney failure. *(Tortora and Anagnostakos, p 54–57; Hole, p 56–62)*

9–12. The answers are 9-C, 10-A, 11-B, 12-C. The bones of the right pelvic girdle and lower extremity are illustrated in the following figure:

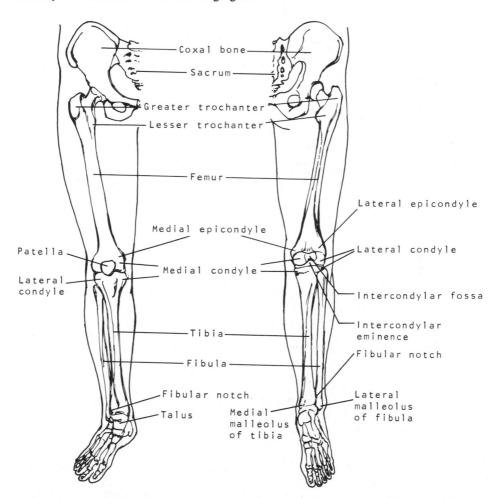

The femur, or thigh bone, is the largest bone in the body. At its upper end is a rounded head, which articulates with the acetabulum of the coxal (pelvic) bone. Below the head is a constricted area, or neck. Where the neck joins the shaft are two large processes, a superior lateral process (greater trochanter) and a lower medial process (lesser trochanter). These large processes attach to muscles in the thigh and buttocks. The shaft represents the long body of the femur, and its distal end gives rise to two rounded processes, called medial and lateral condyles, which articulate with the tibia. Above the condyles are medial and lateral epicondyles, providing attachments for muscles and ligaments of the leg. Between the condyles on the posterior surface of the femur is a depression called the intercondylar fossa, and on its anterior surface between the condyles is the patellar surface. The patella is a triangular sesamoid bone situated anterior to the knee joint. Its upper broad surface is called the base, and its lower pointed end is the apex. The posterior surface of the patella contains two articular facets for the medial and lateral condyles of the femur. The tibia (shinbone), or large medial bone of the lower leg, bears most of the weight of the leg. The upper end of the tibia has expanded processes (medial and lateral condyles); their concave surfaces articulate with the condyles of the femur. The lateral condyle of the tibia also articulates with the head of the fibula. The condyles of the tibia are separated by an upward bony projection called the intercondylar eminence. The distal end of the tibia expands into a medial prominence called the medial malleolus, which articulates with the talus bone of the ankle; on the lateral side of the distal tibia is a depression (fibular notch), which articulates with the fibula. The fibula is the thinner lateral bone of the lower leg. Its upper end, or head, articulates with the tibia, and its lower end gives rise to a prominence called the lateral malleolus, which also articulates with the talus bone of the ankle; the lower fibula also articulates with the fibular notch of the tibia. The fibula does not enter into the knee joint and does not bear weight. *(Hole, p 221–224; Meschan, p 104–109, 115–116; Tortora and Anagnostakos, p 171–174)*

13. The answer is B.   The spinous process, the most posterior portion of the vertebral arch, can often be palpated in the midline through the skin of the back. A typical vertebra consists of a drum-shaped body anteriorly and a ringlike portion called the vertebral arch, which surrounds the spinal cord, posteriorly. The pedicles arise from the upper lateral part of the posterior surface of the body, forming the sides of the vertebral foramen. The laminae are broad and flat and arise from the pedicles posteriorly, where they unite medially, giving rise to the spinous process. The transverse processes project bilaterally and toward the back between the pedicles and laminae. The processes of the vertebrae offer attachment to various ligaments and muscles throughout the spine. *(Ballinger [Vol. 1], p 203; Hole, p 205–206; Tortora and Anagnostakos, p 151–155)*

14. The answer is B.   Urticaria is a skin eruption in the form of hives or raised wheals, which may produce itching. Urticaria is a common allergic reaction that may occur following intravenous injection of radiographic contrast media, as well as other medications. Other causes of urticaria include foreign proteins, contact with irritating substances, foods, and insect bites. Erythema is reddening of the skin, possibly resulting from excessive radiation exposure. Petechiae are small pinpoint hemorrhages due to bleeding into the dermis. Tinea, or ringworm, is a fungus infection of the skin. *(Austrin, p 114, 116; Cawson et al., p 316, 467, 478–479, 482; Wroble, p 223, 232)*

15. The answer is D.   The thyroid, a gland of the endocrine system, is located in the neck inferior and lateral to the thyroid cartilage, which covers the larynx anteriorly. The thyroid secretes two major hormones—thyroxine and triiodothyronine. Thyroid hormones are important in regulating metabolism of proteins, fats, and carbohydrates, along with regulating tissue growth and development and nervous system activity. Thyroid overactivity or hypersecretion (hyperthyroidism) may cause an enlargement of the gland called a goiter and may produce symptoms of restlessness and weight loss due to increased metabolic rate. A goiter may also form in patients with hypothyroidism and thyroiditis. Protrusion of the eyeballs, or exophthalmos, is also a symptom of hyperthyroidism. An *underactive* thyroid does not secrete enough thyroid hormones, resulting in hypothyroidism. Dietary deficiency of iodine may inhibit sufficient production of thyroxine and may lead to hypothyroidism. The thyroid gland also secretes calcitonin, which helps to regulate calcium levels in the blood. *(Cawson et al., p 449–453; Hole, p 451–454; Tortora and Anagnostakos, p 412–415)*

16. The answer is A.   The bony orbit, which forms the cavity around the eyeball, is composed of a few cranial bones, including the frontal, ethmoid, and sphenoid bones, along with several facial bones—the maxilla, zygomatic, palatine, and lacrimal bones. The vomer does not enter into the orbital cavity but does form the inferior part of the bony nasal septum and floor of the nasal cavity. The orbit consists of an upper roof, a lower floor, and medial and lateral walls. The orbits not only secure the eyeballs but also allow for the passage of blood vessels and nerves. *(Ballinger [Vol. 2], p 374–375, 402; Meschan, p 235)*

17. The answer is C.   It is important for the radiologic technologist to be able to recognize various skull types, as alterations in positioning of the skull may be necessary in order to demonstrate various structures radiographically. The mesocephalic skull is considered to be the average contour. It is relatively oval in shape, narrower in the front than the back, with the upper border of its petrous pyramids opening medially and anteriorly, at an angle of about 47° to the midsagittal plane. The brachycephalic skull is wide from side to side, short form front to back, and short from top to bottom. The internal cranial structures of this type of skull tend to be higher in position than in the mesocephalic skull, and the superior ridge of its petrous pyramids form an angle of about 54° to the midsagittal plane. The dolichocephalic skull has a long, narrow contour; its anterior-posterior measurement is greater than that of the mesocephalic and brachycephalic types. The upper border of the petrous pyramids in the dolichocephalic skull forms a 40° angle to the midsagittal plane, and its anterior cranial structures are lower in position than in the other skull types. An abnormally large head in relation to the rest of the body is described as macrocephalic and is usually a congenital anomaly. *(Ballinger [Vol. 2], p 377–379; Thompson, p 234–236)*

18. The answer is B.   Compact bone is different from spongy bone in that it is arranged in a pattern of concentric rings called lamellae, which surround the haversian canals (longitudinal passageways for blood capillaries). Lacunae are found between the lamellae and contain bone cells called osteocytes. Tiny canaliculi, which extend outward from these lacunae, connect other lacunae and then merge with the haversian canals, forming a microscopic network, or haversian system, through which nutrients and wastes can pass. Compact bone is strong and dense and is found mainly in the wall of the diaphysis of bones. Spongy (cancellous) bone does not have haversian systems but contains trabeculae, spicules of bone forming a latticework throughout which red marrow is sometimes contained. Spongy bone is not as dense as compact bone and is found in epiphyses of long bones and between compact bone of the type that is short, flat, and irregular. *(Hole, p 177–178; Tortora and Anagnostakos, p 126–127)*

19. The answer is B.   The parotid glands are the two large salivary glands situated below and anterior to the ears. The parotid glands secrete saliva, which passes down the Stensen's duct and opens into the mouth. The other major salivary glands include the submandibular (submaxillary) glands, which are located on the floor of the mouth, internal to the mandible, and the sublingual glands, which are found under the tongue on the floor of the mouth. The submandibular and sublingual glands also secrete saliva, which is conveyed to the oral cavity by way of the Wharton's and Bartholin's ducts, respectively. Saliva contains materials that help dissolve food, along with salivary amylase, an enzyme that begins the breakdown of starch. The parotid gland is mainly responsible for this enzyme secretion. Salivary secretions are controlled by the nervous system, which receives stimuli from food (the taste, smell, sight, sound, and feel of it). The duct of Santorini is the accessory pancreatic duct, which enters the duodenum. *(Ballinger [Vol. 2], p 525; Chaffee et al., p 438, 448; Hole, p 488–489)*

20. The answer is C.   The large intestine does not contain villi, distinguishing it from the small intestine. The first portion of the large intestine is the cecum, which joins it to the last segment of the small intestine at a point called the ileocecal valve. The taenia coli are the longitudinal muscle bands that exert tension on the large intestine, creating a sacculated appearance of folds called haustra. Water and electrolytes are absorbed by the large intestine, although most absorption in the gastrointestinal tract occurs in the small intestine through numerous villi. *(Hole, p 515–518; Tortora and Anagnostakos, p 618–620; Chaffee et al., p 441–442, 453–454)*

21. The answer is A. The retina contains two types of visual receptor cells, rods and cones. Rods allow us to see in dim light as they are hundreds of times more sensitive than the cones. The rods do not perceive color; this is a function of the cones. The rods are not responsible for perception of image sharpness; they only allow us to visualize general outlines of objects, distinguishing their function from the cones. *(Tortora and Anagnostakos, p 382–383; Hole, p 423–426; Chaffee et al., p 271)*

22. The answer is C. Ischemia is the lack of blood supply to body tissues as a result of circulatory obstruction. Obstruction of a blood vessel may be caused by formation of blood clots (thrombosis), embolus, extrinsic pressure, or atherosclerosis. Ischemia can lead to an infarction, or death of tissue. Anemia is a condition in which there is an abnormally decreased amount of hemoglobin (an essential component of RBCs) in the circulating blood. This may result from increased rate of RBC destruction, underproduction of hemoglobin or RBCs, or hemorrhage. Erythropenia is a deficiency in the number of RBCs present. *(Cawson et al., p 174–175, 185)*

23. The answer is A. The chordae tendineae are the fibrous strands that originate from the papillary muscles of the left and right cardiac ventricles and attach to the atrioventricular valve leaflets, serving to secure closure of these valves when appropriate. The sinoatrial node, also called the pacemaker, is located in the right atrial wall; its cells are responsible for initiating impulses 60 to 80 times per minute and stimulating cardiac muscle contraction. These impulses eventually reach the atrioventricular node, located near the interatrial septum, and then travel to the bundle of His (atrioventricular bundle), located in the interventricular septum. The bundle of His gives off left and right bundle branches, which eventually give rise to the Purkinje's fibers, which conduct impulses to terminal cardiac fibers in the myocardium (muscle wall of the heart) and cause the ventricles to contract. *(Hole, p 655, 663–664; Tortora and Anagnostakos, p 463–464; Chaffee et al., p 317–318)*

24. The answer is C. The visceral cranium contains 14 facial bones. Of these, two are zygomatic (malar) bones and two are palatine bones. The facial bones give the face shape and provide attachment sites for muscles involved in chewing and facial expressions. The remaining bones of the visceral cranium include two of each of the following: nasal, lacrimal, maxillae, and inferior nasal conchae (turbinates), along with one mandible and the vomer. The ethmoid is a bone of the cranial vault, or calvaria; it is one of eight bones that form a protective shell around the brain. *(Ballinger [Vol. 2], p 362–375; Hole, p 197–203; Tortora and Anagnostakos, p 138–150)*

RADIOGRAPHIC POSITIONING AND PROCEDURES

25. In the PA and oblique projections of the hand, the central ray is directed

A. perpendicular to the navicular bone
B. perpendicular to the third metacarpophalangeal joint
C. at an angle of 5° toward the wrist through the third proximal interphalangeal joint
D. at an angle of 20° toward the fingers through the navicular bone

26. The average difference between the orbitomeatal (radiographic) line and the infraorbito-meatal (Reid's) line is

A. 5°
B. 7°
C. 8°
D. 10°

27. Which of the following statements regarding the use of radiographic contrast agents is FALSE?

A. Atomic number is a factor in the choice of agents
B. Rapid absorption or excretion by the body is advantageous
C. Similar density to the radiographed organ enhances contrast
D. Hollow organs require the use of contrast media

28. Which of the following projections would best demonstrate the tail of the breast?

A. Axillary
B. Craniocaudal
C. Mediolateral
D. Lateromedial

29. The pulmonary apices may be demonstrated below the level of the clavicular shadows in which of the following projections?

1. AP lordotic
2. PA axial
3. AP axial

A. 1 only
B. 1 and 2
C. 1 and 3
D. 2 and 3

30. The central ray is directed 15° caudad and 15° anterior in the cranial radiography method developed by

A. Caldwell
B. Law
C. Hickey
D. Valdini

31. In an AP projection of the cervical vertebrae, the mouth may be opened in order to

A. visualize the fourth through seventh cervical vertebrae
B. open up the intervertebral foramina
C. demonstrate the atlas and axis
D. demonstrate the posterior elements of the upper cervical vertebrae

32. The cause of stress incontinence in females may be accurately evaluated by which of the following radiographic examinations?

A. Chain cystourethrography
B. Retrograde cystography
C. Double-contrast cystography
D. Percutaneous nephrostomy

33. The odontoid process may be demonstrated radiographically by which of the following methods?

1. AP projection, chin extended, central ray perpendicular
2. PA projection, head resting on extended chin, central ray perpendicular
3. Tomography

A. 1 and 2
B. 1 and 3
C. 2 and 3
D. 1, 2, and 3

34. Supine chest radiographs are often performed when patients are too ill or incapacitated to be positioned erect. Which of the following statements comparing PA erect versus AP supine positions of the chest is FALSE?

A. The thoracic organs will be more compressed in the AP projection/supine position
B. Air-fluid levels will not be demonstrated on the AP projection/supine position
C. Heart magnification will be greater on the PA projection/erect position
D. The clavicles will assume a higher position in the AP projection/supine position

35. The technique most often employed for selective catheter introduction for aortography is that developed by

A. Dotter
B. Seldinger
C. Gruntzig
D. Franklin

36. Which of the following methods and projections would produce the skull radiograph shown below?

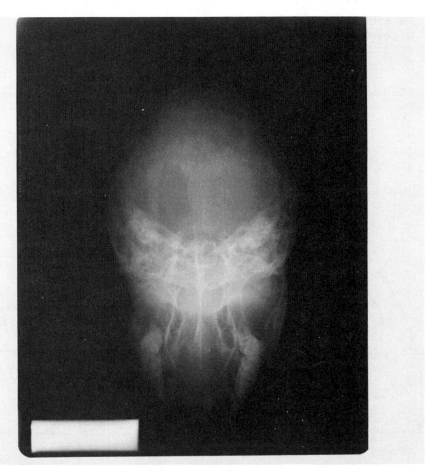

    A. PA axial projection/Caldwell method
    B. Semiaxial AP projection/Towne, or Grashey, method
    C. PA projection/Waters method
    D. Submentovertex projection/Schüller method

37. Of all the carpal bones, the navicular is most often fractured. In order to demonstrate the navicular free of superimposition, it is necessary to

       1. rotate the hand laterally to assume ulnar flexion
       2. direct the central ray at an angle of 20° toward the elbow
       3. rotate the hand medially to assume radial flexion

    A. 1 and 2
    B. 1 and 3
    C. 2 and 3
    D. 1, 2, and 3

38. Medial or lateral displacement of fractures of the nasal bones are best demonstrated in which of the following projections?

  A. Lateral
  B. Superoinferior axial
  C. Transcranial
  D. Semiaxial

39. The diagram pictured below demonstrates which of the following projections and/or methods?

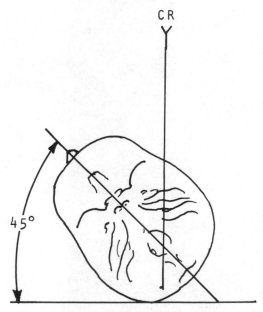 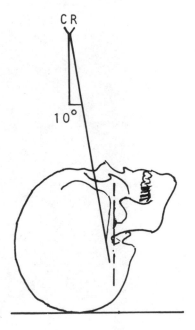

Table radiography

  A. Anterior profile/Arcelin method
  B. Chaussé III method
  C. Parietotemporal/Low-Beer method
  D. Axiolateral oblique/Mayer method

40. Intravenous cholangiography is performed using

          1. aqueous iodinated contrast
          2. biliary compression
          3. tomography

  A. 1 and 2
  B. 1 and 3
  C. 2 and 3
  D. 1, 2, and 3

41. The apophyseal joints of the thoracic spine are best demonstrated by positioning patients in

    A. a true lateral position
    B. an oblique position, rotating them 45° from the supine position
    C. an AP erect position
    D. a steep 70° oblique position

42. The best position for an unobstructed view of the rectum is

    A. LPO
    B. lateral
    C. PA angle shot
    D. prone

43. When radiographing the joint space of the knee for an AP projection, the central ray is directed at what angle through the joint?

    A. 0°
    B. 5° cephalad
    C. 7° caudad
    D. 15° cephalad

44. The sternoclavicular joints are radiographed with the patient positioned

    A. from the prone position, they are obliqued so that the affected side is down
    B. laterally, with the affected side down
    C. supine and prone
    D. from the prone position, they are obliqued so that the affected side is up

45. Which of the following types of contrast media are employed in myelography?

    1. Negative—gaseous medium
    2. Positive—aqueous iodinated medium
    3. Positive—oily iodinated medium

    A. 1 and 2
    B. 1 and 3
    C. 2 and 3
    D. 1, 2, and 3

Questions 46–48. For each position or projection listed below, select the radiographic study in which it is most often used. Each lettered heading may be used once, more than once, or not at all.

    A. Small bowel series
    B. Hypotonic duodenography
    C. Air-contrast barium enema
    D. Rectosigmoid junction

46. Chassard-Lapiné position

47. Decubitus position

48. Interval films

PRETEST—RADIOGRAPHIC POSITIONING AND PROCEDURES
ANSWERS, EXPLANATIONS, AND REFERENCES

25. The answer is B. For both PA and oblique projections of the hand, the central ray is directed perpendicular to the film through the third metacarpophalangeal joint. For the PA projection, the hand is placed palm down with the forearm in contact with the table. This projection demonstrates the carpals, metacarpals, and phalanges of the distal upper extremity and the lower portions of the radius and ulna. For the PA oblique projection of the hand, the metacarpophalangeal joints are positioned so that they form a 45° angle to the film, with the fifth finger side down. The oblique projection is often used as a routine projection of the hand and wrist in addition to the PA and lateral projections. *(Ballinger [Vol. 1], p 122, 125; Bontrager and Anthony, p 86)*

26. The answer is B. The difference between the orbitomeatal (radiographic) line and the infraorbitomeatal (Reid's) line is an average of 7°. The orbitomeatal line runs from the outer canthus of the eye to the external auditory meatus, and the infraorbitomeatal line is located inferior to this, running from the infraorbital margin to the external auditory meatus. These localization lines are used extensively in radiographic positioning of the skull. Various radiographic projections specify the relationship of these anatomic lines (or the planes they represent) in relation to the plane of the central ray or the film. The following diagrams represent various localization lines. *(Ballinger [Vol. 2], p 377; Bontrager and Anthony, p 194):*

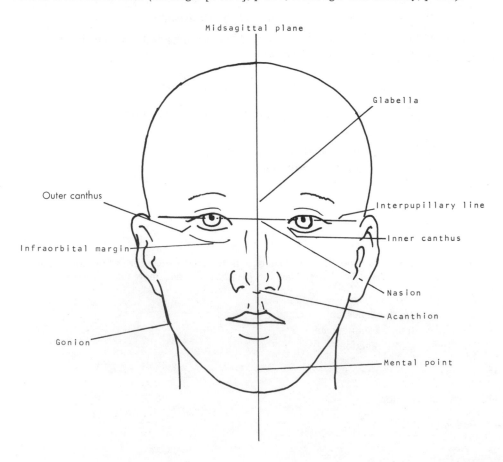

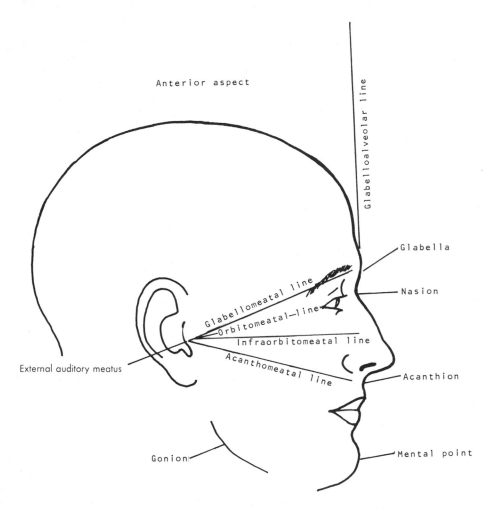

27. The answer is C. Contrast agents used for radiography should be of greater or lesser density than the organs in which they are employed, to allow maximum visualization of the organ radiographically. The reason for using contrast agents is based on the fact that some organs and tissues do not have sufficient density or provide adequate contrast to adjacent tissues to be visualized without the introduction of a positive or negative contrast medium. Ideally, a contrast agent is chosen for demonstration of a body part according to its atomic number, which should be less than or greater than the organ undergoing investigation. For example, if the bronchial lumen is to be radiographed, a positive contrast agent, one with a significantly higher atomic number and density than the wall of the bronchi and the air within its lumen, is needed to demonstrate it radiographically. Hollow organs require the use of contrast agents because they do not produce a significant density shadow themselves as compared with the adjacent tissue. Contrast agents should be of minimal toxicity and should not alter body function, and they should be absorbed, excreted, or easily removed from the body. *(Chesney and Chesney [1978], p 39–52; Torres and Morrill, p 153–160)*

28. The answer is A. The axillary projection demonstrates the tail of the breast to the best advantage, along with the tissues in the superior outer quadrant and axillary lymph node region. This projection can be performed with the patient recumbent or erect. The image receptor is placed under the side being examined, the arm of that same side is abducted so that it forms a 90° angle to the body, and the patient is rotated slightly toward the side being examined. The central ray is directed perpendicularly. The chest wall and proximal humerus are included in this projection, as well as the entire breast, which should not be compressed. Though the axillary projection is not usually one of the routine projections of the breast, it is often used in addition to the two right-angle projections for supplementary information, especially when the axilla and tail of the breast need to be visualized. *(Ballinger [Vol. 3], p 752; Bontrager and Anthony, p 341)*

29. The answer is C. The AP lordotic and AP axial projections will demonstrate the apices of the lungs below the shadows of the clavicles. In the AP lordotic projection, the patient is positioned erect so that the superior portion of the back is in contact with the film holder and the body is approximately 1 foot in front of the film holder. The central ray is directed perpendicularly to the midsagittal plane and midsternum. The AP axial projection is performed with the patient's back flat against the film holder in either the erect or supine position, and the central ray is directed at an angle of 15 to 20° cephalad, entering the midsagittal plane at the level of the second thoracic vertebra (or about the level of the suprasternal notch). The PA axial projection will demonstrate the pulmonary apices above the level of the clavicular shadows. *(Ballinger [Vol. 3], p 592–594; Bontrager and Anthony, p 49)*

30. The answer is B. The original Law's method requires a true lateral position of the patient's cranium and a 15° caudad and 15° anterior angulation of the central ray for an axiolateral projection of the mastoid cells, portions of the pars petrosa, and superimposition of the internal and external auditory meatuses. This method may be modified to use a single angulation by rotating the patient's head from a true lateral position so that the midsagittal plane is turned 15° toward the film and the central ray is directed 15° caudad, through a point 2 inches superior and posterior to the external auditory meatus. The side nearest to the film is radiographed, and both sides are then examined for comparison. The auricles of the ears are usually taped forward to prevent projecting their dense shadow over the mastoid cells. Law's projection is sometimes used for radiographing the temporomandibular joints. *(Ballinger [Vol. 2], p 430–431; Bontrager and Anthony, p 252, 259)*

31. The answer is C. An AP projection of the cervical spine with the patient's mouth open as much as possible is taken in order to demonstrate the lateral masses of the atlas (C-1) and the body and odontoid process of the axis (C-2). A conventional AP projection of the cervical spine, with the mouth closed, will not allow for visualization of the upper cervical segments, as the shadow of the mandible superimposes the first and second cervical vertebrae. For an open-mouth AP projection, the patient is placed supine, with the mouth open wide and the head adjusted in order to line up the tips of the upper incisors and mastoid process so that they form a line perpendicular to the film, or to displace the radiological baseline 5 to 10° cephalad. The central ray is directed at right angles to the film, through the middle of the open mouth. The exposure is taken as the patient phonates and the head and neck are kept motionless. *(Ballinger [Vol. 1], p 212; Bontrager and Anthony, p 314)*

32. The answer is A. Chain cystourethrography is a radiographic study of the relationship of the urinary bladder floor to the urethrovesical angle during relaxed and straining states. This examination involves the installation of a metallic bead chain and introduction of an opaque iodinated contrast medium by way of a catheter, through the urethra and into the bladder. The superior portion of the chain rests on the bladder floor, and the lowermost portion of the chain is secured to the thigh. Following installation of the chain and contrast medium, the catheter is removed and lateral and PA projections are taken, usually with the patient erect, while straining (bearing down as in the Valsalva maneuver) and relaxed. This examination is useful in demonstrating the anatomic changes of the bladder and urethra associated with stress incontinence (involuntary voiding during increased abdominal stress as induced by coughing, sneezing, and laughing). Retrograde cystography and double-contrast cystography are radiographic examinations of the urinary bladder following introduction of contrast via a catheter. The urethra is not demonstrated in either of these examinations unless the patient voids the contrast during radiography. Percutaneous nephrostomy is a special procedure performed to relieve an obstruction in the collecting system of a kidney. Following antegrade pyelography, a needle is placed through the posterolateral aspect of the back and directed into the upper collecting system of the affected kidney. A guide wire and catheter may then be placed into the collecting system for introduction of contrast media or for urinary drainage, or a ureteral stent (special perforated catheter tubing) may be installed for drainage and relief of obstruction in a ureter. *(Ballinger [Vol. 3], p 710–715; Bontrager and Anthony, p 514–515; Katzen, p 132–135)*

33. The answer is D. The odontoid process can be radiographically demonstrated by various methods. An AP projection (Fuchs method), with the chin extended and central ray directed perpendicular to a point just inferior to the chin and midsagittal plane will demonstrate the odontoid process within the foramen magnum shadow. A PA projection (Judd method) with the patient prone and the head resting on the extended chin so that the nose is about an inch from the table, with the central ray directed through the occiput at right angles to the film, will again show the odontoid process within the shadow of the foramen magnum. These AP and PA projections are not recommended for patients with a suspected or diagnosed fracture or degenerative disease of the cervical region. Tomography is useful in demonstrating the odontoid and other areas of the spine and can be performed relatively easily on patients with suspected or diagnosed injury or disease. Tomography enables superimposing structures to be blurred out of the plane of interest and helps to bring fractures more clearly into view for more accurate localization. Other projections that may be used to demonstrate the odontoid and upper cervical spine include AP with open mouth, wagging jaw, and oblique projections. *(Ballinger [Vol. 1], p 212–217)*

34. The answer is C. Heart magnification is greater on an AP projection/supine position of the chest because of the usual shorter focus-film distance (FFD) employed, as well as the greater distance of the object (heart) from the film plane. The heart is located more anteriorly in the body, so the patient should be positioned with the anterior aspect closest to the film, as in a PA projection. Increased object-film distance (OFD) and decreased FFD contribute to increased magnification. Ideally, chest radiographs should be taken at a long FFD (72 inches or greater), and the patient should be positioned for a PA erect position. The PA projection/erect position will reduce compression of the thoracic organs because the diaphragm can drop to its lowest position; the clavicles and shoulders will assume a lower position, and the horizontal x-ray beam will allow demonstration of air-fluid levels. *(Ballinger [Vol. 3], p 591; Bontrager and Anthony, p 37–38)*

35. The answer is B. The Seldinger technique is most frequently used for catheter aortography. It requires the use of a specially designed needle for percutaneous arterial puncture. Following this puncture, a guide wire is introduced through the needle and into the artery. The needle is then removed, and a catheter is passed over the guide wire and manipulated into the desired vessel location under fluoroscopic control. Once the catheter is in the proper place, the guide wire is removed and contrast medium is injected, followed by serial filming. Dotter and Gruntzig are the eponyms used for describing two techniques of transluminal angioplasty, and Franklin is the eponym used for a type of film changer and head unit for radiography. Most techniques were named after the individuals who brought them into use for radiography. *(Ballinger [Vol. 3], p 804, 806; Tortorici, p 141–142, 146–149, 280; Snopek, p 205–206)*

36. The answer is B. The radiograph that accompanies the question represents the semiaxial AP projection of the skull using the Towne, or Grashey, method. For this projection, the patient is positioned supine or erect, with the orbitomeatal line and midsagittal plane at right angles to the film. The central ray is directed at an angle of 30° caudad, entering a point approximately 3 to 4 cm above the nasion and through the midsagittal plane. This projection demonstrates the occipital bone, petrous pyramids, and the posterior foramen magnum, with the posterior clinoid processes within its shadow. *(Ballinger [Vol. 2], p 386–387; Bontrager and Anthony, p 204; Meschan, p 232)*

37. The answer is A. In order to project the navicular, or scaphoid, bone free of superimposition, the hand is placed palm down and turned laterally so that ulnar flexion may be achieved. The central ray can be directed perpendicular to the film, with the hand elevated at an angle of 20° incline to the horizon. Alternatively, the central ray may be directed at an angle of 20° toward the elbow, with the hand and film horizontal. *(Ballinger [Vol. 1], p 133, 135; Bontrager and Anthony, p 89)*

38. The answer is B. Superoinferior axial or tangential projections of the nasal bones will demonstrate medial and lateral displacement of fractured nasal bones to the best advantage. This projection, however, may not yield visualization of the nasal bones in all patients, especially those with small noses, prominent foreheads, and/or protruding upper front teeth. Superoinferior axial or tangential projections are performed with an occlusal (nonscreen) film placed in the patient's mouth or a cassette placed under the patient's chin. The central ray is directed perpendicular to the film, passing through the glabella and midsagittal plane. Lateral projections usually are routinely performed in examination of the nasal bones; although the nasal bone nearest to the film is well seen, medial or lateral displacement is not. Because the Waters projection (parietoacanthial) is often employed in the radiographic examination of the facial bones, it is also useful in demonstrating the nasal septum. Transcranial and semiaxial projections are not usually employed in routine radiography of the nasal bones. *(Ballinger [Vol. 2], p 468, 474–477; Bontrager and Anthony, p 226–228)*

39. The answer is A. The diagram that accompanies the question represents the anterior profile projection using the Arcelin method. This projection may be used to demonstrate a profile image of the pars petrosa, as well as the mastoid process, tympanic cavity, internal auditory canal, and petrous ridge. It is the reverse of the Stenvers posterior profile projection and produces similar radiographic results. In the Arcelin method, the supine patient is rotated away from the side being examined so that the midsagittal plane of the cranium forms an angle of 45° to the film plane and the infraorbitomeatal line is placed perpendicular to the film. The central ray is directed 10 to 12° caudad, entering a point about 1 inch in front and three-quarters of an inch above the uppermost external auditory meatus. *(Ballinger [Vol. 2], p 449; Bontrager and Anthony, p 262)*

40. The answer is B. Intravenous cholangiography is performed after intravenous injection (bolus or infusion) of aqueous iodinated contrast medium. This special contrast medium passes through the liver, where it is excreted along with bile, thereby opacifying the biliary ductal system. Tomography is most often employed in conjunction with this procedure in order to enhance visualization of the sometimes minimally opacified ducts. Tomography enables better visualization of details in the objective plane by blurring out superimposing gas, bone, and soft-tissue structures. The patient is placed in a 15 to 30° RPO position for the examination period, and films of the right upper quadrant are taken at various intervals following contrast injection. Compression is not applied to the bile ducts, but an immobilization device may be applied to the patient to secure the position and prevent motion. *(Ballinger [Vol. 3], p 624–627; Bontrager and Anthony, p 488, 496)*

41. The answer is D. In order to demonstrate the thoracic apophyseal joints, the body must be placed in a steep 70° oblique position from the horizontal. From the lateral position, the patient is rotated 20° forward for the RAO and LAO; this will demonstrate the apophyseal joints closest to the film. For the RPO and LPO, the patient is rotated 20° backward from the lateral position in order to demonstrate the apophyseal joints farthest from the film. The patient can be placed into any of these positions while standing or recumbent. A steep oblique position is required for the demonstration of the thoracic apophyseal joints, as they form about a 70° angle, opening forward to the midsagittal plane of the body. The true lateral position is used in order to demonstrate the intervertebral foramina of the thoracic spine, as they lie perpendicular to the median or midsagittal plane of the body. *(Ballinger [Vol. 1], p 207, 233–234; Bontrager and Anthony, p 307)*

42. The answer is B. The lateral position demonstrates the rectum without superimposition of other bowel segments and for this reason is usually included in the routine barium enema examination. The patient is adjusted to a true lateral recumbent position, both legs together and knees slightly flexed. The central ray is directed perpendicularly to a point 2 inches behind the midaxillary or midcoronal plane and about 2 inches above the symphysis pubis. The rectum, rectosigmoid junction, and presacral region can be seen on this projection. *(Ballinger [Vol. 3], p 683; Bontrager and Anthony, p 475)*

43. The answer is B. In the AP projection of the knee joint, the central ray is directed to a point just below the patellar apex at an angle of 5° cephalad. The patient is placed in the supine position, and the leg is extended. The proximal tibia and fibula, distal femur, and joint space are demonstrated in this projection. The knee joint can also be radiographed with the patient prone for a PA projection; the central ray is directed perpendicular to the joint for this projection. *(Ballinger [Vol. 1], p 67–68; Bontrager and Anthony, p 160)*

44. The answer is A. PA oblique projections (RAO and LAO positions) are most often used as part of the routine examination of the sternoclavicular joints. The patient is placed in the prone position and rotated so that the affected side is down, close to the film. The central ray is directed perpendicular to the joint and film at about the level of the fourth thoracic vertebra. Both the LAO and RAO positions are performed so that both joints can be examined and compared. A similar projection can be obtained with the patient prone and the central ray angled obliquely (from the side) about 15° toward the midline, through the sternoclavicular joint of interest. Only a slight amount of obliquity or angulation is usually required to project the sternoclavicular joints away from the vertebral shadows. *(Ballinger [Vol. 1], p 192)*

45. The answer is D. Myelography is the radiographic study of central nervous system structures within the spinal canal. For this examination, a contrast agent is injected by way of a direct puncture into the subarachnoid space. A variety of contrast agents may be employed for this study, including gas (gas myelography), aqueous iodinated (opaque myelography), or oily iodinated (opaque myelography). One contrast agent is used for each myelogram. Each contrast agent has its advantages and disadvantages. Oily iodinated provides excellent opacification but should be removed from the subarachnoid space after the radiographic examination. Aqueous, or water-soluble, contrast is less viscous than the oily and provides better delineation of the nerve roots; it does not have to be removed, as it is absorbed and excreted by the body. Because the aqueous iodinated agents are absorbed quickly, filming must be expedited. Gaseous agents do not have to be removed, and their position within the subarachnoid space is dependent on body position. *(Ballinger [Vol. 3], p 764–767; Bontrager and Anthony, p 539; Meschan, p 155–162)*

46–48. The answers are 46-D, 47-C, 48-A. The Chassard-Lapiné position is used for demonstration of the rectosigmoid junction following opacification of the large intestine with positive contrast medium. For this position, patients are seated on the side of the radiographic table, with their thighs abducted, their upper body bent over to assume a knee-to-chest position, and their hands grasping their ankles. The central ray is directed perpendicularly through the lumbosacral region and midline. This axial projection demonstrates the rectum, uncoiling of the sigmoid, rectosigmoid junction, and anterior and posterior walls of the lower colon.

Decubitus positions with the patient lying on the left and right sides are employed routinely in double-contrast (air-contrast) studies of the large intestine. A double-contrast barium enema employs both positive (barium sulfate) and negative (air) contrast agents in an effort to coat the walls of the colon and distend its lumen with air so that small lesions will not be hidden by a large amount of barium as in single-contrast barium enema studies. As the patient is placed in the lateral decubitus positions, barium (the heavier agent) will gravitate to the dependent portions of the colon, or the side down, and air (the lighter contrast agent) will rise to the uppermost portions of the colon, or the side up. The central ray is directed at right angles to the film (in a grid cassette), which is placed behind the patient. The x-ray tube is horizontal.

Interval films are taken during study of the small bowel in order to evaluate small intestinal anatomy and motility. Positive contrast medium is administered orally (or through an intubation tube), and films are taken at various time intervals (usually every half hour or hour) until barium has reached the end of the small intestine and beginning of the large intestine (ileocecal junction). At that time, fluoroscopic spot films are often taken of the terminal ileum and ileocecal valve and points of interest. *(Ballinger [Vol. 3], p 664–667, 674–684; Bontrager and Anthony, p 460, 470–471, 478, 480)*

RADIOGRAPHIC EXPOSURE AND PROCESSING

49. For the technologist, probably the most important characteristic of any grid is the ratio. Grid ratio is defined as the

    A. height of the lead strip to the width of the interspacer material
    B. thickness of the lead strip to the width of the interspacer material
    C. height of the interspacer material to the thickness of the lead strip
    D. thickness of the lead strip to the height of the lead strip

50. The response of film to radiation and subsequent processing is referred to as the photographic effect. Which of the following is the formula that combines the factors that produce that effect (where FFD stands for focus-film distance and s stands for seconds)?

    A. $\dfrac{mA \times s \times kV^2}{FFD^2}$

    B. $\dfrac{FFD \times kV}{mA \times s}$

    C. $\dfrac{mA \times s \times FFD}{kV^2}$

    D. $\dfrac{mA \times kV \times FFD^2}{s}$

51. The sharpness with which the details of the radiographic image are recorded will be influenced by

        1. film-screen contact
        2. screen speed
        3. FFD

    A. 1 and 2
    B. 1 and 3
    C. 2 and 3
    D. 1, 2, and 3

52. The technologist can use many methods to increase radiographic density, and each one has a slightly different effect on image quality. Which of the following will have the same density effect as doubling the mAs?

    A. Decreasing intensifying screen speed from rare earth to high speed
    B. Reducing FFD by 50%
    C. Increasing kVp by 15%
    D. Removing the added filtration in the primary beam

53. A radiograph is a two-dimensional image representing a three-dimensional subject. Stereoscopy (stereoradiography) is a radiographic method that imitates normal stereoscopic vision. What is the relationship between tube shift and focus-image distance (FID) in making a stereoradiographic pair of images?

A. 1:5
B. 1:10
C. 1:25
D. 1:50

54. Which of the following factors will decrease radiographic contrast the most?

A. A reduction in the effective energy of the primary beam
B. Increasing intensifying screen speed
C. Lack of collimation
D. Increasing grid ratio

55. In addition to the simple linear unit, dedicated tomographic systems use a number of complex multidirectional movements of tube and cassette to suit every situation. Maximum image blurring occurs when the direction of tube movement

A. follows the structure's axis
B. is within 20° of the structure's axis
C. is within 45° of the structure's axis
D. is 90° to the structure's axis

56. In order to make a magnification radiograph magnifying the object three times, how far from the image plane must the object be placed if a FID of 48 inches is to be used?

A. 3 inches
B. 16 inches
C. 22 inches
D. 32 inches

57. Some aspects of CT equipment are identical to those of conventional radiography, and some are unique to the computer-based system. Which of the following is essential only to the CT system?

A. An especially warm environment, above 75°F
B. Either gas or scintillation radiation detectors
C. A stationary anode, as anode heat requirements are low
D. Variable source-to-detector distance to control slice thickness

58. Although most diagnostic x-ray tubes are of the diode vacuum type credited to Coolidge, some used in special situations are constructed quite differently. The field emission tube differs from the diode vacuum tube in that

A. it is water cooled
B. the anode is surrounded by the cathode
C. it is considerably larger and more expensive to manufacture
D. the filament circuit provides twice the heating potential

59. The "line-focus" principle, which has been used in the manufacture of x-ray tubes for about 50 years, is slightly disadvantageous in that the effective focal spot size varies across the beam. At which point in the beam does the effective focal spot appear smallest?

    A. At the anode edge of the beam
    B. At the central ray
    C. Between the central ray and the cathode side
    D. At the cathode edge of the beam

60. Which method of recording the fluoroscopic image retains the dynamic visualization plus offers the best image quality (although at the highest dose)?

    A. Videotape
    B. Cassette spot films
    C. Cinefluorography
    D. 70-mm strip spot

61. Which of the following statements regarding the anode cooling curve below are true?

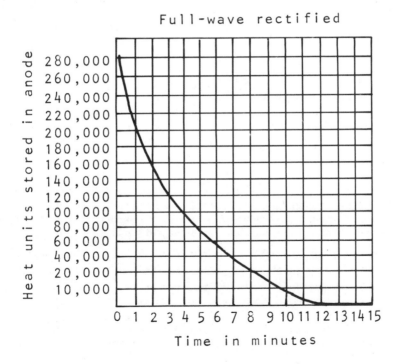

Full-wave rectified

    1. To cool from 80,000 to 40,000 takes less than 2 minutes
    2. To cool from 280,000 to 180,000 takes more than 1 minute
    3. To cool from 160,000 to 20,000 takes more than 7 minutes

    A. 1 and 2
    B. 1 and 3
    C. 2 and 3
    D. 1, 2, and 3

62. Radiographic density, the response of the film emulsion to x-ray exposure, is the black metallic silver of the processed image. Radiographic contrast, an equally important image characteristic, is less easily described. The function or purpose of radiographic contrast is to

A. describe the film's range of diagnostically acceptable density variations
B. diminish the scale of tissue density represented
C. represent the penetrability of the primary x-ray beam
D. facilitate the visualization of detail in the image

63. The factors set on the control panel are often thought of in terms of their ultimate effect on the qualities of the finished radiograph instead of how they control the equipment that first must produce the x-ray beam. Varying the kVp adjustment on the control console actually affects the

A. number of turns in the secondary side of the autotransformer
B. tube current
C. speed at which the anode will rotate
D. incoming line voltage

64. "Quality assurance" testing in the diagnostic x-ray department is an excellent way of monitoring equipment performance variations that can result in wasted material and unnecessary exposure of patients and personnel. Which of the following tests yields information regarding tube output and beam quality?

1. kVp check
2. mR/mAs linearity and repeatability
3. Exposure timer accuracy and repeatability

A. 1 and 2
B. 1 and 3
C. 2 and 3
D. 1, 2, and 3

65. In everyday radiographic situations, the many variables that affect optical density must be weighed and compared carefully to achieve a correctly exposed radiograph. Of the four groups of exposure parameters listed below, which would provide the greatest optical density on the finished radiograph (where SID stands for source-image distance)?

A. 100 mA, 0.4 second, 89 kVp, 36 inches FFD/SID
B. 150 mA, 0.2 second, 65 kVp, 36 inches FFD/SID
C. 200 mA, 0.2 second, 76 kVp, 40 inches FFD/SID
D. 400 mA, 0.75 second, 65 kVp, 72 inches FFD/SID

66. Radiographic density is the result of exposure modified by patient and imaging factors. Which of the following tissue conditions would *decrease* expected density if exposure and imaging factors remained the same?

A. Osteoporosis
B. Osteonecrosis
C. Osteomalacia
D. Osteosclerosis

67–69. For each function or action listed below, select the developer chemical with which it is most closely associated. Each chemical may be used once, more than once, or not at all.

A. Phenidone
B. Hydroquinone
C. Potassium bromide
D. Sodium carbonate

67. Reduces exposed silver halide crystals to black metallic silver, slowly producing black tones in the image

68. Activates emulsion, making it swell and become porous

69. Inhibits fogging and prevents development of unexposed silver halide crystals

70. When a technique chart has to be constructed for a new radiographic unit, specific rules must be used to calculate exposure values for centimeter measurements other than the one measurement derived from the phantom. When constructing a variable-kVp, medium-contrast, general radiographic technique chart, varying tissue volumes are accommodated by

1. varying FFD, or by inverse square law
2. adding 2 kVp/cm of additional tissue
3. increasing mAs by 25 to 30% for each 3 to 4 cm of tissue

A. 1 and 2
B. 1 and 3
C. 2 and 3
D. 1, 2, and 3

71. Radiographic film manufacturing is a very precise, quality-controlled procedure that takes place in a strictly clean environment. Film used for radiography is constructed of

1. polyester
2. silver halide
3. gelatin

A. 1 and 2
B. 1 and 3
C. 2 and 3
D. 1, 2, and 3

72. It may be interpreted from the graph that follows that

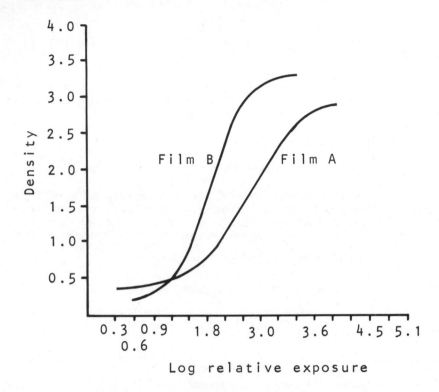

A. film A has the highest contrast and film B has the greatest speed
B. film B has the highest contrast and film A has the greatest speed
C. film A has the highest contrast and greatest speed
D. film B has the highest contrast and greatest speed

PRETEST—RADIOGRAPHIC EXPOSURE AND PROCESSING
ANSWERS, EXPLANATIONS, AND REFERENCES

49. The answer is A.   Grid ratio is defined as the height of the lead strip divided by the thickness of the interspace material. Ratio is an important characteristic in that higher-ratio grids absorb more scatter than lower-ratio grids, because the permissible angle of deviation is smaller for a higher-ratio grid. A 5:1 grid absorbs about 80 to 85% of scatter, whereas a 16:1 grid may be able to absorb as much as 95 to 97%. *(Bushong, p 199–200; Selman, p 383–392)*

50. The answer is A.   The response of film to radiation and subsequent processing is called radiographic density or photographic effect. The factors that produce radiographic density are the factors controlling generation of the beam and the distance between the point at which x-ray photons are generated and the image or film plane. The mA and seconds are directly proportional to density. Density is only approximately proportional to the square of the kVp used. Radiographic density is inversely proportional to the square of the FFD. *(Selman, p 338–340; Thompson, p 165–171)*

51. The answer is D.   When the intensifying screens hold the film with uniform pressure in the closed cassette, the light burst from the phosphor covers the smallest possible area of film, creating a sharp image. As the speed of the screen increases, several factors are at work to decrease the resulting sharpness. For any constant object-image distance (OID), increasing the FFD will actually increase focus-object distance (FOD), reduce magnification, and increase overall sharpness. *(Selman, p 327–330, 335–337)*

52. The answer is C.   There is a direct relationship between mAs and radiographic density—doubling mAs doubles radiographic density. Increasing beam energy increases the efficiency of x-ray production, resulting in both more photons and higher-energy photons. A 15% increase in kVp results in the same density increase as doubling mAs. Reducing FFD by 50% would result in a fourfold increase in radiographic density. Decreasing intensifying screen speed to any extent will decrease radiographic density. Removing added filtration will probably not affect image density at all. *(Bushong, p 149, 150; Selman, p 339–340)*

53. The answer is B.   Stereoradiography is an attempt to duplicate the normal facility for depth perception that our two eyes possess by seeing objects from two slightly different points. The x-ray focus is analogous to a single eye, so stereoscopy must image the subject from two different points, at a distance relative to the distance at which the radiographs will be viewed. The average distance between the pupils of the eyes is about 2.5 inches, and the average radiograph viewing distance is roughly 25 inches. This relationship is translated to a 1:10 ratio between the position of the focal spot for each exposure (tube shift) and the viewing distance of the focal spot from the image (focus-image distance [FID]). *(Bushong, p 307–310; Selman, p 411–415)*

54. The answer is C.   An uncollimated radiograph, which demonstrates an irradiated area of tissue that is larger than necessary, will show decreased contrast as a result of increased scatter production. Lowering the kVp level, or reducing the effective energy of the primary beam, will reduce scatter production and increase radiographic contrast. Increasing intensifying screen speed also tends to increase radiographic contrast. When grid ratio is increased, more scattered radiation is absorbed by the grid, less is transmitted to the film, and overall contrast is enhanced. *(Bushong, p 182, 186, 200; Selman, p 392–393)*

55. The answer is D.   The clarity of the tomographic image is directly related to the amount of blurring of structures that are outside the in-focus plane, and maximum blurring occurs when the direction of tube travel is oriented perpendicular, or 90°, to the structure's axis. When tube direction is most similar to the structure's axis, no blurring occurs, regardless of how far from the in-focus plane the structure is located. Linear tomography produces streaking in the image, as well as incomplete blurring, when tube direction is close to the structure's axis. *(Curry et al., p 246; Selman, p 428–429)*

56. The answer is D.   The magnification factor (MF) is equal to the ratio of FID to FOD, or MF = FID/FOD. For the example given in the question, where the MF is 3,

$$3 = \frac{48}{X} \rightarrow 3X = 48 \rightarrow X = 16.$$

FOD is 16 inches. The object will be placed 32 inches from the image plane. *(Bushong, p 272–273; Selman, p 356)*

57. The answer is B.   Unlike conventional radiography, in CT systems the remnant radiation beam is registered on a series of detectors of the scintillation (cesium iodide or cadmium tungstate) or gas (xenon or xenon-krypton) type. The variations in radiation intensity of the remnant beam are stored in numeric form in the computer and finally reconstructed to form an image. The computer room must be maintained at a cool temperature, below 70 °F. The speed at which the unit can complete an examination is partially dependent on the heat capacity of the anode. A high-speed rotating anode is used in all current units. Slice thickness is controlled by prepatient collimators. *(Bushong, p 372–375; Chesney and Chesney [1984], p 486–488)*

58. The answer is B.   The field emission x-ray tube is an application of the principle that electrons can be liberated from an unheated metal by the application of a very powerful electric field. The cathode, or electron emitter, in a field emission tube is a series of needle-thin projections surrounding a cone-shaped stationary anode. X-rays are emitted from a small area at the tip of the cone. There is no filament-heating circuit required, and water is not used as a coolant. The glass insert tube is about a third or a quarter the size of a conventional x-ray insert tube and is proportionally less expensive. Field emission tubes are being used mainly in very high-kVp chest radiography units and in some mobile units, in which limited size and weight are very advantageous. *(Selman, p 273–275)*

59. The answer is A.   The line-focus principle has proved to be effective in providing a reasonably large target area for rapid heat dissipation while retaining a smaller apparent focus for good detail sharpness. That portion of the anode that is the target area for cathode electrons is angled in such a way that, from the perspective of the filament, it is considerably larger than when viewed from beneath, from the perspective of the imaging system. The effective, or apparent, focal spot is smallest at the anode edge of the beam. This variation in image sharpness is only visible when the entire beam is used at a 40-inch FFD *(Bushong, p 117–118; Selman, p 213–215)*

60. The answer is C.   A cinefluorographic camera records the image directly from the output phosphor of the image intensifier onto film. It may use either 16-mm or 35-mm film, the larger film format requiring larger patient exposure. This high-detail/high-dose recording system (better image quality than any other mode except cassette spot films) is used almost exclusively now for imaging cardiac catheterizations. This movie film can be speeded up and slowed down without significant loss of detail, as well as run at the normal recording speed. Videotape recording also takes the image from the output phosphor of the image intensifier tube, but the magnetic tape system is inferior in quality to that of film and can only be run at the speed at which it was recorded. Dose is considerably lower for videotape recording. Cassette spots and strip spots take only single "still" images. *(Bushong, p 302; Chesney and Chesney [1984], p 398–399)*

61. The answer is A. On the graph that accompanies the question, find 80,000 on the vertical axis and follow the line across to the cooling curve; move straight down to the horizontal axis and read the time: 5 minutes. Next find 40,000 on the vertical axis and follow it across to the cooling curve; move directly down to the horizontal axis and read the time: about 6½ minutes. Cooling from 80,000 to 40,000 takes 6½ − 5 minutes, or about 1½ minutes. Find 280,000 on the vertical axis; it intersects with the cooling curve at 0 minutes. Now find 180,000 on the vertical axis and follow the line across to the point at which it meets with the cooling curve; move straight down to the horizontal line and read the time: about 1¼ minutes. Cooling from 280,000 to 180,000 takes 1¼ − 0 minutes, or about 1¼ minutes. Find 160,000 on the vertical axis and follow it across to where it intersects the cooling curve; now move down to the horizontal and read the time: 2 minutes. Next find 20,000 on the vertical axis; move across to the cooling curve, drop down to the horizontal, and read the time: 8 minutes. To cool from 160,000 to 20,000 takes 8 − 2 minutes, or 6 minutes. *(Bushong, p 136–137)*

62. The answer is D. When viewing the radiographic image as a whole, contrast can be described as the differences in the amounts of black metallic silver as distributed over various areas of the emulsion, and its function is to promote the visualization of anatomic detail by accentuating the differences between adjacent structures. The range of diagnostically acceptable density variations that can be produced by any film describes the film's latitude. The penetrability of the primary x-ray beam is controlled by kVp. *(Selman, p 345–351)*

63. The answer is A. An autotransformer has only one winding around it, and connections are made on the coil's secondary side to vary the voltage through to the maximum, using the same number of turns as on the primary side. The autotransformer supplies the variable voltage to the high-voltage transformer, where it is stepped up for use by the x-ray tube. The selection of kVp on the control console directs the activity of the autotransformer's secondary side. Tube current, or the number of electrons moving from cathode to anode, is regulated through filament temperature by mA station selection on the control panel. The speed at which the anode rotates is programmed into tube construction and usually varies automatically as the cooling requirements of the tube demand. The incoming line voltage is the responsibility of the power company; it may vary according to its capacity or because of varying use requirements of the institution. In any case, most x-ray units compensate automatically for small variations in the incoming line voltage. *(Bushong, p 99–100, 121–122; Chesney and Chesney [1984], p 51–55)*

64. The answer is D. All three tests listed in the question monitor the factors that control the amount and quality of radiation reaching the patient and the image receptor. The kVp should be accurate to 5% or less, an error too small to affect image quality perceptibly, and can be cheaply and easily checked with the Wisconsin (or other) test cassette and a densitometer. Once kVp accuracy is determined, then mA and exposure time are the remaining variables that affect tube output. The accuracy and, more important, the repeatability of the timer can be checked inexpensively with a spinning top test if the generator is single phase or with the motorized timers for three-phase generators. The ability of the generator to reproduce closely the total output for a specific kVp and mAs on any mA station is known as mR/mAs linearity and repeatability guarantees that same output every time. When the performance variations in these factors are controlled, the technologist can increase or reduce exposure time as necessary or change contrast or dose with confidence, knowing that radiographic density will be consistent. *(Chesney and Chesney [1984], p 571–592, 602–604; Gray et al., p 95–101)*

65. The answer is A. Of the choices given in the question, 100 mA, 0.4 seconds, 89 kVp, 36 inches FFD/source-image distance (SID) will produce the greatest optical density on the finished radiograph. This can be shown in the following steps: *Step 1:* Multiply mA times seconds; mAs is directly proportional to optical density, or in choice **A**, 40 mAs; choice **B**, 30 mAs; choice **C**, 40 mAs; and choice **D**, 300 mAs. *Step 2:* kVp is related to optical density in that increasing kVp by 15% doubles optical density; reducing kVp by 15% halves optical density. Increasing kVp by 15% *and* halving mAs or decreasing kVp by 15% *and* doubling the mAs will keep optical density constant. For **a,** reduce the original kVp of 89 by 15% (this equals 76). Double the original mAs of 40, to 80. Again, reduce the kVp by 15%, to 65, and double the mAs again, to 160. Optical density has remained constant. For **c,** reduce the original kVp of 76 by 15%, to 65. Double the original mAs of, 40 to 80. Optical density has remained constant. To summarize **A:** 160 mAs, 65 kVp; **B:** 30 mAs, 65 kVp; **C:** 80 mAs, 65 kVp; and **D:** 300 mAs, 65 kVp. *Step 3:* Optical density varies inversely with the square of FFD/SID. Halving FFD/SID will quadruple optical density. Use the mAs/distance equation to keep optical density proportional as FFD/SID is changed:

$$\text{For } \mathbf{C,} \quad \frac{\text{mAs}_1}{\text{mAs}_2} = \left(\frac{D_1}{D_2}\right)^2 \rightarrow \frac{80}{X} = \left(\frac{40}{36}\right)^2 \rightarrow \frac{80}{X} = \frac{1,600}{1,296} \rightarrow 1,600X = 103,680 \rightarrow$$

$$X = 65 \text{ mAs.}$$

$$\text{For } \mathbf{D,} \quad \frac{\text{mAs}_1}{\text{mAs}_2} = \left(\frac{D_1}{D_2}\right)^2 \rightarrow \frac{300}{X} = \left(\frac{72}{36}\right)^2 \rightarrow \frac{300}{X} = \frac{5,184}{1,296} \rightarrow 5,184X = 388,800 \rightarrow$$

$$X = 75 \text{ mAs.}$$

Final summary:
A. 160 mAs, 65 kVp, 36 inches FFD/SID
B. 30 mAs, 65 kVp, 36 inches FFD/SID
C. 65 mAs, 65 kVp, 36 inches FFD/SID
D. 75 mAs, 65 kVp, 36 inches FFD/SID
When all factors are reduced to the same terms, they can be easily compared. It can be seen that the radiograph having the greatest optical density is **A**.

66. The answer is D. Any tissue condition that increases radiopacity or effective atomic number will decrease expected radiographic density if exposure and imaging factors remain the same. Osteoporosis (decreased bone mineralization and volume) increases radiographic density, as do osteonecrosis (death of bone tissue) and osteomalacia (decreased or absent mineralization). In osteosclerosis, an increase in the atomic density or the hardness of the bone matrix, more radiation is absorbed and less is transmitted, resulting in a decrease in radiographic density. *(Bushong, p 162; Selman, p 347)*

67–69. The answers are 67-B, 68-D, 69-C. The developer solution used in processing radiographs contains a variety of chemicals whose combined actions produce a visible or manifest image in the emulsion of an exposed film. Both phenidone and hydroquinone are reducing agents that change exposed silver halide crystals to black metallic silver; phenidone works quickly to build up the gray tones in the image, whereas hydroquinone works slowly to produce the blackest film densities. Sodium carbonate or sodium hydroxide are used as activators (accelerators), which make the developer pH alkaline and cause the emulsion to swell and become porous so that the other developer chemicals (reducing agents) can get in at the individual crystals. Potassium bromide is added to the developer as a fog inhibitor, or restrainer, which prevents the reducing agents from attacking unexposed silver halide crystals and therefore, prevents chemical fog. If restrainer is not added to the developer solution, even those silver halide crystals that did not receive exposure would be reduced to black metallic silver. A preservative such as sodium sulfite is also added to the developer to prevent oxidation of the developing agent and to maintain chemical balance. The developing solution of an automatic processor also contains a hardening agent to keep the emulsion from becoming too soft as a result of the higher temperatures used in rapid processing. Glutaraldehyde is the usual hardening agent used to serve this function. The solvent used for dissolving chemicals for use in processing is water. Film development is a chemical reaction that is governed by time, temperature, and concentration of the developer chemicals. When any of these factors change adversely, the resultant radiograph may be incorrectly developed and may exhibit unacceptable contrast and density. *(Bushong, p 226–230; Chesney and Chesney [1981], p 129–136; Selman, p 310–313; Thompson, p 259–261)*

70. The answer is C.   A variable-kVp technique chart results in slightly higher contrast for any particular body part than does the fixed-kVp method. For each additional centimeter of tissue, 2 kVp are added, starting from a base kVp of 30 or 40. (The base selected will vary total contrast slightly and should be appropriate for the calibration of each individual unit and for the intensifying screens selected.) For each body part, size is generally specified as "small," "medium," or "large," and tissue differences of between 3 and 4 cm may require an increase in mAs of 25 to 30% in addition to the kVp increases already noted. For example, an abdomen of 16 cm might require 72 kVp and 40 mAs and an abdomen of 20 cm might require 80 kVp and 52 mAs, using this system. FFD or SID is not used as a variable because of the undesirable changes in the amount of magnification that would be apparent between radiographs. *(Thompson, p 110–122, 222–226)*

71. The answer is D.   Radiographic film consists of two major parts, the emulsion and the base. Film emulsion contains finely precipitated silver halide crystals (usually silver bromide and silver iodide) suspended in gelatin. Emulsion is the most important component of film, as it interacts with light and x-rays and records the image of the part being radiographed. Emulsion is coated on one or both sides of a polyester base. The function of the base is to support the emulsion and allow for flexibility in handling. The polyester base is essentially lucent, with a blue tint added to enhance viewing. Between the emulsion and the base, an adhesive layer is added to ensure good contact between these essential parts during chemical processing. On the emulsion surface is a protective layer or supercoating, which helps guard the emulsion from the effects of rough handling. *(Bushong, p 212–215; Chesney and Chesney [1981], p 15–17; Thompson, p 18–20; Selman, p 277–278)*

72. The answer is D.   In the graph that accompanies the question, film B has the highest degree of contrast and the greatest speed compared with film A. It takes less exposure to produce a certain density on film B than on film A. Film B's curve is located further to the left of the graph than film A's curve, making film B faster. The slope steepness of film B is greater than that of film A, so film B has a higher degree of contrast than film A. Film A has wider latitude, less contrast, and is not as fast as film B. *(Bushong, p 261–272; Chesney and Chesney [1981], p 56–79; Thompson, p 37–43)*

PHYSICS AND EQUIPMENT

73. Which of the following statements are true concerning the constituents of an atom?

      1. Protons are found in the nucleus and carry a positive charge
      2. Electron mass is less than that of a proton
      3. The maximum number of electrons in the L shell of an atom is 18

  A. 1 and 2
  B. 1 and 3
  C. 2 and 3
  D. 1, 2, and 3

74. X-rays are similar to heat, radio waves, and visible light in that they all

  A. have the same frequency
  B. vibrate at 10^{19} Hz
  C. have the same speed
  D. have identical electric charge

75. The life of an x-ray tube can be as short as a few months or as long as several years, depending on the type of use it is subjected to. Tube life tends to be increased by

      1. running the rotor for long time periods before making the exposure
      2. warming the anode with small exposures before heavy use
      3. keeping fluoroscopic time to less than 2 minutes

  A. 1 only
  B. 2 only
  C. 3 only
  D. 1, 2, and 3

76. If a transformer has 320,000 turns on its primary winding (coil) and 400 turns on its secondary winding (coil), and 110 V and 0.2 A are supplied to the primary side, the secondary current will be

  A. 0.00025 A
  B. 0.1375 A
  C. 80 A
  D. 160 A

77. In an x-ray unit that produces pulsed radiation, a simple device called a spinning top can be used to check the accuracy of the exposure timer. How many "dots" or "dashes" should appear if an exposure of 0.2 second is made on a full-wave rectified unit?

  A. 2
  B. 12
  C. 24
  D. 36

78. When a diagnostic x-ray tube is operating at a potential between 80 and 100 kVp, approximately what percentage of the primary beam generated will be made up of photons produced by the characteristic process?

    A.   1%
    B.   10%
    C.   60%
    D. 90%

79. In a rotating anode x-ray tube, two essential circuits are required to heat the filament and to propel electrons across the tube. Which of the following represents the numeric value for the filament current?

    A.   100 to 300 mA
    B.   300 to 600 mA
    C.   3 to 6 A
    D.   28 to 50 A

80. X-ray photons interact with matter in one of five basic ways. Which non-ionizing interaction is common when photon energy is less than 40 kVp?

    A. Photoelectric absorption
    B. Thompson, or coherent, scattering
    C. Pair production
    D. Compton effect

81. Which of the following statements is NOT true concerning medical x-ray film?

    A. Film latitude is inversely proportional to film contrast
    B. Crossover is decreased with thinner film base and the addition of dye
    C. Sensitivity specks are potential development centers located on the silver halide crystal
    D. Film speed varies directly with the amount of dye added to the emulsion

Questions 82 and 83 consist of four lettered headings followed by a list of numbered words or phrases. For each description that follows, select the imaging modality with which it is most closely associated. Each heading may be used once, more than once, or not at all.

    A. Fiberoptics
    B. Cinefluorography
    C. Spot film camera
    D. Cassette spot film

82. Essential in cardiac catheterization

83. Contributes to reduced dose in fluoroscopy

84. Xeroradiography is the process of producing an electrostatic image after exposure to x-rays. All of the following are part of the xeroradiographic system EXCEPT

    A. film
    B. conditioner
    C. toner
    D. fuser

PRETEST—PHYSICS AND EQUIPMENT
ANSWERS, EXPLANATIONS, AND REFERENCES

73. The answer is A.   The smallest part of any element that cannot be broken down by simple means is an atom. The fundamental particles of the atom are the neutron, proton, and electron. The nucleus of the atom is home for the neutron, a particle that does not carry an electric charge, and the proton, a particle that is nearly equal in mass to a neutron but carries a positive charge. Around the nucleus are various energy levels, or electron shells, where negatively charged particles called electrons exist. The number of electrons present in any energy level, or shell, depends on its distance from the nucleus. Shells are lettered alphabetically, from the innermost level closest to the nucleus outward, starting with the K shell. Using the formula $2n^2$ (where n represents the numeric position of the shell from the nucleus), one can determine the maximum number of electrons that any of the shells can contain; therefore, the L shell, being the second energy level from the nucleus, can contain no more than eight electrons: $2 \times 2^2 = 8$. The mass of an electron is approximately $\dfrac{1}{1,828}$ that of a proton. *(Bushong, p 36–40; Selman, p 40–43)*

74. The answer is C.   All electromagnetic radiations travel at the same speed (the speed of light, 3×10^8 meters/second); what differentiates them is their wavelength. The speed at which electromagnetic radiation travels is equal to frequency times wavelength; as wavelength decreases, frequency increases. Frequency refers to the number of crests or cycles per second and is measured in hertz; only x-rays have a frequency of 10^{19} Hz. All electromagnetic radiations are associated with electric and magnetic fields, but not all have electric charge. *(Bushong, p 53–56; Selman, p 155–157)*

75. The answer is B.   Warming the anode with small exposures avoids the sudden stress of a large exposure on a cold anode, which can cause the anode to crack. Running the rotor prepares the filament for exposure by low-level heating. This causes evaporation, which can plate out on the insert and lead to arcing or simply to thinning, which can eventually cause it to break. Both filament thinning and arcing can lead to decreased tube life. Fluoroscopy uses low mA, usually less than 5 mA. This relatively low level of heat generation does not affect tube life. *(Bushong, p 133–134; Selman, p 229–230)*

76. The answer is D.   The transformer law can be applied to current in the opposite way as for voltage but in a similar proportion. That is, if voltage is increased in the secondary winding, current decreases; if voltage decreases, then current increases. The ratio of current in the secondary winding of a transformer to the current in the primary winding is inversely proportional to the ratio of turns in the secondary winding to the number of turns in the primary winding, or

$$\frac{I_s}{I_p} = \frac{N_p}{N_s},$$

where I_s is the current in the secondary winding, I_p is the current in the primary winding, N_p is the number of turns in the primary winding, and N_s is the number of turns in the secondary winding. To determine the current in the secondary winding (I_s) when the current in the primary winding (I_p) = 0.2 A, the number of turns in the primary winding (N_p) = 320,000, and the number of turns in the secondary winding (N_s) = 400, the following calculations are used:

$$\frac{I_s}{0.2} = \frac{320,000}{400} \rightarrow I_s = I_p\left(\frac{N_p}{N_s}\right) \rightarrow I_s = 0.2\ \text{A}\left(\frac{320,000}{400}\right) \rightarrow I_s = 0.2\ \text{A}\left(\frac{800}{1}\right) \rightarrow I_s = 160\ \text{A}$$

The transformer described in this example is a step-down type because the number of turns in the secondary winding is less than the number of turns in the primary winding. In this type of transformer, the voltage would be stepped down, or decreased, in the secondary winding, but the current or amperage would be stepped up, or increased, on the secondary side of the step-down transformer.

The following equation symbolizes the transformer law and the relationships between turns ratio, voltage, and current:

$$\frac{V_s}{V_p} = \frac{N_s}{N_p} = \frac{I_p}{I_s}$$

V_s refers to voltage in the secondary winding, and V_p refers to voltage in the primary winding. *(Bushong, p 98–99; Selman, p 124–127)*

77. The answer is C.   A full-wave rectified x-ray unit operating on 60 cycles per second current produces 120 pulses of current per second, resulting in 120 pulses of x-ray output per second. A 1-second exposure of a spinning top would demonstrate 120 "dots" or "dashes" on the processed film. An exposure of 0.2, or one-fifth, of a second would therefore demonstrate only 24 "dots" or "dashes". *(Bushong, p 125–127; Selman, p 242–244)*

78. The answer is B.   The characteristic process of x-ray production makes up only a small percentage, about 10%, of the beam emitted from the target in the midrange of energies used in diagnostic x-ray. When the target atom is ionized by removal of a K-shell electron as the result of a collision with the incoming cathode electron, electrons from other shells can fill the space, with the emission of an x-ray photon equal in energy to the difference in the binding energies of the two target atom shells involved. A much greater percentage of the primary beam is composed of bremsstrahlung-generated photons, accounting for the polyenergetic nature of the primary beam. *(Selman, p 163; Bushong, p 142–144)*

79. The answer is C.   Filament circuits require quite high-amperage current between 3 and 6 amperes to produce sufficient thermionic emission for tube currents of up to 1,000 mA, or 1A. Very small increases in filament current raise filament temperatures, causing large increases in the rate at which electrons are emitted, or tube current (mA). The filament-heating circuit requires its own step-down transformer. *(Bushong, p 111, 122; Selman, p 210)*

80. The answer is B.   In the Thompson, or coherent, scattering interaction, the photon interacts with the target atom as a whole, causing it to become excited; a secondary photon of equal energy but traveling in a different direction is immediately released by the atoms. There is no energy transfer and no ionization in this interaction. Pair production occurs only when photon energy is 1.02 meV or greater. Photoelectric and Compton interactions occur throughout the diagnostic x-ray range, with target atom ionization occurring in both cases. *(Bushong, p 156–157; Selman, p 186)*

81. The answer is D.   Film speed is actually inversely related to the amount of dye added to the emulsion of radiographic film. As more dye is added, more light photons are absorbed by the emulsion, decreasing the speed, or sensitivity, of the film. Film speed is also controlled by sensitization of the silver halide crystals. Temperature and processing conditions are other factors that affect film speed. Film latitude increases as film contrast decreases. Latitude refers to a film's response to exposures in the useful diagnostic density regions (somewhere between 0.25 and 2.0 density). On a characteristic curve, a film with increased latitude will have a less-steep straight-line portion than a film with high contrast; the greater-latitude film will cover a wider range of useful densities and responds to a larger range of exposures. Sensitivity specks are important to the silver halide crystals in film emulsion as they serve as sites for latent image formation and potential development centers for exposed crystals. The sensitivity specks located on the crystal's surface usually comprise silver sulfide. Crossover, or cross-talk, refers to the exposure on one side of film emulsion from light given off by the screen in contact with the opposite side of emulsion. Light from the opposite screen actually passes through the film base to expose the opposite emulsion. Crossover exposure tends to produce unsharpness, because the light from the opposite screen diffuses and scatters before reaching the opposite emulsion. In order to reduce crossover or parallax unsharpness, thinner bases are used to bring the double image created on duplitized (double-emulsion) film closer together. A special dye can be added on top of the base to absorb diffused, scattered light photons; however, the addition of dye will decrease film speed. *(Chesney and Chesney [1981], p 8, 68–71; Curry et al., p 126–127, 145–146, 148–149; Thompson, p 19, 21)*

82–83. The answers are 82-B, 83-C. Cardiac catheterization relies heavily on cinefluorography for a sharp and accurate record of the entire procedure. Although dose is relatively high, image quality is very good. The cine strip can be viewed an unlimited number of times and, with careful editing, can be an excellent educational medium. During the procedure, a television monitor and a video disk recorder are used as well as the cine for immediate access and current monitoring of progress.

There are a number of ways to view and record the fluoroscopic image, each differing somewhat in convenience of use, image quality, and patient dose. Of those techniques currently in use, the cassette spot film is probably still the most widely used because of its excellent image quality. Dose is reduced, however, when the spot film camera is used. This system records the image on the output phosphor of the image-intensifier tube, whereas the cassette spot film exposes the patient to typically high-mAs factors. *(Bushong, p 302; Selman, p 410–411)*

84. The answer is A. Unlike conventional radiography, xeroradiography does not use film. Instead, a charged selenium-coated metal plate is used to receive the latent image. The conditioner is the part of the xeroradiography system that not only removes residual charges from used Xerox plates but also stores plates and places a positive charge over the surface of the plate, preparing it for exposure. Once the selenium-coated plate has received a uniform positive charge, it is loaded into a light-tight cassette, then removed from the conditioning unit. It must be used (exposed) within 30 minutes or the charge will leak off, decreasing its efficiency and sensitivity. The part to be imaged is placed on top of the xerox plate and cassette and exposed to x-rays. As x-rays strike the photoconductive selenium layer, discharge takes place, causing those positive charges on the plate that receive exposure to dissipate in proportion to the amount of x-rays reaching the plate. Thick body parts absorb more x-rays and do not allow as many to pass through to discharge the positively charged selenium plate; thus more positive charges will remain on the plate in the areas under thick, dense parts. At this point, there is a latent electrostatic image on the plate. Once exposed, the xerox plate and cassette are placed in a special processor, another major component of the xeroradiography system. Here, the plate is removed from the cassette and brought to a development chamber, where a charged blue powder, called toner, is sprayed onto the plate, adhering proportionally to the regions of residual charge on the plate. This toner will produce a visible image on the plate, which must be transferred onto a specially treated paper. Then it is made permanent in the fuser, where the paper is heated, allowing the blue toner to seep into the paper's specially treated plastic layer. The final image is produced by means of this special process, beginning with conditioning, then x-ray exposure, followed by development with toner, and finally made storable by the fuser, The xerox plate must then be cleared of any residual charge and toner so that it can be used again. *(Bushong, p 318–324; Selman, p 438–441)*

RADIATION PROTECTION
AND RADIOBIOLOGY

85. In the early 1900s, Bergonié and Tribondeau formulated some theories about the radiosensitivity of biologic tissue. The Law of Bergonié and Tribondeau states in part that

A. when metabolic activity is high, radiosensitivity is high
B. stem cells are radioresistant
C. radiation damage to cells can be completely repaired the first time it occurs
D. radiosensitive cells are those that rarely divide

86. The technologist has considerable control over both image quality and patient dose, depending on which materials or methods are selected for each examination. One technique that reduces patient dose and improves image quality at the same time is

A. the use of an automatic exposure control (phototimer)
B. collimating to the area of clinical interest
C. applying gonad shielding whenever possible
D. the use of a maximum-sharpness imaging system

87. The target theory is a concept for clarifying radiation effects at the cellular level. The basis for this theory is that in every cell there is a significant target that, if rendered nonfunctional, will result in death of that cell. Which of the following is that most important molecular target?

A. Water
B. DNA
C. Glycerol
D. Protein

88. Because the size of the field irradiated has such an impact on patient dose, there are many safety regulations regarding collimation. Which of the following are National Council on Radiation Protection recommendations?

    1. Collimators must attenuate the beam to the same level as the tube housing
    2. Field size indication and x-ray field/light field congruence are required to be accurate to 1 inch at a 6-foot FFD
    3. Fluoroscopic automatic collimation may not exceed the diameter of the input phosphor

A. 1 and 2
B. 1 and 3
C. 2 and 3
D. 1, 2, and 3

89. The maximum permissible cumulative dose for occupationally exposed individuals permits a certain annual exposure maximum that can be received throughout one's working life. The maximum permissible cumulative dose for a 43-year-old radiation worker is

A. 75 rem
B. 100 rem
C. 125 rem
D. 150 rem

90. A patient with an internal source is emitting 50 mR/hour measured at a point 3 feet from the patient. At what distance would the exposure rate fall to 10 mR/hour?

A. 6.7 feet
B. 1.3 feet
C. 5.0 feet
D. 9.0 feet

91. The dose-response, or dose-effect, relationships derived from radiobiologic research and clinical use of ionizing radiation have proved useful in

      1. planning therapeutic treatment schedules
      2. estimating the effects of low-dose irradiation
      3. setting standards for high-dose accidental exposure

A. 1 and 2
B. 1 and 3
C. 2 and 3
D. 1, 2, and 3

92. Three units are used extensively in diagnostic radiology to measure dose from different perspectives. Which unit is used to measure output (or intensity) of an x-ray machine?

A. Rem or sievert
B. Roentgen
C. Rad or gray
D. Becquerel

93. The cells that compose any tissue system in the body respond to radiation relative to the cell's degree of differentiation and level of metabolic activity, among other factors. Which of the following cell types is highly radiosensitive?

A. Chondrocytes
B. Intestinal crypt stem cells
C. Muscle cells
D. Nerve cells

94. Radiation detection and measuring devices perform a variety of functions, from personnel monitoring to portable surveying. Which of the following instruments has a wide range, is very accurate, and can be used for personnel, patient, and area monitoring?

A. Proportional counter
B. Scintillation detector
C. Thermoluminescent dosimeter
D. Cutie pie

95. Apart from biologic factors, certain physical factors relative to the radiation itself affect the response of a cell to irradiation. Which of the following represents the measure of the rate at which energy is deposited by ionizing radiation in tissue?

    A. Relative biologic effectiveness
    B. Linear energy transfer
    C. Quality factor
    D. Distribution factor

96. The $LD_{50/30}$ is a measure of the ability of ionizing radiation to produce death in a population. It is that dose of radiation to the whole body that will produce death in 50% of the population within a period of 30 days. Which of the following ranges represents the $LD_{50/30}$ for humans?

    A. 150 to 300 R
    B. 300 to 450 R
    C. 500 to 750 R
    D. 800 to 1,000 R

97. A few items of equipment, correctly used, have the inherent capacity to reduce patient dose in diagnostic examinations. Which of the following imaging systems and exposure factor combinations result in reduced patient dose?

    1. Rare earth imaging system, 20 mAs, 70 kVp
    2. High-speed imaging system, 20 mAs, 81 kVp
    3. Par-speed imaging system, 40 mAs, 81 kVp

    A. 1 and 2
    B. 1 and 3
    C. 2 and 3
    D. 1, 2, and 3

Questions 98–100 consist of four lettered headings followed by a list of numbered words or phrases. For each of the radiation exposures during gestation listed below, choose the most likely effect. Each lettered item may be used once, more than once, or not at all.

    A. Acute radiation syndrome
    B. Erythema
    C. Prenatal death
    D. Congenital abnormalities

98. 300 rad at the preimplantation period

99. 200 rad at the fifth week of gestation

100. 100 rad at birth

PRETEST—RADIATION PROTECTION AND RADIOBIOLOGY
ANSWERS, EXPLANATIONS, AND REFERENCES

85. The answer is A.   When the metabolic activity of a cell is high—that is, intracellular events are occurring rapidly and oxygen is being consumed—then the radiosensitivity of that cell is high. Stem cells (undifferentiated, or precursor, cells) the immmature cells of any tissue, are more radiosensitive than the mature cells of that same tissue. The degree of repair following irradiation is not a subject dealt with by the Law of Bergonié and Tribondeau. Radiosensitivity is directly related to the proliferation rate, or the rate at which a cell divides. *(Bushong, p 438)*

86. The answer is B.   Collimating to the area of clinical interest reduces the volume of tissue exposed, thereby reducing patient dose. When less tissue volume is exposed, less scattered radiation is produced, so the radiograph will exhibit greater contrast. Automatic exposure controls regulate only the amount of mAs used for any exposure; there is no inherent improvement of image quality. Gonad shielding similarly does not affect image quality. A maximum-sharpness imaging system is a slow system, and its use increases patient dose. *(Bushong, p 547; Frankel, p 102)*

87. The answer is B.   DNA is the significant target molecule because of its responsibilities for correct functioning of the cell and also because there are no other molecules that can perform the functions of DNA. Damage to DNA can result in abnormal metabolic activity, changes in the normal mitotic rate, and in a germ cell, a genetic mutation. Individual glycerol, protein, and water molecules are not unique in their functioning and so are not of such great importance. *(Bushong, p 454; Frankel, p 16-17)*

88. The answer is D.   The collimator can be a source of leakage radiation in the same way that the tube housing can, and both of these components are required to reduce such stray radiation to a specific level. When automatic collimation is not in use, the technologist relies on the field size indication on the front of the collimator to restrict the beam accurately. Both the field size indicator and light field/x-ray field congruence must be accurate to within 1 inch over a 6-foot FFD. The fluoroscopic tube collimator must not be able to be opened to a larger diameter than that of the input phosphor, the image receptor. The recommendations set forth by the National Council on Radiation Protection (NCRP) are very useful in limiting nonproductive exposure to patients. *(Bushong, p 512-513; NCRP [No. 33], p 8, 12-13)*

89. The answer is C.   The formula 5 $(N - 18)$, where N is the age in years, indicates that 5 rem of radiation exposure is the permissible dose for each working year that follows the 18th birthday. Therefore, 5 $(43 - 18)$ indicates a permissible cumulative exposure of 125 rem for a 43-year-old person. It is also permissible for this 43-year-old person to receive more than 5 rem/year, providing that the cumulative $5(N - 18)$ is not exceeded. This is not likely to occur in diagnostic radiology, because most individual exposures are generally less than 0.5 rem/year. *(Bushong, p 510)*

90. The answer is C.   The inverse square law of radiation states that radiation intensity is inversely proportional to the square of the distance from the source. The formula to solve problems involving inverse square law is as follows:

$$\left(\frac{\text{Intensity}_1}{\text{Intensity}_2} \right) = \left(\frac{\text{Distance}_2}{\text{Distance}_1} \right)^2.$$

In the example given in the question, Intensity$_1$ is 50 mR/hour, the original exposure rate. Intensity$_2$ is 10 mR/hour, the new exposure rate. Distance$_2$ is the unknown new distance.

Distance$_1$ is 3 feet, the original distance. The following calculations will yield the new distance. *(Bushong, p 64):*

$$\frac{50}{10} = \frac{X^2}{3} \rightarrow \frac{50}{10} = \frac{X^2}{9} \rightarrow 10X^2 = 450 \rightarrow X^2 = 45 \rightarrow X = 6.7 \text{ feet.}$$

91. The answer is A. The planning of treatment methods and schedules for patients with malignant disease relies heavily on information gained from dose-response relationships. The dose-response curves show quantitative relationships between dose and response and whether or not the response has a threshold level. These dose-response relationships also define the quality of the response, which can be either linear or nonlinear. Dose-response relationships derived from high-dose exposures (such as in the survivors of the Japanese atomic bomb) can be used to extrapolate safety maximums in low-dose exposure. There are no standards for accidental exposure; by definition, they cannot be planned. *(Bushong, p 443-446; NCRP [No. 39], p 55-58)*

92. The answer is B. X-ray quantity, exposure, or output intensity of a diagnostic x-ray machine is measured in roentgens or milliroentgens. The roentgen is a measurement of the number of ion pairs produced in a specific air volume by a certain quantity of x-rays. The rem or sievert is the unit of dose equivalent used mainly to specify dose limits. The rad or gray is the unit of absorbed dose. The becquerel is the Systeme International d'Unités (SI) unit of radionuclide activity. *(Bushong, p 21-22, 173; Selman, p 168)*

93. The answer is B. The intestinal crypt cells are very specialized cells, secreting digestive enzymes and absorbing nutrients from the intestinal tract. These cells are highly differentiated and are quite radiosensitive. Chondrocytes, muscle cells or fibers, and nerve cells (neurons or neuroglia) are among the least radiosensitive body cells. *(Bushong, p 437)*

94. The answer is C. The thermoluminescent dosimeter is replacing the film badge for personnel monitoring in some institutions. It has a wider range than the film badge, can also be used to measure dose received for a particular examination or to a specific location, and is accurate to as low as 10 mrad. The proportional counter is a laboratory instrument, and the cutie pie is a portable survey instrument; both are gas detectors. The scintillation detector is used in nuclear medicine as the basis for a gamma camera and is also used in many CT scanners. *(Bushong, p 519-527; Noz and Maguire, p 50)*

95. The answer is B. Linear energy transfer (LET) is the rate at which energy is deposited in soft tissue. The unit of LET is keV/μm of track length, or energy deposited per unit of track length. High LET radiation produces more biologic damage than does low LET radiation. Relative biologic effectiveness (RBE) in experimental radiobiology differentiates between radiations producing different quantitative biologic effects per unit of absorbed dose. Quality factor and distribution factor are both modifiers of biologic effect. *(Bushong, p 439; NCRP [No. 39], p 29)*

96. The answer is B. The LD$_{50/30}$ for humans is 300 to 450 R. The lower number indicates the midline absorbed dose in tissue, and the higher number represents the dose measured at the skin. Individuals can survive larger whole-body doses of radiation if they receive intense clinical support. On the other hand, most sensitive individuals in the group could suffer death from doses below this range if no support were available. *(Bushong, p 469; NCRP [No. 39], p 46)*

97. The answer is A. Rare earth phosphors (compared with other phosphors used in medical radiography) are a group of materials that have a far greater x-ray photon to light photon conversion efficiency; that is, fewer x-ray photons are required to produce a given number of light photons. This type of imaging system can obviously reduce patient dose because it requires fewer x-ray photons to produce a given optical density. Many different combinations of mAs and kVp can produce very similar radiographic densities. For example, 20 mAs and 70 kVp produce roughly the same density with the rare earth imaging system as does 20 mAs and 81 kVp with the high-speed imaging system. Patient dose is slightly increased with the high-speed system. The par-speed system requires 40 mAs and 81 kVp to reach the same radiographic density; however, this increase in mAs more than doubles patient dose over the rare earth imaging system. *(Bushong, p 546-547; Frankel, p 108)*

98–100. The answers are 98-C, 99-D, 100-A. Preimplantation is that period between fertilization of the ovum and the attachment of the blastocyst to the endometrium. In humans, this occurs within 7 to 10 days following fertilization. A very large dose of radiation (e.g., 300 rad) during this period of rapid cell division will result in death of the blastocyst and a spontaneous abortion. Congenital abnormalities are associated with a large radiation dose (e.g., 200 rad) at the fifth week of gestation. After implantation and until the end of the second month of gestation, the embryo is developing organs and organ systems. A large dose of radiation during this period would interfere with organogenesis, hampering its normal completion. This effect would be visible as a congenital defect in whichever system was developing at the time of exposure. A dose of 100 rad delivered at once to the whole body of newborn infants, who are much more sensitive than adults, could result in a response known as the acute radiation syndrome. The acute radiation syndrome is an immediate or early effect with late sequelae which could be genetic or somatic. *(Bushong, p 499-501)*

BODY

ANATOMY AND PHYSIOLOGY
(including Medical Terminology and Pathology)

1. Which of the following statements are true concerning the cellular components of blood?

    1. Phagocytosis is a function of leukocytes, or WBCs
    2. Erythrocytes, or RBCs, transport essential gases
    3. Thrombocytes are compounds consisting of iron and protein

  A. 1 and 2
  B. 1 and 3
  C. 2 and 3
  D. 1, 2, and 3

2. Which of the following statements is (are) true concerning fetal circulation?

    1. Oxygenated blood is brought to the fetus by way of the umbilical vein
    2. The ductus arteriosus serves to bypass the liver
    3. The foramen ovale lies in the interventricular septum of the heart, serving to bypass the lungs

  A. 1 only
  B. 2 only
  C. 3 only
  D. 1, 2, and 3

3. The colon is supplied with blood by branches of the

    1. inferior mesenteric artery
    2. superior mesenteric artery
    3. celiac artery

  A. 1 only
  B. 1 and 2
  C. 1 and 3
  D. 1, 2, and 3

Questions 4–7 consist of four lettered headings followed by a list of numbered words. For each of the numbered structures listed below, select the cranial bone with which it is most closely associated. Each lettered heading may be used once, more than once, or not at all.

  A. Ethmoid
  B. Frontal
  C. Occipital
  D. Parietal

4. Cribiform plate

5. Foramen magnum

6. Crista galli

7. Glabella

8. All of the following are part of the lymphatic system EXCEPT the

A. spleen
B. thoracic duct
C. tonsils
D. pancreas

9. A transverse fracture of the distal radius with posterior displacement of the distal fragment is called a

A. Pott's fracture
B. boxer's fracture
C. greenstick fracture
D. Colles' fracture

10. Which of the following conditions or problems may be associated with the occurrence of jaundice?

    1. Stone in the common bile duct
    2. Tumor of the pancreas
    3. Stone in the cystic duct

A. 1 and 2
B. 1 and 3
C. 2 and 3
D. 1, 2, and 3

11. The cerebral hemispheres are connected by a bundle of white matter called the

A. falx cerebri
B. corpus callosum
C. longitudinal fissure
D. tentorium cerebelli

12. The trachea is correctly described as

    1. situated anterior to the esophagus
    2. extending from the level of the sixth cervical vertebra to the fifth thoracic vertebra
    3. composed of incomplete cartilaginous rings

A. 1 only
B. 2 only
C. 3 only
D. 1, 2, and 3

13. All of the following are part of the sphenoid bone of the skull EXCEPT the

A. styloid processes
B. foramina rotundum
C. sella turcica
D. optic canals

14. The point of union of the coronal and sagittal sutures of the skull is called the

A. nasion
B. lambda
C. inion
D. bregma

15. The term that means "difficult or painful swallowing" is

A. dyspepsia
B. dysphagia
C. pyrosis
D. dystocia

16. Spermatazoa are conducted from the testes to the prostatic portion of the urethra by way of the

A. epididymis—ductus deferens—seminal vesicle—ejaculatory duct
B. seminal vesicle—ductus deferens—membranous urethra
C. ductus deferens—ejaculatory duct—membranous urethra
D. ejaculatory duct—seminal vesicle—ductus deferens

17. The gastric glands secrete

    1. pepsinogen, which is converted into pepsin in order to break down proteins
    2. mucus and alkaline fluid, which help prevent the stomach from digesting itself
    3. secretin, which helps to break down carbohydrates

A. 1 and 2
B. 1 and 3
C. 2 and 3
D. 1, 2, and 3

18. Inspired air is conveyed to the alveoli of the lungs by which of the following routes?

A. Nose—nasal cavity—pharynx—larynx—trachea—mainstem bronchi—bronchi— bronchioles
B. Mouth—oral cavity—trachea—mainstem bronchi—bronchioles
C. Nose—nasal cavity—sinuses—trachea—mainstem bronchi—bronchioles
D. Mouth—oral cavity—sinuses—pharynx—larynx—mainstem bronchi—bronchi— bronchioles

19. The detrusor muscle is responsible for

    A. flexing the arm at the elbow joint
    B. contracting the bladder for urination
    C. flexion and extension of the neck
    D. contracting the gallbladder for expulsion of bile

20. According to the ABO blood grouping system, persons who are theoretically considered to be universal donors for blood transfusions are those with blood type

    A. A
    B. B
    C. AB
    D. O

21. The mandible is a large facial bone forming the lower jaw. Which of the following are true concerning its structure?

    1. Its coronoid processes articulate with the temporal bones bilaterally
    2. The condyles are posterior processes arising from the rami
    3. Its alveolar arch gives rise to teeth

    A. 1 and 2
    B. 1 and 3
    C. 2 and 3
    D. 1, 2, and 3

22. In an effort to maintain homeostasis in the body, the cells and tissues provide an inflammatory response when needed. Tissue inflammation is characterized by

    1. heat
    2. edema
    3. redness

    A. 1 and 2
    B. 1 and 3
    C. 2 and 3
    D. 1, 2, and 3

23. Elevated blood urea nitrogen (BUN) and creatinine levels may be indicative of

    A. pregnancy
    B. kidney malfunction
    C. obstruction of the bile ducts
    D. appendicitis

24. Which of the following statements concerning the ribs are true?

    1. The first seven pairs of ribs are called true ribs because they are attached directly to the sternum by costal cartilage

    2. Floating ribs attach to vertebrae but not to the sternum

    3. The facets of the ribs articulate with facets of the vertebrae

    A. 1 and 2
    B. 1 and 3
    C. 2 and 3
    D. 1, 2, and 3

25. All of the following statements are true concerning the gallbladder EXCEPT that

    A. the mucosa of the gallbladder secretes cholecystokinin in the presence of fats
    B. the neck of the gallbladder joins the cystic duct
    C. concentration of bile occurs in the gallbladder by reabsorption of water
    D. inflammation of the gallbladder may occur with cholelithiasis

26. Movement of a body part toward the central axis of the body is called

    A. flexion
    B. inversion
    C. adduction
    D. supination

27. The wrist consists of eight short bones, called carpals, located between the distal forearm and proximal ends of the metacarpals. Four of the carpals form the proximal row, and the other four the distal row. Which carpal bone is located in the proximal row on the thumb side?

    A. Greater multangular (trapezium)
    B. Pisiform
    C. Navicular (scaphoid)
    D. Hamate (unciform)

28. Which of the following types of body habitus has a short, wide thorax and long abdomen with viscera located high and laterally?

    A. Hyposthenic
    B. Sthenic
    C. Hypersthenic
    D. Asthenic

29. Oliguria is best defined as

    A. excessive secretion and output of urine
    B. scanty urine output
    C. uncontrolled discharge of urine or bed-wetting
    D. total suppression of urine formation by the kidneys

30. Adult blood cells are produced in the

       1. red bone marrow
       2. spleen
       3. lymph nodes

  A. 1 and 2
  B. 1 and 3
  C. 2 and 3
  D. 1, 2, and 3

31. A bone that is broken into small fragments is best described as having a

  A. compound fracture
  B. comminuted fracture
  C. complicated or complex fracture
  D. capillary fracture

Questions 32–36 refer to the anatomic sketch below, which illustrates the hepatobiliary system and pancreas. Certain parts of the figure are labeled with numbers. Each question is followed by four suggested labels or answers. For each question select the one best answer.

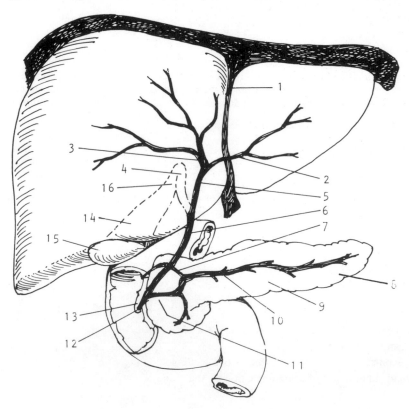

32. The fundus of the gallbladder is designated by the number

    A. 4
    B. 14
    C. 15
    D. 16

33. The common hepatic duct is designated by the number

    A. 3
    B. 5
    C. 6
    D. 7

34. The common bile duct is designated by the number

    A. 1
    B. 3
    C. 5
    D. 6

35. The cystic duct is designated by the number

    A. 2
    B. 3
    C. 4
    D. 7

36. The duct of Wirsung is designated by the number

    A. 2
    B. 6
    C. 7
    D. 10

37. An abnormal lateral curvature of the spine is called

    A. lordosis
    B. kyphosis
    C. scoliosis
    D. spondylosis

38. A painful disease affecting the nerve that innervates the thigh and leg muscles, possibly a result of compression by a herniated disk, is

    A. Bell's palsy
    B. paraplegia
    C. trigeminal neuralgia
    D. sciatica

39. The transparent mucous membrane lining the anterior surface of the eyeball and inner eyelid surface is called the

A. sclera
B. lacrimal sac
C. cornea
D. conjunctiva

40. Which of the following statements are true concerning the female reproductive system?

1. The entire amount of potential ova are present at birth
2. Fertilization of an ovum normally takes place in the uterine cavity
3. Estrogen is secreted by the ovaries and maintains female reproductive organs and secondary sex characteristics

A. 1 and 2
B. 1 and 3
C. 2 and 3
D. 1, 2, and 3

41. All of the following are part of the axial skeleton of the body EXCEPT the

A. skull
B. pelvic girdle
C. thoracic cage
D. vertebral column

42. Which of the following statements concerning the circulation are true?

1. The abdominal aorta bifurcates in the lower abdomen into the common iliac arteries
2. The coronary sinus empties deoxygenated blood from the myocardium into the right atrium
3. The great saphenous vein originates in the knee area and extends to the groin

A. 1 and 2
B. 1 and 3
C. 2 and 3
D. 1, 2, and 3

43. All of the following are cell organelles (structures that perform specific functions necessary for the cell survival) EXCEPT the

A. Golgi complex
B. centriole
C. cytoplasm
D. nucleus

44. Which of the following glands are found in the integumentary system and secrete sweat?

    A. Sudoriferous glands
    B. Sebaceous glands
    C. Ceruminous glands
    D. Bartholin's glands

45. Abnormal architectural changes with thickening and weakening of the bones, especially those of the pelvis, skull, and extremities, characterize the bone disorder known as

    A. multiple myeloma
    B. osteoporosis
    C. rickets
    D. Paget's disease

46. The thymus gland is correctly described as

    1. a part of the lymphatic system that plays an active role in the immune response
    2. achieving its maximum size during puberty
    3. located superior to the thyroid gland

    A. 1 and 2
    B. 1 and 3
    C. 2 and 3
    D. 1, 2, and 3

47. The substance that grows between the ends of broken or fractured bones and is eventually changed into osseous tissue in the healing process is known as

    A. callus
    B. cicatrix
    C. collagen
    D. diploë

Questions 48–53 consist of four lettered headings followed by a list of numbered items. For each of the following structures, choose the bone with which it is associated. Each lettered item may be used once, more than once, or not at all.

    A. Scapula
    B. Humerus
    C. Ulna
    D. Radius

48. Coracoid process

49. Glenoid cavity

50. Medial styloid process

51. Olecranon process

52. Capitulum

53. Deltoid tuberosity

Questions 54–58 refer to the anatomic sketch of the skull below. Certain parts of the sketch are labeled with numbers. Each question is followed by four suggested labels or answers. For each question select the one best answer.

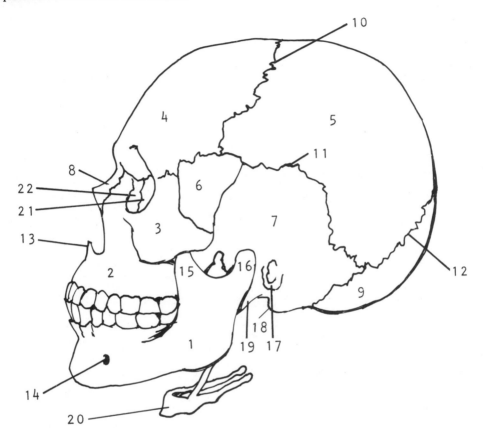

54. The temporal bone is designated by the number

    A. 3

    B. 5

    C. 6

    D. 7

55. The lambdoidal suture is designated by the number

    A. 5

    B. 10

    C. 11

    D. 12

56. The zygomatic bone is designated by the number

    A. 2
    B. 3
    C. 6
    D. 15

57. The ethmoid bone is designated by the number

    A. 6
    B. 8
    C. 21
    D. 22

58. The styloid process is designated by the number

    A. 13
    B. 18
    C. 19
    D. 20

59. The main portion, or shaft, of a long bone is called the

    A. epiphysis
    B. endosteum
    C. diaphysis
    D. metaphysis

60. When performing single-rescuer cardiopulmonary resuscitation, the ratio of cardiac compressions to ventilations on an adult victim is

    A. 5:1
    B. 12:4
    C. 15:2
    D. 20:1

61. A reduced number of RBCs or a decreased hemoglobin level characterizes the condition known as

    A. anemia
    B. Hodgkin's disease
    C. polycythemia
    D. hemophilia

62. A long process of a neuron that conducts impulses away from a cell body to body tissue or another neuron is called

    A. an axon
    B. a dendrite
    C. a Nissl body
    D. a synapse

63. The portal vein is formed by the union of the

    A. splenic and superior mesenteric veins
    B. hepatic and inferior mesenteric veins
    C. splenic and gastric veins
    D. superior mesenteric and cystic veins

64. Cerebrospinal fluid (CSF) passes from the choroid plexuses of the brain to the subarachnoid space by way of the

    A. lateral ventricles→cerebral aqueduct → third ventricle → fourth ventricle → foramina of Luschka and Magendie → subarachnoid space
    B. cerebral aqueduct → lateral ventricles → foramina of Luschka and Magendie → third ventricle → fourth ventricle → subarachnoid space
    C. lateral ventricles → interventricular foramen → third ventricle → cerebral aqueduct → fourth ventricle → foramina of Luschka and Magendie → subarachnoid space
    D. foramina of Luschka and Magendie → lateral ventricles → interventricular foramen → third ventricle → cerebral aqueduct → fourth ventricle → subarachnoid space

65. The ridge of cartilage at the tracheal bifurcation is the

    A. glottis
    B. carina
    C. cricoid
    D. conchae

66. The abdomen is clinically considered as divided by two horizontal and two sagittal planes into nine regions. The regions that lie bilaterally in the lowest part of the abdomen are referred to as the

    A. hypochondriac
    B. inguinal (iliac)
    C. lumbar
    D. hypogastric

Questions 67–71 refer to the following radiograph, which is an AP projection of the colon during a barium enema. Certain parts of the radiograph have been labeled with numbers. Each of the following questions is followed by four suggested labels or answers. For each question, select the one best answer.

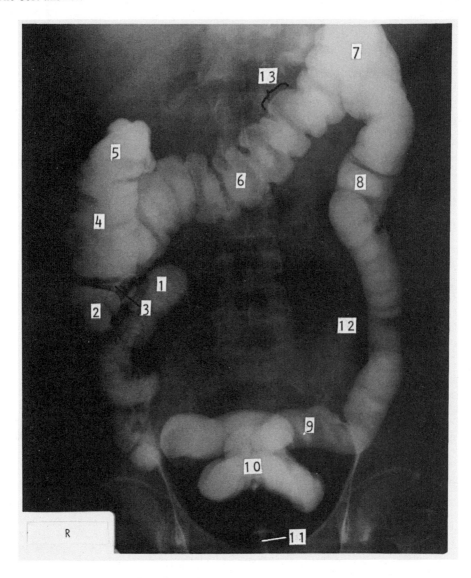

67. The cecum is the structure labeled with the number

A. 1
B. 2
C. 7
D. 9

68. The sigmoid is the structure labeled with the number

A. 6
B. 8
C. 9
D. 10

69. The hepatic flexure is the structure labeled with the number

A. 1
B. 5
C. 6
D. 7

70. The descending colon is the structure labeled with the number

A. 4
B. 6
C. 7
D. 8

71. The ileum is the structure labeled with the number

A. 1
B. 6
C. 10
D. 12

72. Cancer refers to a group of malignant diseases that have similar characteristics and effects on body cells and tissues. Which of the following are characteristic of cancer?

1. Hyperplasia
2. Anaplasia
3. Metastasis

A. 1 and 2
B. 1 and 3
C. 2 and 3
D. 1, 2, and 3

BODY—ANATOMY AND PHYSIOLOGY
ANSWERS, EXPLANATIONS, AND REFERENCES

1. The answer is A.   Blood consists of a liquid portion called plasma and cellular components called erythrocytes (RBCs), leukocytes (WBCs), and thrombocytes (platelets). RBCs consist of an iron and protein compound, hemoglobin, which is responsible for the transportation of essential gases, oxygen and carbon dioxide, throughout the body. WBCs help to combat disease through their phagocytotic function and also provide immunity. Thrombocytes are fragments of cells that play an active role in the clotting of blood, thereby preventing blood loss. Blood is essential to human viability: It provides a route by which vital nutrients and gases can be transported to and from cells, helps provide important defense mechanisms against disease, and helps to maintain a stable internal environment. *(Hole, p 612-624; Tortora and Anagnostakos, p 437-442)*

2. The answer is A.   Oxygenated blood from the placenta is brought to the fetus by way of the umbilical vein, which lies within the umbilical cord. This vessel enters the umbilicus of the fetus and continues to the liver, where it divides into two branches. One branch joins with the portal vein, and the other branch becomes the ductus venosus, which bypasses the fetal liver (as it does not contribute to digestive function) and enters the inferior vena cava. The foramen ovale is an opening that exists in the interatrial septum, between the right and left atria of the heart during fetal life. It shunts approximately one-third of the blood from the right side of the heart to the left, bypassing the pulmonary circulation (as the lungs are not functional in fetal life). The remainder of the blood, which does go from the right atrium into the right ventricle and pulmonary artery, will be shunted away from the lungs by the ductus arteriosus, which joins the pulmonary artery to the aorta of the fetus. *(Tortora and Anagnostakos, p 510-511; Hole, p 871-873; Chaffee et al., p 352-354)*

3. The answer is B.   The colon, or large intestine, is supplied with blood by branches of the inferior and superior mesenteric arteries. Branches of the superior mesenteric artery (SMA) supply the right side of the colon and most of the small intestine with oxygenated blood, and branches of the inferior mesenteric artery (IMA) supply the left side of the colon, sigmoid, and rectum with blood. Both the SMA and IMA arise directly off the front of the abdominal aorta. The celiac artery (axis) also arises off the abdominal aorta; but its branches supply the stomach and upper digestive tract, spleen, liver, and pancreas with blood. *(Hole, p 692; Tortora and Anagnostakos, p 498-499)*

4–7. The answers are; 4-A, 5-C, 6-A, 7-B.   The ethmoid is a small bone located between the orbits and behind the nose in the cranium. It consists of a cribiform plate, which transmits many nerves of smell (olfactory nerves) through its numerous foramina. This horizontal plate gives rise to a midline projection known as the crista galli on its anterosuperior aspect. Other parts of the ethmoid include the perpendicular plate, the superior and middle nasal conchae (turbinates), and the ethmoid air sinuses.
    The frontal bone forms the anterior part of the skull, upper orbital walls, forehead, and part of the upper nasal cavity. The glabella is a bony prominence of the frontal bone, located between the bony ridges of the eyebrows in the midline. This is often used as a positioning landmark in skull radiography. The frontal air sinuses are located in the squama of the frontal bone.
    The occipital bone forms part of the posterior (back) and inferior (base) of the cranium. The foramen magnum, a large opening in the basilar portion of the occipital bone, allows for passage of the medulla oblongata (part of the brain stem) through the cranial cavity. Other areas of the occipital bone include the squama and lateral portions. The occipital bone articulates with the first cervical vertebra at the atlantooccipital joints.
    The parietal bones form a great part of the sides and roof of the skull and articulate with the frontal bone in front, occipital bone behind, and temporal and sphenoid bones laterally. The biparietal diameter is a measurement of the widest width of the skull between the two parietal

bones laterally; this measurement may be employed in radiography and ultrasonography to help determine skull size and fetal age. *(Ballinger [Vol. 2], p 362-369; Tortora and Anagnostakos, p 141-148)*

8. The answer is D.   The pancreas is not considered to be a constituent of the lymphatic system; however, it is both an endocrine and exocrine gland, secreting the hormones insulin and glucagon along with digestive juices. The spleen, tonsils, and thoracic duct, as well as the lymph nodes, vessels, and thymus are all parts of the lymphatic system. The lymphatic system accompanies the circulatory system, picking up escaped plasma proteins from the interstitial spaces throughout the body and circulating them through lymphatic vessels. These eventually unite with lymph nodes, which then filter the lymph prior to its ultimate return to the blood vascular system. The lymphatic system also helps to defend the body against pathogenic organisms. The spleen is the largest organ of the lymphatic system and is responsible for storing blood, producing lymphocytes, and performing phagocytosis. Tonsils are masses of lymphatic tissue situated in the pharynx area. The thoracic duct is the large lymphatic vessel that receives lymph from all parts of the body except the right side of the head and thorax and delivers it to veins in the upper chest. *(Hole, p 499-500, 718-729; Tortora and Anagnostakos, p 520-526, 604-606)*

9. The answer is D.   A Colles' fracture involves the distal radius, with its distal fragment being displaced posteriorly and usually accompanied by a fracture of the ulnar styloid process; this is a common type of fracture of the wrist, occurring with trauma. A Pott's fracture involves the lower fibula, with injury to the distal tibial articulation. A boxer's fracture involves the neck of a metacarpal, with volar displacement of the head of the metacarpal. A greenstick fracture is most often encountered in younger patients and is characterized by an incomplete break accompanied by bowing. *(Tortora and Anagnostakos, p 133; Austrin, p 74)*

10. The answer is A.   An obstruction of the common bile duct may cause bile pigment (bilirubin) to back up into the liver and into the bloodstream (hyperbilirubinemia), causing a yellowish discoloration of the skin and of the sclera of the eye. Obstruction of the common bile duct may result from a gallstone lodged in the duct or from a tumor or stricture. Tumors, such as carcinoma of the head of pancreas, may produce extrinsic pressure on the common bile duct's opening into the duodenum, causing obstruction to the flow of bile and producing jaundice (icterus). Other causes of jaundice include dysfunction of the liver cells and increased RBC destruction. A stone in the cystic duct does not usually produce jaundice, as the bile could still flow from the liver to the duodenum. Other problems such as inflammation of the gallbladder (cholecystitis) and biliary colic (severe pain in the right upper quadrant of the abdomen) may, however, result from a stone obstructing the cystic duct. *(Cawson et al., p 369-370; Tortora and Anagnostakos, p 608-609)*

11. The answer is B.   The corpus callosum is a mass of white matter fibers that connect the two cerebral hemispheres internally. The falx cerebri is also located between the cerebral hemispheres but it is not composed of white matter; instead, it is an extension of the outer cranial meninx, the dura mater. The tentorium cerebelli is another extension of the cranial dura mater; it separates the cerebellum from the inferior portion of the cerebrum. The longitudinal fissure is a deep groove located between the two cerebral hemispheres. *(Hole, p 347-348; Tortora and Anagnostakos, p 324, 331)*

12. The answer is D.   The trachea is a fibrous and muscular tube located in front of the esophagus, extending from the larynx (C-6 verteba) to about the fifth thoracic vertebra, where it then bifurcates into the right and left mainstem bronchi. The rigid wall of the trachea consists of 16 to 20 incomplete cartilage rings. The trachea is flattened on its posterior wall, where smooth muscle connects the ends of the incomplete cartilage rings, allowing the esophagus to expand into the trachea during swallowing. The rigid cartilage walls of the trachea help to prevent inward collapse and airway obstruction. *(Hole, p 573-575; Tortora and Anagnostakos, p 546-550)*

13. The answer is A.   The styloid processes are not part of the sphenoid bone; instead, they are located on the undersurface of the temporal bone, bilaterally. The sphenoid bone forms part of the base of the skull and contains numerous foramina and processes. Its main parts are the body, greater and lesser wings, and pterygoid processes. The body of the sphenoid gives rise to a saddle-like depression called the sella turcica, which houses the pituitary gland. The sphenoid contains two sphenoidal air sinuses, the posterior clinoid processes, and the dorsum and tuberculum sellae. The greater wings of the sphenoid contain the foramina ovale, spinosum, and rotundum, which are situated bilaterally and transmit cranial blood vessels and nerves. The lesser wings contain the superior orbital fissures, optic canals, and anterior clinoid processes. The undersurface of the sphenoid bone gives rise to two pterygoid processes bilaterally. *(Ballinger [Vol. 2], p 366-367, 370; Chaffee et al., p 96-97; Meschan, p 222-226; Tortora and Anagnostakos, p 144-145)*

14. The answer is D.   The bregma is the point where the coronal and sagittal sutures of the skull meet. The nasion is the point of union between the frontal and nasal bones. The inion (external occipital protruberance) is the bony prominence in the back of the skull in the midline, above the foramen magnum of the occipital bone. The lambda is the point where the sagittal and lambdoidal sutures of the skull meet. *(Ballinger [Vol. 2], p 363-364, 366; Meschan, p 220)*

15. The answer is B.   *Dysphagia* is the term that means "difficult or painful swallowing." It is often a primary symptom of patients with esophageal abnormalities. *Dyspepsia* means "difficulty digesting" (indigestion), and *pyrosis* is the medical term for heartburn, or a burning sensation experienced in the lower esophagus and stomach. *Dystocia* means "difficulty in giving birth," abnormal labor. *(Cawson et al., p 331, 335; Frenay and Mahoney, p 187, 192, 260; Hole, p 519; Tortora and Anagnostakos, p 625)*

16. The answer is A.   The testes, or male gonads, produce spermatazoa, which travel through two excretory channels, one from each testis. The excretory channel begins in the epididymis, an oblong structure consisting of tiny convoluted ductules (seminiferous tubules). These tubules emerge from each testis and convey spermatazoa to the ductus (vas) deferens, a long tube (16 to 18 inches in length) that ascends through the scrotum and lower abdomen to the lower surface of the urinary bladder, where it meets the seminal vesicles. The seminal vesicles, pouch-like structures lying on the lateral posterior aspect of the bladder, secrete an alkaline fluid that helps to maintain viability of the spermatazoa. The ejaculatory ducts are formed by the union of the ductus deferens and seminal vesicles and are responsible for ejecting spermatazoa into the prostatic urethra, which passes through the prostate gland, receiving more alkaline fluid secretion from this gland. The fluid secretions and spermatazoa are collectively called semen, which will pass from the prostatic urethra to the membranous and spongy urethra, eventually being externally passed through the urethral orifice. *(Ballinger [Vol. 3], p 718-719; Hole, p 812-818; Tortora and Anagnostakos, p 703-706)*

17. The answer is A.   Glands in the mucosa of the stomach contain several kinds of cells that secrete various constituents of gastric juice. Chief cells of these glands secrete pepsinogen, which is converted into pepsin by other gastric juices, to break down proteins. Mucous cells of the gastric glands secrete mucus and alkaline fluid, which help to protect the mucosal wall of the stomach from being digested by pepsin. Other secretions of the gastric glands include hydrochloric acid, which provides an acid environment for pepsinogen to be converted into active pepsin, and gastrin, a hormone that stimulates the secretion of hydrochloric acid and pepsinogen. Gastric juice is the fluid combination of all of these secretions. Secretin is not secreted by the stomach but is secreted by the duodenal mucosa; this hormone stimulates pancreatic secretions. *(Hole, p 494-496, 500; Tortora and Anagnostakos, p 598-602, 606)*

18. The answer is A.   Air inspired through the nose or mouth will normally pass into the nasal cavity (if entering through the nose) or into the oral cavity (if entering through the mouth). It then passes into the pharynx (throat), which lies behind the nasal and oral cavities and above the trachea. After passing through the pharynx, it goes through the larynx, into the trachea. The trachea branches off into two mainstem, or primary, bronchi, one to each lung; air passes through these bronchi into smaller lobar and segmental bronchi. Bronchi eventually merge into smaller channels, called bronchioles (terminal, then respiratory bronchioles), which eventually enter into the alveoli (air sacs) of the lungs through tiny ducts. In the alveoli, inspired air passes through the alveolar-capillary membrane and permits the exchange of gases between the respiratory and circulatory systems. *(Hole, p 568-579; Tortora and Anagnostakos, p 542-556)*

19. The answer is B.   The detrusor muscle forms the muscular wall of the urinary bladder and participates in the urination (micturition) reflex. The detrusor muscle is innervated by the parasympathetic nervous system as the bladder distends with urine. During urination, the detrusor muscle contracts, along with some of the pelvic and abdominal muscles, and the external urethral sphincter (band of muscle) relaxes. *(Hole, p 772; Tortora and Anagnostakos, p 678)*

20. The answer is D.   Persons with type O blood are considered to be universal donors and can theoretically have their blood transfused to persons with any other blood type (O, A, B, AB), as type O will not agglutinate the other types. Persons with type AB blood are theoretically considered to be universal recipients and can receive all other blood types. In practice, however, only matched blood types are used for transfusion in order to minimize any adverse reactions. *(Tortora and Anagnostakos, p 447-449; Hole, p 634-637)*

21. The answer is C.   The mandible consists of a horizontal body and two vertical extensions called rami. The superior part of the body gives rise to the alveolar process, or arch, which receives the roots of the lower teeth. Each of the two bilateral rami extends upward and divides into two processes, an anterior coronoid process, which attaches to muscle, and a posterior condyle, which articulates with the temporal bone above to form the temporomandibular joint. Between the condyles and coronoid processes is a mandibular notch. Other characteristic components of the mandible include the mental protruberance, mental foramina, and symphysis menti. The mandible is an important facial bone because it is the only one that moves, enabling chewing action and speech formation. Fractures of the mandible often involve parts of the mandibular body and processes of the rami. *(Ballinger [Vol. 2], p 376-377; Hole, p 200-202; Tortora and Anagnostakos, p 150)*

22. The answer is D.   Body tissues respond to injury through inflammation, which is usually characterized by heat, edema, redness, and pain. When tissue injury is severe enough, normal function may be lost as well. The inflammatory response occurs in various stages, producing these characteristic symptoms as it tries to restore homeostasis in the body. After tissue injury, blood vessels in the injured area dilate and become more permeable so that more blood and needed substances can get to the affected area. As the blood vessels become more permeable, fluid moves out of the blood and accumulates in the injured tissue spaces, producing edema or swelling. Heat and redness are also produced after vascular dilation and increased permeability, as more warm blood accumulates in the injured area. Pain is produced when nerve fibers are injured, when edema produces increased pressure in the area, and when microorganisms cause irritation to tissues. Besides vasodilation and increased vascular permeability, other inflammatory response stages include phagocytotic function, nutrition to the cells, clot formation, and pus formation. The inflammatory response is an important defense mechanism for maintaining the body's internal environment and promoting healing. *(Cawson et al., p 46-65; Hole, p 116-117, 136, 620-621; Tortora and Anagnostakos, p 98-101)*

23. The answer is B.   Blood urea nitrogen (BUN) levels are a measurement of urea (nitrogenous waste) in the blood. Protein is metabolized in the liver, and urea is the by-product that is normally carried through the bloodstream to the kidneys, where it is excreted. If the kidneys are malfunctioning as a result of disease, then urea may not be filtered and excreted by the kidneys as it should be, leaving excess urea in the blood. Creatinine is the by-product of muscle metabolism. It is another nitrogenous waste that is also filtered out of the blood and excreted by the kidneys. The amount produced and excreted per day is relatively constant for each individual. If the blood level of creatinine increases, however, then kidney dysfunction may be suspected. BUN and blood creatinine determinations can be very useful to radiologists prior to intravenous urography using positive contrast agents, as they indicate not only kidney function but also efficacy of the examination. Together these laboratory evaluations are sensitive indicators of kidney function. (Normal levels of BUN are approximately 0.8 to 18 mg/100 ml of blood, and of creatinine, approximately 0.6 to 1.2 mg/100 ml of blood.) (*Frenay and Mahoney, p 445, 446; Hole, p 87, 627, 769; Tortora and Anagnostakos, p 675*)

24. The answer is D.   There are twelve pairs of ribs, which help to form the thoracic cage. Each rib has a superior and inferior facet and articulates with a thoracic vertebra (facet) posteriorly. The first seven pairs of ribs are called true ribs because each attaches directly to the sternum by costal cartilage. The other five pairs of ribs do not attach directly to the sternum; therefore, they are called false ribs. The eighth, ninth, and tenth pairs of ribs are joined by their costal cartilage, which then attaches to the costal cartilage of the seventh rib. The 11th and 12th pairs of ribs are not attached in any way to the sternum anteriorly; hence, the name floating ribs has been given to them. The ribs, along with the sternum, provide protection to the vital internal organs of the thoracic cavity. (*Hole, p 209-211; Tortora and Anagnostakos, p 159-160*)

25. The answer is A.   The gallbladder contracts in response to the hormone cholecystokinin, which is secreted by the duodenal mucosa when fats are present in the small intestine. The neck of the gallbladder is constricted and joins the cystic duct, which then empties bile into the common bile duct. The gallbladder stores and concentrates bile many times by reabsorbing water. The presence of stones in the gallbladder (cholelithiasis) may produce inflammation of the mucosa of the gallbladder (cholecystitis). (*Austrin, p 183, 185; Chaffee et al., p 445-449; Hole, p 504-506; Tortora and Anagnostakos, p 610, 624*)

26. The answer is C.   Adduction refers to the movement of a body part toward the central axis, or midline, of the body, such as bringing an extended arm or leg back toward the body. The opposite of adduction is abduction, or drawing a body part away from the midline of the body, such as extending the arms or legs straight out from the shoulders or hips. Flexion is the bending of a joint; its opposite is extension, or straightening a joint. Inversion is the turning inward of a body part (extremity); its opposing motion is eversion, turning outward. Supination is turning upward, such as turning the palm of the hand up or turning the body, face, and ventral aspect up. All of these terms denoting movement are used to describe body positioning for radiography of various anatomic parts. (*Austrin, p 69; Ballinger [Vol. 1], p 14; Gylys and Wedding, p 185-186; Wroble, p 174-175*)

27. The answer is C.   The navicular, or scaphoid, bone is the first carpal bone in the proximal row, distal to the radius on the thumb side. The navicular bone must sometimes be radiographed using special projections of the wrist in order to free its borders from the other carpal bones. Of all the carpal bones, the navicular is most commonly fractured. The greater multiangular bone, or trapezium, is the first carpal bone in the distal row on the thumb side. The pisiform is located in the proximal row on the ulnar side, and the hamate is in the distal row, also on the ulnar side. Other carpal bones include the lunate, triquetral (triangular), lesser multangular (trapezoid), and capitate (os magnum). From the thumb, or lateral, side to the medial side, the eight carpals are arranged as follows: proximal row—navicular, lunate, triquetral, and pisiform; and the distal row—greater multangular, lesser multangular, capitate, and hamate. (*Ballinger [Vol. 1], p 118-119; Chaffee et al., 109-110; Hole, p 216; Tortora and Anagnostakos, p 166-167*)

28. The answer is C.   The hypersthenic body habitus is one in which the thorax is broad and deep, the thoracic cavity is shallow, the lungs are short, the heart is short and wide, and the diaphragm is high, creating a long abdomen. The stomach and gallbladder occupy high, almost horizontal positions. The colon is also high and courses around the periphery of the abdominal cavity. The sthenic habitus represents the predominant body build and is a modification of the hypersthenic. The abdomen and thorax tend to be more equal in size. The asthenic habitus is one of an extremely slender body, with a thorax that is narrow and shallow, long thoracic cavity and lungs, and a long and narrow heart and low diaphragm, creating a short abdominal cavity. The stomach and gallbladder are low, vertical, and nearer to the midline of the body, with the colon folding upon itself and occupying a low, medial position. The hyposthenic body build is not as extreme as the asthenic type, falling between it and the sthenic build. *(Ballinger [Vol. 3], p 570-571)*

29. The answer is B. Oliguria refers to scanty urine output in relation to fluid intake. It may be due to electrolyte and fluid imbalance, kidney pathology, or urinary tract obstruction. Excessive secretion and output of urine are referred to as polyuria, and uncontrolled urination or bed-wetting is called enuresis. Anuria is total suppression of urine formation and secretion. Most of these terms are used to describe symptoms of urinary tract pathology or other problems. *(Austrin, p 220; Frenay and Mahoney, p 218, 224; Gylys and Wedding, p 222)*

30. The answer is D. Blood cell production takes place in several hematopoietic (blood-forming) organs and tissues, including the red bone marrow, spleen, lymph nodes, and tonsils. RBCs (erythrocytes), which are important in transporting gases between the circulatory system and cells throughout the body, are produced primarily in the red bone marrow, as are platelets (thrombocytes), which play a role in clotting blood. WBCs (leukocytes) are formed in two different types of tissues: Those WBCs with granules in their nucleus (neutrophils, basophils, and eosinophils) are only formed in the red bone marrow; those without granules in their nucleus (lymphocytes and monocytes) are produced in both red bone marrow and lymphoid tissue of the spleen, lymph nodes, and tonsils. WBCs play an important part in defending the body against pathogenic organisms and in the immune response. *(Hole, p 615, 726-729; Tortora and Anagnostakos, p 436-442)*

31. The answer is B. A bone that is broken or splintered into small fragments is said to have a comminuted fracture. In a complicated or complex fracture, a broken bone may injure nearby tissues or an organ (e.g., a pelvic fracture that tears the urinary bladder). A capillary fracture is a hairline break in a bone, and a compound (open) fracture is one in which an external wound leads to a broken bone or a bone protrudes through a break in the skin. Fractures commonly occur as a result of trauma and usually require radiographic demonstration before treatment or reduction can be attempted. *(Austrin, p 74; Gylys and Wedding, p 190-191)*

32–36. The answers are 32-C, 33-B, 34-D, 35-C, 36-D. The hepatobiliary system and pancreas, illustrated in the figure that accompanies the question, are considered as accessory organs to the digestive system. The following structures are identified: (1) falciform ligament, (2) left hepatic duct, (3) right hepatic duct, (4) cystic duct, (5) common hepatic duct, (6) common bile duct, (7) accessory pancreatic duct, or duct of Santorini, (8) tail of the pancreas, (9) body of the pancreas, (10) duct of Wirsung, or main pancreatic duct, (11) head of the pancreas, (12) ampulla of Vater, or hepatopancreatic ampulla, (13) duodenal papilla, (14) body of gallbladder, (15) fundus of gallbladder, and (16) neck of gallbladder. The hepatobiliary system consists of the liver, bile ducts, and gallbladder. The liver is a very large, solid organ located in the upper abdomen beneath the diaphragm. It is divided by the falciform ligament into two major lobes. The liver cells are responsible for numerous functions, one being the production (secretion) of bile, which helps to digest fats in the small intestine. This bile secretion is carried from the hepatic cells into tiny ducts called canaliculi, which eventually empty into larger ducts. Numerous bile ducts merge from the right and left lobes of the liver into the right and left hepatic ducts, which unite to form a single common hepatic duct. As the common hepatic duct descends, it joins the cystic duct from the gallbladder. The gallbladder functions to store and concentrate bile and release it when needed to emulsify fats in the small intestine. The cystic duct and common hepatic duct unite to form the common bile duct, which empties bile into the descending duodenum. In the majority of individuals, the common bile duct and duct of Wirsung (main pancreatic duct) join at their lower portions to form the ampulla of Vater (hepatopancreatic ampulla), which then enters the descending duodenum. The elevation inside the duodenum where these ducts open is called the duodenal papilla. The duct of Wirsung brings digestive enzymes from the pancreas to the duodenum to help digest carbohydrates, proteins, and fats. The duct of Santorini (accessory pancreatic duct) emerges from the head of the pancreas and usually enters the duodenum about an inch above the ampulla of Vater. Bile and digestive enzymes pass through a sequential ductal system in order to reach the small intestine, where the majority of digestion takes place. In radiography of the hepatobiliary system and pancreas, radiopaque contrast agents are administered in a variety of ways in order to demonstrate the accessory digestive organs and their ductal system. *(Ballinger [Vol. 3], p 604-606; Hole, p 499-506; Tortora and Anagnostakos, p 604-610)*

37. The answer is C. Scoliosis is an abnormal lateral curvature of the vertebral column, often encountered in childhood. The hips or shoulders may be at unequal heights, and thoracic and abdominal organs may be displaced or compressed. Kyphosis ("hunchback") is an abnormal exaggerated convex curvature of the thoracic spine. Lordosis refers to an abnormal exaggerated concave curvature of the lumbar spine, often called "swayback." Abnormal spinal curvatures may be the result of congenital malformations or a variety of disease processes. Spondylosis is a condition characterized by stiffening and/or fixation of the vertebral joints, also called vertebral ankylosis. *(Austrin, p 75; Hole, p 210; Tortora and Anagnostakos, p 160; Bontrager and Anthony, p 265-266)*

38. The answer is D. Sciatica (sciatic neuralgia) is a painful disorder affecting the sciatic nerve, which innervates muscles in the thigh and leg. Compression of this nerve by pathology such as a herniated intervetebral disk or tumor in the lower spine region results in excruciating pain that radiates through the buttocks and thigh to the leg. Bell's palsy is an acute neurological condition affecting muscles of the face, usually on one side. Trigeminal neuralgia (tic douloureux), is a disorder affecting the facial area innervated by the trigeminal nerve. Attacks of severe pain occur along the area where the trigeminal nerve is distributed and last for a few seconds but may recur. Paraplegia is paralysis or loss of sensory or motor function affecting the lower extremities and possibly involving lower back and abdominal muscles. Paraplegia may be the result of spinal cord compression or trauma. *(Boyd and Sheldon, p 462; Cawson et al., p 528-529; Frenay and Mahoney, p 72; Tortora and Anagnostakos, p 305; Wroble, p 522, 529)*

39. The answer is D. The conjunctiva lines the eyelid (palpebral conjunctiva) and reflects over the anterior surface of the eyeball (bulbar conjunctiva). The sclera is the opaque white portion of the eye forming the posterior part of the outer fibrous tunic. The cornea is transparent and is continuous with the sclera, forming the anterior portion of the outer fibrous tunic. The lacrimal sac is located medial to the eye, deep in the lacrimal bone; it receives tears from the lacrimal ducts. *(Tortora and Anagnostakos, p 377-380; Hole, p 411-414; Chaffee et al., p 267-269)*

40. The answer is B. Females are born with approximately 200,000 primary follicles enclosing potential ova in each ovary. Every month, some of these follicles begin to develop until one matures and expels an ovum into the pelvic cavity. After this, those follicles that began to develop will atrophy and die. Follicle growth is governed by various hormonal secretions. Estrogen and progesterone are secreted by endocrine glands within the ovaries; estrogen is responsible for growth and maintenance of the female reproductive organs along with secondary sex characteristics. Progesterone and estrogen prepare the uterine lining for implantation of a fertilized ovum and also prepare the breasts for lactation (milk production). Fertilization (union of ovum and sperm) normally occurs in the distal portion of the fallopian tube after the fimbriae (ends) of the tubes sweep the expelled ovum (after ovulation) from the pelvic cavity through the tube and toward the uterus. Implantation normally takes place in the uterine cavity; if, however, fertilization does not take place, the ovum will decompose and another menstrual cycle begins. *(Hole, p 837-838; Tortora and Anagnostakos, p 709-718, 735)*

41. The answer is B.   The pelvic girdle is not part of the axial skeleton but is part of the appendicular skeleton, which also includes the free bony appendages of the upper and lower extremities, along with the shoulder (pectoral) girdle. There are 126 bones in the appendicular skeleton and 80 bones in the axial skeleton. The skull, thoracic cage, and vertebral column, along with the auditory ossicles and hyoid bone, form the axial skeleton, those bones surrounding the body's axis. *(Hole, p 191-192; Tortora and Anagnostakos, p 138, 141)*

42. The answer is A.   At about the level of the fourth lumbar vertebra, the abdominal aorta bifurcates in the abdomen into the right and left common iliac arteries. Each common iliac descends and then divides into the internal and external iliac arteries. The external iliacs continue through the groin to become the femoral arteries, and the internal iliac (hypogastric) arteries give off branches that supply the pelvic organs and muscles. The coronary sinus, a large venous structure located on the posterior aspect of the heart, receives blood from the cardiac veins that drain the myocardium. The coronary sinus carries blood that contains carbon dioxide and wastes to the right atrium of the heart, where it will eventually be pumped into the pulmonary circulation for reoxygenation. The great saphenous vein is a long superficial vein extending from the foot to the groin area in each leg. It brings blood that is rich in carbon dioxide and wastes from the superficial tissues of the lower extremities to the femoral vein. The great saphenous vein communicates with the deep veins of the leg through numerous tributaries. The small saphenous vein, another superficial vein of the leg, extends from the foot to the knee area. The superficial veins of the lower extremities are often subject to varicosity because the force of gravity exerts pressure on the blood that is flowing upward in these veins. This condition is generally caused by standing for long periods and breaking down or weakening the valves within these veins. The saphenous veins are also frequently used as grafts for coronary bypass surgery. *(Hole, p 659, 698, 706-707; Tortora and Anagnostakos, p 467-468, 500-501, 508-509)*

43. The answer is C.   Cytoplasm is not a cell organelle; it is a fluid found within the cell membrane and external to the cell nucleus. This fluid is the substance within which chemical reactions occur. Organelles are located within the cell's cytoplasm and are responsible for specific roles in growth, maintenance, repair, and control. Organelles include the following structures: the nucleus, endoplasmic reticulum, ribosomes, lysosomes, mitochondria, Golgi complex, centrosomes and centrioles, microtubules, flagella, and cilia. *(Tortora and Anagnostakos, p 58-64; Hole, p 44-53; Chaffee et al., p 33-39)*

44. The answer is A.   The sudoriferous (sweat) glands are distributed throughout the skin and secrete perspiration (sweat). The function of these glands is to eliminate wastes and to help maintain body temperature. The sebaceous glands, also located in the dermis, secrete an oily substance called sebum, which helps to keep the skin soft and moist and prevents the hair from becoming dry and brittle. Ceruminous glands, found in the external auditory meatus of the ear, secrete cerumen, a waxy secretion that helps to prevent foreign objects from entering the ear. Bartholin's (vestibular) glands, small glands that lie in the vestibule of the female vulva, secrete a lubricating fluid into the vagina. *(Tortora and Anagnostakos, p 113, 387, 389, 720; Hole, p 131, 132, 401, 830)*

45. The answer is D.   Paget's disease (osteitis deformans) is a common bone disorder characterized by increased bone resorption and formation of new bone that is abnormal in architecture. Thickening and weakening of the affected bones may cause distortion under stress. This disease primarily affects individuals older than 50 years and may affect the bones of the skull, pelvis, and extremities. Besides the deformities that may result, pathological fractures, osteogenic sarcoma, and compression of the cranial nerves may occur. Multiple myeloma is a malignant bone disease characterized by multiple tumors occurring throughout the skeletal system. Osteoporosis is a condition of increased bone porosity due to abnormal mineralization, most often accompanying the aging process. Rickets, a bone disorder that affects children, is caused by abnormal mineralization of bone accompanied by softening and deformity. The nutritional deficiency of vitamin D and lack of sunlight are thought to be contributing factors.

Radiographic examination of the bones may reveal any of the above diseases and their characteristic architectural abnormalities. *(Cawson et al., p 410-414, 424; Tortora and Anagnostakos, p 131-133)*

46. The answer is A. The thymus gland consists of two lobes and is located in the superior mediastinum, behind the sternum. This gland is relatively large in infants and continues to grow, achieving its maximum size at puberty, after which the gland atrophies. The lymphatic tissue of the thymus gland plays a role in immunity, as it helps to produce lymphocytes that work to destroy foreign organisms in the body. The cells that the thymus processes are called T cells; they eventually leave the thymus and enter lymphoid tissue throughout the body, where they can be activated by foreign antigens. The thymus gland also stimulates production of B-cell lymphocytes, which also play a role in the immune response. *(Hole, p 466, 726, 731; Tortora and Anagnostakos, p 425-426, 525-526, 533-535)*

47. The answer is A. Callus is the substance that grows between fractured ends of bones during healing and is an important constituent in the stabilization of broken bones. It is eventually changed into hard osseous tissue after bone repair, binding the fractured ends together. Bony callus can usually be demonstrated radiographically. Thickened, hardened skin as a result of chronic friction or pressure is also known as callus. Diploë is the spongy bone found in the cranium; cicatrix is scar tissue; and collagen is the substance present between the fibers of connective tissue throughout the body. *(Austrin, p 116; Cawson et al., p 61; Wroble, p 154, 184)*

48. The answer is A. The coracoid process is a projection off the anterior surface of the scapula (shoulder blade) on the lateral end of its superior border, serving as an attachment for muscles. In radiographing the shoulder joint, the coracoid is the point to which the central ray of the x-ray beam is directed in the AP projection. The coracoid should not be confused with the coronoid process, which projects anteriorly from the proximal portion of the ulna at the elbow joint. *(Tortora and Anagnostakos, p 164-166; Hole, p 213-214; Meschan, p 79-82)*

49. The answer is A. The glenoid cavity is the depression on the head of the scapula that articulates with the head of the humerus (upper arm bone) to form the shoulder joint. The coracoid process arises internal to the glenoid cavity and projects forward. The acromion process is the lateral extension of the spine of the scapula; it articulates with the clavicle to form the acromioclavicular joints. Subluxations and dislocations of the shoulder may occur as a result of trauma and separation of the humerus from its normal position in the glenoid cavity. *(Hole, p 213; Meschan, p 79-83; Tortora and Anagnostakos, p 164-166)*

50. The answer is C. The medial styloid process is located at the distal end of the ulna (medial bone of the forearm). This medial styloid process can be palpated along with the lateral styloid process of the distal radius (lateral bone of the forearm) when positioning a patient for radiographs of the wrist and forearm. Both medial and lateral styloid processes serve as attachments for ligaments of the wrist. *(Hole, p 216; Meschan, p 64-70; Tortora and Anagnostakos, p 166)*

51. The answer is C. The olecranon process forms the bony posterior prominence of the proximal end of the ulna, providing an attachment for the muscle that straightens the arm at the elbow joint. The olecranon process is the most prominent bony projection of the elbow. Between the olecranon and the coronoid process (anterior prominence of the proximal ulna) is a curved opening called the semilunar, or trochlear, notch, which articulates with the trochlea of the humerus. Above the trochlea are two fossae—the olecranon fossa, posteriorly, and the coronoid process, anteriorly. As the elbow is straightened, the olecranon fossa receives the olecranon process; and as the elbow is bent or flexed, the coronoid fossa will receive the coronoid process. Both processes, as well as fossae, are important in normal movement of the elbow joint. *(Hole, p 214-216; Meschan, p 69-75; Tortora and Anagnostakos, p 164-167)*

52. The answer is B. The capitulum is a rounded, knob-like part on the lateral side of the distal humerus. It articulates with the head of the radius at the elbow joint. The trochlea, a pulley-shaped prominence, is located medial to the capitulum on the distal humerus and articulates with the ulna at the elbow joint. Other names for the trochlea and capitulum are the medial and lateral condyles, respectively. The elbow is radiographed in the AP, oblique, and lateral positions in order to evaluate these bony prominences. *(Hole, p 214-215; Meschan, p 69-75; Tortora and Anagnostakos, p 164-167)*

53. The answer is B. The deltoid tuberosity is a V-shaped area on the midshaft of the humerus, serving as an attachment for the deltoid muscle of the upper arm. This muscle connects the scapula and clavicle to the lateral side of the humerus and helps to raise the arm horizontally to the side. *Deltoid* means "shaped like a delta or triangle." *(Tortora and Anagnostakos, p 164-167; Hole, p 214-215, 275; Meschan, p 76)*

54–58. The answers are 54-D, 55-D, 56-B, 57-C, 58-C. The anatomic sketch that accompanies the question identifies the following skull structures: (1) mandible, (2) maxilla, (3) zygomatic bone, (4) frontal bone, (5) parietal bone, (6) sphenoid bone, (7) temporal bone, (8) nasal bone, (9) occipital bone, (10) coronal suture, (11) squamosal suture, (12) lambdoidal suture, (13) anterior nasal spine, or acanthion, (14) mental foramen of mandible, (15) coronoid process of mandible, (16) condyle of mandible, (17) external acoustic meatus, (18) mastoid process, (19) styloid process, (20) hyoid bone, (21) ethmoid bone, and (22) lacrimal bone. The skull encloses and protects the brain and gives rise to muscle attachments of the face. There are 22 bones in the skull; 8 make up the cranial vault, and 14 form the face. There is only one movable bone in the skull, the mandible. The eight cranial bones that cover the brain are the two parietal bones, two temporal bones, one sphenoid, one ethmoid, one occipital, and one frontal bone.

The sphenoid bone forms part of the base of the skull and articulates with the seven other cranial bones. The ethmoid bone is found between the orbits and forms the anterior floor of the cranium. The occipital bone lies posterior and forms the posterior floor of the cranial base. The frontal bone lies anterior and forms the forehead and part of the cranial floor. The two parietal bones form the sides and roof of the skull, and the two temporal bones are located near the ears, inferior to the parietal bones, and form the lower sides of the skull. The temporal bones give rise bilaterally to the styloid processes, which project forward and provide attachment sites for muscles and ligaments. The zygomatic processes are also part of the temporal bones bilaterally; they articulate with the zygomatic, or malar, bones.

Cranial bones are joined together at sutures, which are the immovable joints of the skull. Four of the major sutures are the coronal, sagittal, lambdoidal, and squamosal. The lambdoidal suture lies between the parietal and occipital bones, posteriorly, and the coronal suture lies between the frontal and parietal bones. The sagittal suture lies between the two parietal bones, and the squamosal suture joins the parietal and temporal bones, bilaterally.

The bones of the anterior skull, or face, include two nasal, two maxillae, two inferior nasal conchae, two palatine, two lacrimal, one vomer, one mandible, and two zygomatic bones. The zygomatic bones form the cheeks and part of the orbital floors. *(Ballinger [Vol. 2], p 362-376; Hole, p 195-202; Tortora and Anagnostakos, p 138-151)*

59. The answer is C. The diaphysis, or shaft, of a long bone is formed from the primary center of ossification. It is located between the articular ends, or epiphyses, of long bones. The endosteum is the lining of a long bone's medullary cavity, which surrounds the bone marrow. The metaphysis is that part of a long bone between the diaphysis and epiphysis. Other major portions of a long bone include the periosteum, the outer protective covering surrounding most of the bone except the epiphysis, and the articular cartilage, which covers the epiphysis of a bone at a joint. *(Hole, p 176-177; Tortora and Anagnostakos, p 125)*

60. The answer is C. In the performance guidelines set up by the American Heart Association, 15 compressions over the lower sternum at a rate of 80 compressions per minute followed by two rescue breaths are recommended for single-rescuer cardiopulmonary resuscitation (CPR) on an adult victim. This cycle is begun after the rescuer has determined a lack of response, breathing, and pulse in a victim and after the rescuer has performed the tasks of establishing an open airway, correctly positioning the victim, and requesting emergency help. Infants and small children require a more rapid cardiac compression rate of 100 or 80/minute, respectively, with a rescue breath administered after every five compressions. Hand positioning also changes for infants and small children. Two-rescuer CPR uses a 5:1 ratio of compressions to ventilations in an adult victim. *(Montgomery and Herrin, p 22-31, 44-47; Tortora and Anagnostakos, p 571-574)*

61. The answer is A.   Anemia is a blood disorder characterized by lack of RBCs or decreased hemoglobin concentration. Persons afflicted with this disorder may appear pale and tired because their oxygen-carrying capacity is reduced. Some of the various types of anemia are aplastic, hypochromic, hemolytic, hemorrhagic, and pernicious. Polycythemia is an abnormal blood condition in which too many RBCs exist in the bloodstream, causing the blood to thicken and producing a resistance to blood flow. Hodgkin's disease is a malignant disorder of the lymphatic system characterized by the presence of abnormal lymphocytes (a type of WBC), enlargement of lymph nodes, and lymphoma. Hemophilia is a hereditary blood disease characterized by abnormal bleeding due to deficient clotting mechanisms. *(Hole, p 618, 633; Tortora and Anagnostakos, p 75, 440, 445-446)*

62. The answer is A.   Neurons, or nerve cells, are essential in the conduction of impulses between various parts of the body and central nervous system. Neurons consist of three main parts—a cell body (perikaryon), an axon, and dendrites. The cell body is composed of a nucleolus and nucleus surrounded by cytoplasm containing organelles, Nissl bodies, and neurofibrils. Proteins and other essential substances are synthesized in the cell body, and the cytoplasmic processes, axons, and dendrites are involved with conduction of nerve impulses. An axon is a long, narrow process that extends from the cell body of a neuron and is responsible for carrying impulses away from the cell body to body tissues or other neurons. Dendrites are thick, branch-like extensions of a cell body; they conduct impulses toward the cell body from another neuron or tissue. A synapse refers to the junction between neurons over which impulses are transmitted. Impulses are usually transmitted from the dendrites or cell body of a neuron to its axon and then across a synaptic junction to the dendrites or cell body of another neuron. *(Hole, p 310-311, 320; Tortora and Anagnostakos, p 269-271, 278)*

63. The answer is A.   The splenic and superior mesenteric veins unite to form the portal vein, which brings venous blood from the spleen and gastrointestinal tract to the liver for processing. The splenic vein drains the spleen and receives the gastric veins (which drain the stomach), pancreatic veins (which drain the pancreas), inferior mesenteric veins (which drain the left side of the colon), and other venous tributaries. The cystic vein (from the gallbladder) enters the portal vein just before the portal vein enters the porta hepatis of the liver. Ultimately, blood from the portal vein passes through liver sinusoids and into the hepatic veins, which drain blood into the inferior vena cava. *(Tortora and Anagnostakos, p 510; Hole, p 704-705; Chaffee et al., p 351-352)*

64. The answer is C.   Cerebrospinal fluid (CSF) is a clear, protective fluid formed in the choroid plexuses of the brain. It circulates through the ventricular system into the subarachnoid space surrounding the brain and spinal cord, helping to absorb shock (injury) to these important parts of the central nervous system. Most CSF passes into the two lateral ventricles (one in each cerebral hemisphere) from the choroid plexuses. From the lateral ventricles, it passes through the interventricular foramen (or foramen of Monro), which opens into the third ventricle (below and between the lateral ventricles). From the third ventricle, CSF passes through the cerebral aqueduct (or aqueduct of Sylvius) through the midbrain, into the upper portion of the fourth ventricle. From the fourth ventricle, CSF passes through two lateral openings (foramina of Luschka) and one medial opening (foramen of Magendie), which communicate with the subarachnoid space. Once in this space, CSF can bathe the brain and spinal cord, providing both nutrients and protection. Some CSF is produced in the choroid plexuses of the third and fourth ventricles; its passage begins at a lower point in the ventricular system but travels the remainder of the course as described above. CSF is produced continuously as it is absorbed into the bloodstream following its circulation. CSF pressure should be constant; however, pathological changes can cause it to increase, creating abnormal and potentially dangerous increased intracranial pressure. *(Ballinger [Vol. 3], p 762-763; Hole, p 354-357; Tortora and Anagnostakos, p 310-313)*

65. The answer is B.   The carina is the ridge within the trachea where bifurcation into the left and right primary bronchi occurs. Abnormal widening and distortion of the carina may be indicative of pathology, especially carcinoma. An instrument called a bronchoscope allows visual examination of this area and other aspects of the tracheal and bronchial lumen. The glottis is the opening between the true vocal cords in the larynx through which air passes. The cricoid is a ring of cartilage located below the larynx and attached to the first tracheal cartilage. Conchae are the scroll-like bones that form part of the lateral walls of the nasal cavity. *(Tortora and Anagnostakos, p 150, 545-549; Hole, p 572-575)*

66. The answer is B.   The nine abdominal regions are illustrated in the following figure:

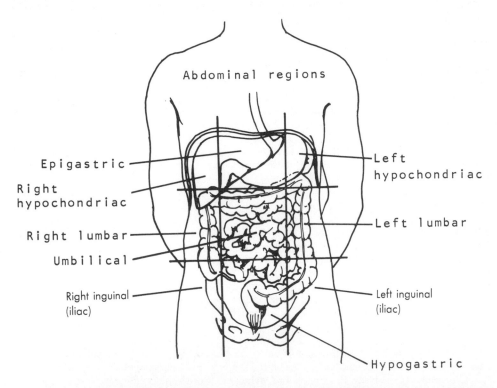

The inguinal, or iliac, regions are the lower, lateral portions of the abdomen comprising the groin area, bilateral to the hypogastric region (middle portion of lower abdomen). The upper sides of the abdomen bilateral to the epigastric region (middle region of the uppermost abdomen) are known as the hypochondriac regions. The lumbar regions are described as the area between the inguinal and hypochondriac regions on the sides of the abdomen. The lumbar regions are bilateral to the umbilical region, which lies in the center of the abdomen between the epigastric region (above) and hypogastric region (below). *(Austrin, p 53; Ballinger [Vol. 3], p 569; Hole, p 154; Tortora and Anagnostakos, p 13-20)*

67–71. The answers are 67-B, 68-C, 69-B, 70-D, 71-A.   The radiograph that accompanies the question represents a barium enema examination after insertion of radiopaque contrast medium via an enema tube placed in the rectum. The following structures are shown: (1) ileum, (2) cecum, (3) vermiform appendix, (4) ascending colon, (5) hepatic flexure, (6) transverse colon, (7) splenic flexure, (8) descending colon, (9) sigmoid, (10) rectum, (11) anus, (12) ilium bone, and (13) haustra. Contrast is administered retrograde in order to fill all portions of the large intestine (colon). The large intestine is so named because its diameter is greater than that of the small intestine. It is approximately 5 feet in length, beginning in the right lower quadrant of the abdomen where the ileum (the last segment of the small intestine) joins the cecum (first portion of the large intestine). The small and large intestines join at the ileocecal valve. The cecum is a blind pouch that hangs down below the ileocecal valve. Attached to the cecum is a wormlike process called the vermiform appendix. The cecum opens into the ascending colon, which ascends up the right side under the liver then turns, creating the right colic, or hepatic, flexure. Where the colon continues across the abdomen, it is named the transverse colon. When it reaches the left side, it curves downward under the spleen, creating the left colic, or splenic, flexure. This flexure merges into the descending colon, which travels down the left side of the abdomen to the region of the iliac crest. The sigmoid colon begins at this area, projecting medially and curving downward where it terminates at the rectum. The rectum is approximately 8 inches long, the last inch comprising the anal canal. The opening of the colon to the exterior is the anus, which is guarded by an internal and an external sphincter. Normally, the anus remains closed except during the evacuation of the waste products of digestion. Three longitudinal muscle bands run the length of most of the large intestine. Contractions of these bands cause the colon to gather into a series of pouches called haustra, which give the colon a puckered or sacculated appearance. The large intestine prepares the end products of digestion for eventual evacuation by absorbing water and electrolytes. Its only significant secretion is mucus, and absorption is generally limited to electrolytes and water. *(Tortora and Anagnostakos, p 618-620; Hole, p 515-519; Meschan, p 485; Ballinger [Vol. 3], p 645, 670-674)*

72. The answer is D.   Hyperplasia, anaplasia, and metastasis are common manifestations of cancer. Hyperplasia refers to uncontrolled multiplication of cells caused by increased cell division. Anaplasia refers to abnormal form and appearance of cells—cells that have lost differentiation and do not resemble those of the tissues from which they originated. Metastasis refers to the spread of cancer cells or disease from their original (primary) site to another (secondary) site. Two common routes by which metastasis can occur are the bloodstream and lymphatic system. Metastasis is of great clinical importance as it often dictates the prognosis. *(Cawson et al., p 145-158; Hole, p 70)*

RADIOGRAPHIC POSITIONING
AND PROCEDURES

73. In order to achieve a true lateral projection of the elbow joint, the patient must be positioned with the

    1. elbow flexed 90°
    2. forearm and humerus in the same plane
    3. thumb up

  A. 1 and 2
  B. 1 and 3
  C. 2 and 3
  D. 1, 2, and 3

74. For an AP axial projection of the clavicle, with the patient standing straight upright or lying supine, the central ray is directed through the midshaft of the clavicle

  A. perpendicularly
  B. cephalad
  C. caudad
  D. medially

75. Which of the following statements is FALSE regarding radiography of the temporomandibular joints?

  A. Projections are taken with the mouth open and closed
  B. Tomography affords a more detailed image
  C. Only the affected joint is radiographed
  D. AP axial and transcranial projections are useful in demonstrating the condyloid process and mandibular fossa

76. Gastroesophageal reflux can be demonstrated fluoroscopically following ingestion of opaque contrast media by performing the

  A. Valsalva maneuver
  B. Mueller maneuver
  C. water siphonage test
  D. Chassard-Lapiné position

77. Which of the following single projections will demonstrate all four paranasal sinuses and their superoinferior dimensions?

  A. Parietoacanthial
  B. Verticosubmental
  C. Lateral
  D. PA

Questions 78–80. For each given amount of patient rotation or central ray angulation listed below, choose the anatomic part for which it would be employed in radiography. Each anatomic part may be used once, more than once, or not at all.

A. Kidneys
B. Urinary bladder
C. Pelvic outlet
D. Prostate gland

78. 30° obliquity

79. 60° obliquity

80. 15° caudal angulation

81. Which of the following statements does NOT correctly describe the radiograph below?

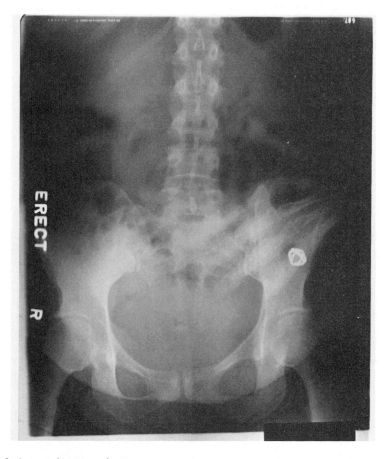

A. Motion unsharpness is present
B. The x-ray beam was positioned perpendicular to the horizon
C. The film was not centered properly to the x-ray beam
D. A patient artifact is seen

82. Ketoacidosis may occur in a patient who

    A. has just received an intravenous injection of iodinated contrast media
    B. is diabetic and has not received insulin
    C. has hypoglycemia
    D. has aspirated a bolus of food

83. A weight-bearing axial projection of the entire foot is performed by

    1. directing the central ray 15° posteriorly, with the x-ray tube in front of the patient
    2. directing the central ray 25° anteriorly through the ankle, with the x-ray tube behind the patient
    3. directing the central ray perpendicular through the metatarsals

    A. 1 and 2
    B. 1 and 3
    C. 2 and 3
    D. 1, 2, and 3

84. Axiolateral oblique positions of the mandible are most useful in demonstrating the

    1. symphysis menti
    2. condyloid processes
    3. mandibular body

    A. 1 and 2
    B. 1 and 3
    C. 2 and 3
    D. 1, 2, and 3

85. Which of the following statements is FALSE concerning laryngography?

    A. Phonation during exposure causes adduction of the vocal cords
    B. The larynx is radiographed with negative or positive contrast medium
    C. The Valsalva maneuver will demonstrate opening of the glottis
    D. Quiet inspiration during exposure causes abduction of the vocal cords

86. The best position to demonstrate the gallbladder free of superimposition is the

    A. LAO
    B. LPO
    C. left lateral decubitus
    D. prone

87. The position of the patient in the following radiograph of the abdomen is

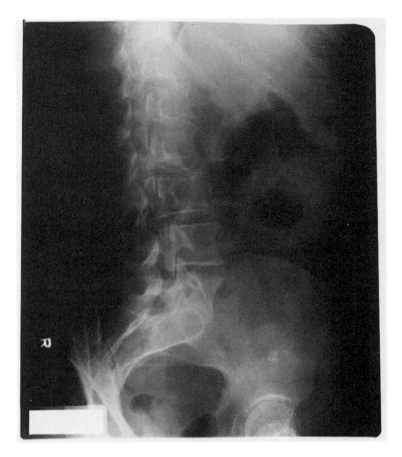

A. RPO
B. LPO
C. LAO
D. supine

88. Which of the following eponyms describe methods of pelvimetry and cephalometry?

　　1. Fletcher
　　2. Colcher-Sussman
　　3. Ball

A. 1 and 2
B. 1 and 3
C. 2 and 3
D. 1, 2, and 3

89. Which of the following projections is most often used for pediatric bone age studies?

    A. Lateral projection of the left knee

    B. AP projection of the left foot and ankle

    C. AP projection of the left femur

    D. PA projection of the left hand and wrist

90. Which of the following eponyms describes a method of examining the temporal bone without angular distortion?

    A. Haas

    B. Lysholm

    C. Mayer

    D. Valdini

91. Functional studies of the cervical spine are obtained by

    A. AP projections while bending the head from side to side

    B. oblique projections with the patient supine and erect

    C. lateral projections while flexing and extending the head and neck

    D. AP and lateral projections while bearing weights

92. In which of the following examinations is tomography often employed?

        1. Intravenous cholangiography

        2. Intravenous urography

        3. Peripheral venography

    A. 1 and 2

    B. 1 and 3

    C. 2 and 3

    D. 1, 2, and 3

93. What is the position of the patient in the following radiograph?

    A. Supine

    B. Prone

    C. Erect

    D. Left lateral decubitus

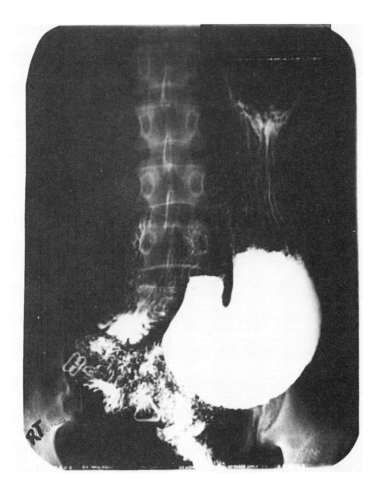

94. Many patients who come to the radiology department for an x-ray examination have various types of intravenous tubing, drainage tubes and bags, and other apparatus. Which of the following statements is NOT correct in regard to the care of these patients?

    A. Intravenous lines should be kept above the level of the vessel in which they are inserted

    B. Urinary drainage bags should be kept below the level of the urinary bladder

    C. Drainage apparatus from the pleural cavity should be kept at a level equal to the chest

    D. Nasogastric intubation apparatus should be secured to the patient to avoid unintentional withdrawal

95. For a PA projection of the heart and aorta, the central ray is directed perpendicular to the midsagittal plane at

    A. the level of the fourth thoracic vertebra

    B. the level of the fifth thoracic vertebra

    C. the level of the sixth thoracic vertebra

    D. none of the above levels

96. The diagrams below represent which of the following projections and methods?

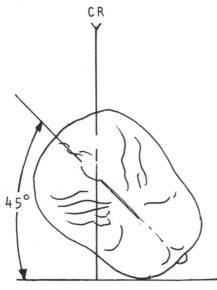

Table radiography

    A. Anterior profile—Arcelin
    B. Axiolateral oblique—Mayer
    C. Axiolateral oblique—Owen-Pendergrass
    D. Posterior profile—Stenvers

97. The angle between the intervertebral foramina of the lumbar spine and the midsagittal plane is

    A. 20°
    B. 45°
    C. 70°
    D. 90°

98. A radiographic method used for examining the blood vessels that supply the myocardium of an adult patient is

    A. angiocardiography
    B. selective coronary arteriography
    C. peripheral angiography
    D. celiac arteriography

99. Which of the following imaging modalities is based on heat emission from the subjects being examined?

   A. Thermography
   B. Nuclear magnetic resonance
   C. Nuclear medicine scanning
   D. Xeroradiography

100. If a RAO position of the chest could not be obtained, which of the following positions might give an equally informative demonstration of the same anatomy?

   A. RPO
   B. LPO
   C. LAO
   D. Right lateral decubitus

101. Oblique positions are sometimes required for additional information regarding the lungs. What degree of rotation is employed for chest obliques?

   A. 35°
   B. 45°
   C. 55°
   D. 65°

102. In order to localize accurately the position of an intrathoracic lesion, which of the following positions should be taken?

   A. LAO and RAO
   B. PA and lateral erect
   C. Left and right lateral decubitus
   D. PA and LAO erect

103. In the carpal canal position, the central ray is

   A. angled 10° toward the navicular bone
   B. angled 15° toward the elbow
   C. angled 30° toward the elbow
   D. perpendicular through the metacarpophalangeal joint

104. The coronoid process is best demonstrated by the

   A. AP projection of the elbow
   B. internal oblique position of the elbow
   C. external oblique position of the elbow
   D. AP projection of the shoulder

105. In a routine lateral projection of the skull, the central ray is directed perpendicular to the sagittal plane of the skull at or to a point

   A. ¾ inch anterior to and superior to the external auditory meatus
   B. 2 inches anterior to the external auditory meatus at the level of the acanthion
   C. 2 inches posterior to the outer canthus of the eye at the level of the mastoid process
   D. 1 inch posterior to and inferior to the outer eye canthus

106. Enteroclysis is a radiographic method of

A. examining the small and/or large intestine following the administration of a positive contrast agent through an abdominal stoma
B. examining the small intestine via a special catheter tube
C. obtaining a double-contrast study of the duodenum following injection of a drug that reduces peristalsis
D. examining the small intestine quickly following barium sulfate ingestion and cold saline

107. Possible adverse reactions to intravascularly injected iodinated contrast media include

1. urticaria
2. dyspnea
3. hypotension

A. 1 and 2
B. 1 and 3
C. 2 and 3
D. 1, 2, and 3

108. In order to best visualize the intervertebral disk spaces of the thoracic vertebrae without the use of positioning aids, with the patient in the lateral recumbent position, the central ray is directed

A. 5 to 10° caudad
B. 10 to 15° cephalad
C. 15 to 20° cephalad
D. perpendicular

109. Which of the following projections/positions are most often performed in the evaluation of the hip of a traumatized patient?

A. AP and cross-table lateral
B. PA and oblique of affected side
C. PA and frog lateral
D. AP and frog lateral

110. The proximal humerus in a patient who has received trauma can be projected laterally by

A. performing an inferosuperior transaxillary projection with the affected arm abducted
B. abducting the affected arm and flexing the elbow 90°
C. performing a transthoracic lateral projection
D. performing a Bennett projection

111. In order to open up the articulation between the talus and fibula in the AP projection of the ankle, the foot is

A. straight upright, with the plantar aspect at right angles to the film
B. flat, with the plantar aspect in contact with the film
C. everted
D. inverted

112. The diagram that follows demonstrates an axiolateral projection using the method described by

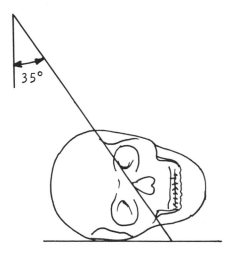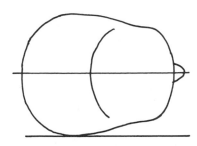

Table radiography

A. Lysholm
B. Law
C. Henschen
D. Schüller

113. Which of the following methods and projections will demonstrate the intercondyloid fossa and tibial spines (eminences)?

    1. Camp-Coventry/PA axial
    2. Béclère/AP axial
    3. Holmblad/PA axial

A. 1 and 2
B. 1 and 3
C. 2 and 3
D. 1, 2, and 3

114. The first projection of the cervical vertebrae required on a patient who has received acute trauma is

A. an AP projection with the mouth open
B. an AP projection with a wagging jaw
C. a cross-table lateral projection
D. a pillar projection

115. A 35 to 45° cephalic angulation of the x-ray tube may be useful during an upper gastrointestinal series with the patient prone in order to

    A. open up a transverse stomach so that the lesser and greater curvatures can be seen

    B. open up jejunal loops and visualize the ligament of Treitz

    C. demonstrate minimal hiatal hernias

    D. demonstrate ulcers of the fundus

116. Which of the following statements are true concerning pneumoencephalography?

    1. A special somersault chair is employed for distribution of the contrast agent

    2. A brow-up position will allow air to fill the occipital horns of the lateral ventricles as well as the posterior third and fourth ventricles

    3. Air is injected by way of a lumbar puncture into the subarachnoid space

    A. 1 and 2

    B. 1 and 3

    C. 2 and 3

    D. 1, 2, and 3

117. The maxillae are best demonstrated by performing which of the following projections?

    A. Lateral

    B. Axiolateral

    C. Intraoral

    D. Extraoral

118. The Chassard-Lapiné projection requires that the

    1. patient be placed in a knee-to-chest position, grasping the ankles

    2. central ray be angled 45° caudally

    3. central ray be directed through the lumbosacral region at the level of the greater trochanters

    A. 1 and 2

    B. 1 and 3

    C. 2 and 3

    D. 1, 2, and 3

119. For the PA oblique projection of the acetabulum (Teufel method), the central ray is directed through the lower coccyx region, 2 inches lateral to the midsagittal plane of the affected side, and

    A. perpendicular to the film

    B. at an angle of 12° cephalad

    C. at an angle of 20° cephalad

    D. at an angle of 38° caudad

120. In order to project the foot in the truest lateral position, it is best to

A. angle the central ray 5 to 10° toward the heel
B. position the foot so that the medial aspect is nearest to the film
C. position the foot so that the lateral aspect is nearest to the film
D. hyperextend the foot at the ankle joint

121. Which of the following projections and positions will best demonstrate narrowing of the knee joint due to arthritis?

A. AP/supine
B. Lateral/recumbent
C. AP/weight-bearing erect
D. Axial/with knee flexed 40°

122. Which of the following radiographic procedures is represented by the radiograph below?

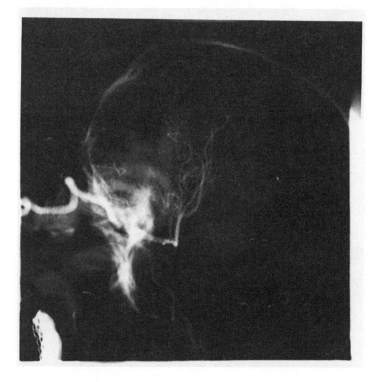

A. External carotid arteriogram
B. Internal carotid arteriogram
C. Vertebral arteriogram
D. Brachiocephalic arteriogram

Questions 123–125. For each type of arteriogram listed below, select the level of the spine at which the central ray would be directed. Each lettered heading may be used once, more than once, or not at all.

A. First lumbar vertebra
B. Third lumbar vertebra
C. Fifth lumbar vertebra
D. First sacral vertebra

123. Selective superior mesenteric arteriogram

124. Selective celiac arteriogram

125. Selective left renal arteriogram

126. In order to prevent superimposition of the bones of the forearm in an AP projection, the hand must be placed in which of the following positions?

A. Lateral
B. Supine
C. Prone
D. Oblique

127. Arthrography is a radiographic examination involving

    1. injection of radiopaque contrast medium into a joint
    2. injection of radiolucent contrast medium into a joint
    3. the study of ligaments, cartilage, and bursae

A. 1 and 2
B. 1 and 3
C. 2 and 3
D. 1, 2, and 3

128. Which of the following statements are true concerning bronchography?

    1. The contrast medium is administered by way of a catheter and is removed through coughing
    2. The flow of contrast medium is facilitated by body positioning
    3. Suppression of the patient's cough and gag reflexes is required throughout the examination

A. 1 and 2
B. 1 and 3
C. 2 and 3
D. 1, 2, and 3

129. A herniated or ruptured intervertebral disk may be demonstrated radiographically by performing

      1. a CT scan
      2. a myelogram
      3. diskography

A. 1 and 2
B. 1 and 3
C. 2 and 3
D. 1, 2, and 3

130. In order to demonstrate the pubic and ischial rami with the patient in the supine position, the central ray is directed

      1. 20 to 35° cephalad
      2. 30 to 45° cephalad
      3. 40 to 55° cephalad

A. 1 only
B. 1 and 2
C. 1 and 3
D. 2 and 3

131. Which of the following projections and methods is essential in routine radiography of the facial bones?

A. Parietoacanthial/Waters
B. PA axial/Caldwell
C. Verticosubmental/Schüller
D. AP axial/Grashey or Towne

132. When examining patients for a questionable acromioclavicular separation, it is best to position them

A. prone
B. supine
C. lateral recumbent
D. erect

133. In a PA axial projection of the cranium for the purpose of demonstrating the superior orbital fissures, the central ray is directed

A. 15° cephalad
B. 20° cephalad
C. 25° caudad
D. 30° caudad

Questions 134–135. For each anatomic part listed below, choose the projection/method that would demonstrate that part to best advantage radiographically. Each lettered heading may be used once, more than once, or not at all.

A. Parietoacanthial projection/Waters method
B. Submentovertex projection/basilar position
C. PA axial projection/Caldwell method
D. Parieto-orbital oblique/Rhese method

134. Optic foramina (canals)

135. Foramina rotundum

136. Which of the following positions are useful in demonstrating free air in the peritoneal cavity (spontaneous pneumoperitoneum)?

　　　1. Erect
　　　2. Lateral decubitus
　　　3. Dorsal decubitus

A. 1 and 2
B. 1 and 3
C. 2 and 3
D. 1, 2, and 3

137. For the lateral projection of the scapula, it is best to position the patient's body

A. in a lordotic position
B. in a true lateral position
C. obliquely, with the affected side away from the film
D. obliquely, with the affected side in contact with the film

138. For angiographic procedures, the use of a J-tipped guide wire may be necessary in order to

　　　1. negotiate tortuous blood vessels
　　　2. safely manipulate through atherosclerotic blood vessels
　　　3. avoid causing embolization

A. 1 and 2
B. 1 and 3
C. 2 and 3
D. 1, 2, and 3

Questions 139–141. For each anatomic structure listed below, select the level of the spine to which it corresponds. Each vertebral level may be used once, more than once, or not at all.

A. Third cervical vertebra
B. Fifth cervical vertebra
C. First thoracic vertebra
D. Third thoracic vertebra

139. Suprasternal notch

140. Gonion

141. Thyroid cartilage

142. Filling of the renal pelvicalyceal system with contrast media is enhanced by

1. placing the patient in the prone position
2. applying ureteric compression
3. employing the Trendelenburg position

A. 1 and 2
B. 1 and 3
C. 2 and 3
D. 1, 2, and 3

143. The sternum is usually radiographed in which of the following positions?

A. AP and RPO
B. LAO and lateral
C. PA and RAO
D. RAO and lateral

144. Which of the following would best demonstrate the entire foramen magnum when performing an AP projection?

A. 0° angulation
B. 30° caudal angulation
C. 37° caudal angulation
D. 50° caudal angulation

BODY—RADIOGRAPHIC POSITIONING AND PROCEDURES
ANSWERS, EXPLANATIONS, AND REFERENCES

73. The answer is D. In order to achieve a true lateral projection of the elbow joint, the patient must be positioned so that the forearm and humerus are resting on the film in the same plane. (The radius and ulna should be parallel to the plane of the film; this can be achieved by elevating the lower end of the forearm approximately ½ inch in order to compensate for its smaller diameter.) The elbow should be flexed 90°, the thumb should be up, and the medial and lateral epicondyles of the humerus should be superimposed. The central ray is directed through the elbow joint at right angles to the plane of the film. The true lateral projection of the elbow demonstrates the distal humerus, proximal ulna, and radius and is usually included as a routine projection in examination of the elbow joint. *(Ballinger [Vol. 1], p 141; Bontrager and Anthony, p 104)*

74. The answer is B. When performing an AP axial projection of the clavicle, the central ray is directed 15 to 25° cephalad through the midclavicular area. Patients can be positioned erect or supine, with their back nearest to the film. An AP axial projection can also be performed with the patient assuming a lordotic position, leaning back with shoulders in contact with the film and the arched body placed about 1 foot away from the film holder. The central ray is directed perpendicularly to the film. A caudal angulation is required for the PA axial projection of the clavicle, with the patient PA erect or prone. This method will decrease magnification of the clavicle and may be preferred over an AP projection. *(Ballinger [Vol. 1], p 172, 175; Bontrager and Anthony, p 123)*

75. The answer is C. Routine examination of the temporomandibular joints includes radiography of both joints for comparison. Routine studies may incorporate AP axial and transcranial projections and/or tomography for demonstration of the condyloid process and mandibular fossa of the temporal bone. Projections are usually taken with the patient's mouth open and closed. A variety of transcranial projections may be used to demonstrate the temporomandibular joints, including the Schüller and Law methods; each requires the patient to be adjusted from a lateral recumbent or erect position and the central ray to be angled through the cranium. AP axial projections are often employed in addition to transcranial or transfacial projections for the demonstration of the condyloid processes and mandibular fossae, bilaterally. Tomography is very useful, as it affords detailed information on the temporomandibular joints by blurring superimposed structures out of the area (level) of interest. *(Ballinger [Vol. 2], p 499–504; Bontrager and Anthony, p 248, 251–252)*

76. The answer is C. The water siphonage test is performed in order to study the gastroesophageal junction after administration of barium sulfate. The patient is placed in the supine or LPO position so that the fundus of the stomach is filled with barium. With fluoroscopy, the radiologist will observe the gastroesophageal junction as the patient swallows water through a straw. Reflux can be demonstrated if barium regurgitates from the stomach up into the esophagus. The Valsalva and Mueller maneuvers are often used to increase intrathoracic and intraabdominal pressure and to help demonstrate esophageal varices fluoroscopically and/or radiographically during upper gastrointestinal examination. The Chassard-Lapiné position is not of much value in examining the upper gastrointestinal tract but is sometimes employed during examination of the lower large intestine. *(Ballinger [Vol. 3], p 651, 683; Bontrager and Anthony, p 426; Meschan, p 426)*

77. The answer is C. The lateral projection will demonstrate all four paranasal sinuses (frontal, ethmoidal, sphenoidal, and maxillary) and their relationship to other structures, as well as their superoinferior dimensions. For radiographs of the paranasal sinuses, the patient is placed in the erect or seated position whenever possible in order to demonstrate air-fluid levels and to differentiate fluid from other pathological shadows. The beam is usually directed horizontally (parallel to the floor). For the lateral projection, the head should be adjusted to a true lateral position, the midsagittal plane should be parallel and the interpupillary line should be perpendicular to the film plane. The central ray is directed perpendicularly to a point about 1 inch behind the outer canthus of the eye. The PA Caldwell projection with the patient positioned erect (whenever possible) and the central ray directed 15° caudad (when the orbitomeatal line is perpendicular to the film) or 23° caudad (when the glabellomeatal line is perpendicular to the film) is used to demonstrate the frontal and anterior ethmoidal sinuses to the best advantage. The parietoacanthial (Waters) projection is used to demonstrate the maxillary sinuses to best advantage, and the verticosubmental (Schüller) projection is most useful in demonstrating the sphenoidal sinuses. *(Ballinger [Vol. 2], p 510–515, 520; Bontrager and Anthony, p 253–257)*

78–80. The answers are 78-A, 79-B, 80-B. When the kidneys and bladder are studied radiographically either by retrograde (ascending) or intravenous (descending) methods, oblique projections are sometimes required. When the kidneys and upper collecting systems are of prime interest, the patient is rotated approximately 30° from the supine position (RPO and LPO). A greater degree of patient obliquity would cause the uppermost kidney and collecting system to be obscured by the vertebrae. When the bladder is of prime interest, the degree of patient obliquity is approximately 40 to 60° from the supine position. This steeper degree of obliquity is required in order to demonstrate the posterolateral walls of the bladder and ureterovesical junctions. A 15° caudal tube angulation is used in conjunction with the supine position in examination of the urinary bladder. Angulation helps to "throw" the symphysis pubis below the inferior portion of the bladder, thereby preventing any overlapping. The reverse angulation (15° cephalic) can be applied when the patient is placed in the prone position. *(Ballinger [Vol. 3], p 710–711; Bontrager and Anthony, p 518, 522)*

81. The answer is B. The radiograph that accompanies the question required a repeat examination because of the numerous technical errors present. The patient was positioned for an AP erect projection of the abdomen with the x-ray beam parallel to the horizon. The film is not centered exactly to the x-ray beam, as demonstrated by the area where film density is absent along the inferior margin of the radiograph. If this were centered properly and collimated smaller than the film size, the upper and lower margins of the film would reveal an equal absence of density across the radiograph. An obvious artifact in the midabdominal region on the left side is that of a ring on the patient's hand, which was placed over the abdomen during the exposure. Unsharpness, also present throughout the abdominal region, is the result of motion during the exposure, most likely because of failure to suspend respiration for the duration of the exposure, along with peristaltic activity. The patient could have been centered more accurately to the film, as demonstrated by the fact that the spine is not centered in the middle of the radiograph.

82. The answer is B. Ketoacidosis is a medical emergency that may result from insufficient metabolism of blood glucose in the absence of adequate insulin. Diabetic patients who have eaten but have not received their normally scheduled insulin administration may experience this problem and may exhibit signs of weakness and drowsiness, along with symptoms such as increased thirst, dry skin, nausea, vomiting, and change in respiratory rate and depth. It is essential that this medical emergency be treated quickly in order to avoid accumulation of ketone bodies in the blood, coma, and possible death. Hypoglycemia is another medical emergency that may be experienced by a diabetic patient, but it is more likely to occur in a patient who has received insulin but not the necessary nourishment to metabolize the hypoglycemic medication. Early recognition of symptoms and emergency treatment are required to avoid coma. Intravenous injections of iodinated contrast agents may produce reactions ranging from mild to severe, and their use requires constant observation of the patient, medical preparedness to treat a reaction, as well as knowledge of the patient's present health and allergy history. Aspiration of a bolus of food may require emergency medical treatment in the event that the airway should become obstructed. Because patients undergo a variety of x-ray procedures that sometimes require a long waiting period, the technologist should be aware of the patient's condition, watch for symptoms of reactions, and be prepared to assist or administer appropriate treatment. *(Torres and Morrill, p 57–66)*

83. The answer is A. The weight-bearing axial projection of the entire foot is performed with the patient standing erect, with the sole of the affected foot resting on the film. Two projections (exposures) are taken without any movement of the affected foot between each. For one exposure, the x-ray tube is brought in front of the patient's foot and the central ray is directed through the navicular (scaphoid) bone at an angle of 15° toward the posterior aspect; the leg and foot not being examined are placed behind. The second exposure is made with x-ray tube behind the affected foot, with the central ray directed through the back of the ankle at an angle of 25° toward the anterior part of the foot. The foot not being examined is brought in front. This method of examining the foot reveals all the bones of the foot free of any superimposition by bones or shadows of the leg. *(Ballinger [Vol. 1], p 51)*

84. The answer is B. Axiolateral oblique positions are usually incorporated as part of the routine examination of the mandible, as they are useful in demonstrating the mandibular body and symphysis menti. In order to best visualize each part, the angulation of the central ray must be adjusted. The patient may be placed in either the erect or recumbent position, with the side of the mandible being examined nearest to the film, the chin extended, and the head adjusted according to the structures to be demonstrated. The head should be adjusted enough to place the long axis of the mandibular body parallel to the film plane, with the central ray angled 25 to 35° cephalad for the demonstration of the side of the mandibular body nearest to the film. The mandibular symphysis may be demonstrated by adjusting the patient's head so that the zygoma, nose, and extended chin rest on the film holder and the central ray is directed approximately 20° cephalad. The condyloid processes and temporomandibular joints are demonstrated to the best advantage by the AP axial projection, with the patient adjusted so that the orbitomeatal line and midsagittal plane are perpendicular to the film plane and the central ray is angled 30 to 35° caudad through the forehead and midsagittal plane and exits the region of the temporomandibular joints. Other projections may be required in order to demonstrate the rami and its processes, such as PA, verticosubmental, and submentovertical. *(Ballinger [Vol. 2], p 490–499; Bontrager and Anthony, p 246–248)*

85. The answer is C. Laryngography is the radiographic study of the larynx employing either negative or positive contrast media and various respiratory and stress maneuvers. AP and sometimes lateral projections are usually taken with the patient erect or recumbent. Negative contrast studies use inspired and expired air to demonstrate the anatomy of the larynx and pharynx. If the patient quietly inspires during exposure, the vocal cords abduct and a continuous column of air is demonstrated. Normal phonation (during the expiratory phase) will cause adduction of the vocal cords. Normal phonation is performed by having the patient take in a deep breath and then exhale slowly while phonating "e-e-e-e" or "a-a-a-h." Inspiratory phonation will also demonstrate adduction of the vocal cords as well as expansion of the laryngeal ventricle. If the exposure is taken after the patient takes in a deep breath and bears down, the glottis will close completely; this is the Valsalva maneuver. Tomography and xerography are often employed with negative laryngographic studies, as both allow the soft-tissue structures in the larynx and pharynx to be brought into better view. Positive contrast studies of the larynx are sometimes performed following mild sedation of the patient, application of topical anesthesia to the throat, and administration of an iodized oil-based contrast medium. Respiratory and stress maneuvers are also employed and monitored with fluoroscopy. The larynx may also be examined with CT. *(Ballinger [Vol. 2], p 538–541)*

86. The answer is A. The LAO position is most useful in demonstrating a gallbladder free of self-superimposition as well as free of the spine. The LAO is usually employed as a routine position following opacification of the gallbladder by oral cholecystography. With the patient's left side down and right side elevated, the gallbladder will move laterally (toward the right), away from the spine. The central ray is directed perpendicularly to the level of the gallbladder (as identified on a preliminary scout film) and the right sagittal plane. The level of the gallbladder varies greatly among various body builds and should therefore be radiographed initially for identification of its location and proper opacification. *(Ballinger [Vol. 3], p 628–629, 632; Bontrager and Anthony, p 493)*

87. The answer is B. The radiograph that accompanies the question demonstrates the abdomen of a patient in a LPO position. In this position, the left side is down (nearest to the table and film) and the posterior aspect is in close relationship to the film; the right side is elevated. This position can be distinguished from a supine position because of the asymmetry of the spine and pelvis. It can also be distinguished from both the RPO and the LAO positions by the appearance of the spine and pelvis. In the LPO, the side of the pelvis closest to the flim (left) appears larger and more open, whereas the side up appears foreshortened. The RPO would demonstrate the opposite effect, and the LAO will appear similar to the RPO. *(Ballinger [Vol. 1], p 11; Bontrager and Anthony, p 20)*

88. The answer is C. The eponyms Colcher-Sussman and Ball describe radiographic methods of pelvimetry and cephalometry. The Colcher-Sussman method employs a centimeter-perforated metal pelvimeter supported by a short metal stand and base, which is always placed parallel to the film plane. This pelvimeter is used to determine the magnification rate so that accurate measurements can be made of pelvic diameters. AP and lateral projections of the pelvis of a pregnant female are taken with the pelvimeter placed at specified levels. For the AP projection, the patient is placed supine on an x-ray table, the knees flexed and thighs slightly abducted. The pelvimeter is adjusted to the level of the ischial tuberosities or 10 cm below the upper border of the symphysis pubis and is placed close to the buttocks. For the lateral projection, the patient is placed in a true lateral position, either recumbent or erect, and the pelvimeter is adjusted to the height of the patient's midsagittal plane and placed against the sacrum. The central ray is directed perpendicularly for both projections; the final radiograph should demonstrate the entire pelvis, the lumbosacral junction, symphysis pubis, and pelvimeter. Radiographic measurements are made of the female pelvis and fetal head to determine whether or not the female pelvis is adequate for normal vaginal delivery of the fetus. The Ball method of pelvimetry does not require any special devices such as a pelvimeter; instead, AP and lateral projections are made, radiographic measurements are taken, and the results are compared with a nomogram (calculator). Fletcher described a method of examining the sigmoid colon, not a method of pelvimetry or cephalometry. *(Ballinger [Vol. 3], p 682, 735–741; Bontrager and Anthony, 189–190)*

89. The answer is D. A PA projection of the left hand and wrist is usually employed exclusively or as part of a routine for pediatric bone age studies. Other methods of studying bone age may incorporate additional projections such as AP and lateral projections of the left knee, foot, and ankle and AP projections of the humerus and clavicle. The femur is not usually radiographed for pediatric bone age evaluation. *(Ballinger [Vol. 1], p 294)*

90. The answer is D. The PA axial projection of the petrous portions of the temporal bones using the Valdini method requires no angulation of the x-ray beam. The central ray is directed perpendicular to the plane of the film through the foramen magnum and midsagittal plane. Because there is no central ray angulation, no angular distortion is produced and an excellent view of the hearing organs is delivered. For the Valdini position, the patient's head is adjusted so that it rests on the upper forehead and the midsagittal plane is perpendicular to the film plane. The infraorbitomeatal line should be adjusted to form an angle of 50° to the film for demonstration of the tympanic cavities, external auditory canals, and eustachian tubes. The Haas, Lysholm, and Mayer methods all require angulation of the central ray of the x-ray beam and therefore will produce radiographs with angular distortion. *(Ballinger [Vol. 2], p 440)*

91. The answer is C. The function of the cervical spine can be studied by radiographing patients in the lateral position and taking two exposures: one as they flex their head and neck and one as they hyperextend their head and neck. The flexion position will show separation of the spinous processes, whereas extension projects them close together. Functional studies may be requested on patients with suspected arthritic changes or other disease processes that may interfere with normal movement. *(Ballinger [Vol. 1], p 219; Bontrager and Anthony, p 312–313)*

92. The answer is A. Tomography, or body section radiography, is useful in demonstrating various anatomic structures by blurring out superimposed structures. Intravenous cholangiography, an opaque contrast study of the biliary ductal system, usually requires tomographic cuts to enhance visualization of details of the ducts by blurring overlying gas, soft tissue, and/or rib shadows. Intravenous urography, a radiopaque contrast study of the kidneys and collecting structures of the urinary system, often incorporates tomography in order to better visualize the renal borders and parenchyma. Peripheral venography is a radiopaque contrast study of the veins in the extremities; it is not necessary to use tomography for this examination, because adequate demonstration of the peripheral vessels following opacification is achieved by routine overhead radiography. *(Ballinger [Vol. 1], p 273–278; Ballinger [Vol. 3], p 624–626, 698, 700–701; Bontrager and Anthony, p 536)*

93. The answer is C. The radiograph that accompanies the question demonstrates the stomach following ingestion of opaque contrast (barium sulfate) while the patient is erect. This is a PA projection with the x-ray beam parallel to the floor. If the patient were supine or prone and the x-ray beam were vertical, air-fluid levels would not be demonstrated as they are in the radiograph, where the barium tends to fall to the lowest portion of the stomach (part of the body and the pylorus) and air rises to the uppermost body and fundus. In the prone position, barium gravitates to the body and the pylorus and air occupies the fundus, and in the supine position, barium gravitates to the fundus and air occupies the lower portion of the stomach. However, a sharp demarcation line between barium (fluid) and air in the stomach would not be seen as in the erect position. A left lateral decubitus position will demonstrate air-fluid levels, but the barium would occupy the left (lower) side of the stomach and air would occupy the right (upper) side of the stomach. *(Ballinger [Vol. 3], p 654, 656, 658–661; Bontrager and Anthony, p 415)*

94. The answer is C. Chest drainage apparatus that has been inserted into the pleural cavity should be kept below the level of the pleural cavity in order for proper drainage to take place. The tubing should be kept free of kinks, and the drainage set or bottle should be approximately 3 feet below the level of the chest. Intravenous lines should be kept above the level of the vein in which they have been inserted, or the medication being administered will not be allowed to run in at the rate prescribed and the patient's blood may back up into tubing. Other precautions to be exercised when caring for patients with intravenous lines include the following: Keep the tubing from being pulled from the patient during transfer procedures; avoid kinking or obstruction of the tubing; and observe the intravenous site for swelling or infiltration. Urinary drainage bags attached to urinary catheters should be kept below the level of the urinary bladder to avoid reflux of urine into the bladder, with the possible danger of inducing infection, and to permit proper drainage of urine. Urinary drainage systems should also be carefully transported with the patient to avoid any kinking, pulling, or tension on the tubing. The system should be kept closed so as not to expose it to pathogenic microorganisms. Nasogastric intubation apparatus is usually secured to the patient (nose area) in order to avoid unintentional withdrawal of the tubing from the stomach; it too should be carefully transferred with the patient, avoiding pulling, kinking, or disconnection. *(Torres and Morrill, p 93, 96, 122–123, 142–143)*

95. The answer is C. In PA projections of the chest, patients are positioned so that their anterior aspect is closest to the film, their hands are positioned with the palms up on the hips, their shoulders are rolled forward, their chin is extended, and the midsagittal plane is centered to the middle of the film. The central ray is directed to the level of the sixth thoracic vertebra for demonstration of the heart and great vessels. Exposure is taken at the end of inhalation in order to demonstrate the maximum area (volume) of the lung fields. Faint visualization of the vertebrae through the heart shadow usually indicates proper exposure for the PA projection. In radiographing the lungs, the central ray is directed to the level of the fourth thoracic vertebra and midsagittal plane and the patient is positioned as previously described. *(Ballinger [Vol. 3], p 584–585; Bontrager and Anthony, p 37-38, 41-42)*

96. The answer is D. The Stenvers method of the posterior profile projection of the petrous portion of the temporal bone is represented in the diagrams that accompany the question. The midsagittal plane of the patient's head must be adjusted to form a 45° angle to the film plane. The patient's head rests on the zygoma, nose, and forehead. The central ray is directed 12° cephalad and exits a point 1 inch in front of the external auditory meatus of the side down. The Stenvers method is often employed in radiography of the mastoid processes and demonstrates a profile view of the pars petrosa, as well as the area of the internal auditory canal, bony labyrinth, tympanic cavity, and petrous ridge. The side nearest to the film is being radiographed, but both sides should be examined and compared. *(Ballinger [Vol. 2], p 448; Bontrager and Anthony, p 260)*

97. The answer is D. The intervertebral foramina of the lumbar spine are situated so that they form a 90° angle to the midsagittal plane. In order to visualize these foramina radiographically, patients undergoing the examination must be placed in a true lateral position (90° rotation to the horizon) so that their midsagittal plane is parallel to the plane of the film. It should be noted, however, that the intervertebral foramina of the last lumbar vertebra are located at a slightly different angle from the first four, requiring a slight obliquity from the lateral position (about 30°) in order to demonstrate them radiographically. *(Ballinger [Vol. 1], p 208, 238–239, 241; Bontrager and Anthony, p 300–301)*

98. The answer is B. Selective coronary arteriography is the radiographic study of the coronary arteries that supply blood to the heart muscle (myocardium) following opacification with an aqueous iodinated contrast medium. This examination is performed to assess the coronary anatomy when there is question of coronary atherosclerosis, chest pain of unknown origin, possible occlusion, and a variety of other pathological problems. A catheter is passed from a peripheral artery to the origin of the aorta and may be further manipulated into the orifice of either the right or left coronary arteries, which arise from the sinuses of Valsalva. Once the catheter is in place, contrast is injected through it and images are recorded by rapid film changers or, more commonly, cinefluorography. The patient is constantly monitored throughout the procedure for any abnormal reaction or physiological change. Angiocardiography is the radiographic examination of the interior chambers of the heart and great vessels following opacification with water-soluble contrast media. Angiocardiography also requires catheterization, but usually a peripheral vein is selectively catheterized to gain cardiac access. Peripheral angiography is the radiographic study of peripheral vessels (arteries or veins of the extremities) following opacification with aqueous iodinated contrast. Femoral arteriograms and leg venograms are common peripheral studies performed. Celiac arteriography is the selective catheterization of the celiac axis by way of a peripheral artery approach to the abdominal aorta. The celiac axis and its branches are opacified with aqueous iodinated contrast medium and serial films are taken. All of these procedures are performed using sterile technique and require that all emergency drugs and equipment be readily available. *(Ballinger [Vol. 3], p 802–811; Bontrager and Anthony, p 531–533, 535; Meschan, p 205–217; Snopek, p 155–169, 171–181, 212–220)*

99. The answer is A. Infrared thermography is a special imaging modality based on the emission of heat from the surface of subjects being examined. The body normally emits heat to achieve equilibrium with its surroundings; this heat can be detected, measured, and recorded by a thermograph. Because various disease processes may interrupt the normal emission of thermal energy from body parts, a thermograph may be used to detect these changes and can often be used as a screening device for medical diagnosis. One of the most common applications of thermography is in examining for breast disease, for which it is mainly used as a screening examination or in combination with physical and radiographic examination. Thermography is also applicable in the study of vascular, skin, bone, and eye disorders. The patient is placed in front of the infrared detector without any interposed objects (clothing) between the subject and detector, the room temperature is strictly controlled, and various positions are employed. A real-time image can be viewed on a television monitor, or permanent images can be recorded on film. *(Ballinger [Vol. 3], p 866–870)*

100. The answer is B. The LPO and RAO positions demonstrate the same anatomy radiographically; therefore, if one could not be obtained, the other position would serve as an alternative. The RPO position corresponds to the LAO position. Obliques of the chest are sometimes requested as additional positions in order to identify or locate intrathoracic lesions and may also be part of a "cardiac series," in which the patient swallows a thick barium paste to opacify the esophagus. The contour and position of the opacified esophagus are examined in relation to the heart and great vessels. *(Ballinger [Vol. 3], p 588–590; Bontrager and Anthony, p 46–47)*

101. The answer is B. Chest obliques are performed with the patient assuming a 45° angle to the plane of the film. For the LAO and RAO the patient is rotated from the PA erect position. The arm of the side farthest from the film is raised up and rests on the vertical holder, and the arm of the side nearest to the film is placed palm down on the hip. The central ray is directed horizontally at the level of the fourth or sixth thoracic vertebra and the sagittal plane of the side up. The LAO is sometimes performed with the patient oblique between 55 and 60° in order to project the heart between the spine and aortic shadow. When the LAO and RAO cannot be used, the RPO and LPO may be employed. (The LAO is equivalent to the RPO, and the RAO is equivalent to the LPO.) *Ballinger [Vol. 3], p 588–590; Bontrager and Anthony, p 46–47)*

102. The answer is B. In order to localize accurately a lesion anywhere in the body, it is most often required to take two projections at right angles to one another. The two projections of the chest required for localization of an intrathoracic lesion are the PA and lateral projections with the patient erect. If a PA cannot be obtained, then an AP projection may be used. The PA and AP projections demonstrate structures from side to side and superiorly to inferiorly, whereas the lateral projection adds depth to the structures visualized by providing a view of structural position from the anterior to posterior aspects of the chest. For example, the PA projection may demonstrate a lesion on the right side, but from this projection alone it would be very difficult to say whether the lesion was anterior, posterior, or somewhere between. A lateral projection would contribute this needed information. LAO and RAO may be requested as additional positions of the chest when more information is needed. *(Ballinger [Vol. 3], p 584–587; Bontrager and Anthony, p 27, 40, 41–43)*

103. The answer is C. The carpal canal position, Gaynor-Hart method is performed with the patient's forearm prone and the affected hand dorsiflexed at the wrist. The inferosuperior projection by this method requires that the palm of the hand be placed as perpendicular to the film as possible and the central ray be angled 25 to 30° toward the elbow, 1 inch distal to the base of the fourth metacarpal. If the superoinferior projection by this method is desired because the patient cannot be positioned for the above, then the palm of the hand is placed in contact with the film, the wrist is dorsiflexed, and the central ray is directed perpendicularly through the canal. The carpal canal position is useful in demonstrating the carpal canal (carpal tunnel), the entire pisiform, hamular process (hook) of the hamate, and various other aspects of the carpal bones. *(Ballinger [Vol. 1], p 136)*

104. The answer is B. The internal oblique position of the elbow demonstrates the coronoid process of the ulna free of superimposition by the radial head. For this position the arm is extended at the elbow joint, the hand is pronated, the elbow rotated to form a 45° angle to the film. The central ray is directed perpendicularly to the film. In the AP projection of the elbow, the coronoid process is not usually seen. The external oblique projection of the elbow shows the coronoid process but is best for demonstrating the radial head and neck area. *(Ballinger [Vol. 1], p 139; Bontrager and Anthony, p 102–103)*

105. The answer is A. For a routine lateral projection of the skull, the patient is positioned erect or recumbent so that the midsagittal plane of the face is parallel to the plane of the film, the interpupillary line is perpendicular to the film. The head should be perfectly straight without any rotation; sponges may be used to support the head in this position. The central ray is directed perpendicularly to a point ¾ inch anterior to and superior to the external auditory meatus (this coincides with the sella turcica). A 10 × 12-inch film is generally used for this projection and is labeled to denote the side of the head (left or right) closest to the film. This projection demonstrates the anterior and posterior clinoid processes, sella turcica, dorsum sellae, and details of the side of the cranium nearest to the film. For accurate assessment of positioning, the shadow of the mandibular sides should be superimposed. *(Ballinger [Vol. 2], p 382–383; Bontrager and Anthony, p 202)*

106. The answer is B. Enteroclysis is a radiographic method of examining the entire small intestine by inserting a special tube (Bilbao or Sellink tube) into the duodenum under fluoroscopic control and injecting a positive contrast agent into the intestinal lumen at a fairly rapid rate in order to visualize the entire small bowel. A negative contrast agent may be injected following positive opacification of the lumen of the small intestine. A double-contrast study of the duodenum following inducement of temporary paralysis of peristalsis by propantheline bromide or glucagon injection is a method called hypotonic duodenography. This examination is performed in order to evaluate duodenal and pancreatic disease. Cold saline or water can be administered following introduction of barium sulfate into the small intestine in order to increase motility so that portions of the small intestine can quickly be examined (within an hour) radiographically. *(Ballinger [Vol. 3], p 666–668; Meschan, p 451)*

107. The answer is D. Numerous chemotoxic or allergic reactions ranging from mild to severe have been reported to occur in response to intravascularly injected contrast agents. Some of the mild reactions that may be encountered include warmth, flushing, nausea, vomiting, metallic taste in the mouth, dizziness, itching, sweating, headache, and local pain in the arm. Moderate reactions may include edema, urticaria, and vasovagal hypotensive responses. Severe responses, which may be life-threatening, include convulsions, pulmonary edema, severe bronchospasm, and laryngeal edema. These may produce dyspnea (difficulty breathing), cardiac arrhythmia, and death. It should be noted that the majority of contrast reactions are minor, and only a small percentage of patients actually experience severe, life-threatening reactions. The causes of reactions to contrast media are still being investigated, but it is thought that certain existing factors may be responsible for increasing the reaction rate. Some of the high-risk factors associated with contrast reactions are the type and temperature of contrast used, the rate and site of injection, and the condition of the patient (iodine sensitivity, severe renal and/or hepatic disease, allergic history, severe heart disease, hypertension). Patients should be questioned about their previous experience with contrast injections and allergy history, and information regarding their health, laboratory evaluation, etc. should be available to the physician and radiologist. During any contrast injection, the patient should be monitored closely for any abnormal response or reaction and emergency drugs, equipment, and medical personnel should be immediately available. *(Ballinger [Vol. 3], p 620, 694; Bontrager and Anthony, p 506–508; Rose, p 12–16; Tortorici, p 158–164)*

108. The answer is B. The thoracic intervertebral disk spaces and intervertebral foramina can be demonstrated by placing the patient in a lateral recumbent or erect position and directing the central ray through the disk spaces. In order for the central ray of the x-ray beam to pass through the thoracic intervertebral disk spaces without using positioning aids such as radiolucent sponges to straighten out the spine, the central ray should be angled to 10 to 15° cephalad through the sixth thoracic vertebrae. If the spine is elevated with sponges so that its long axis is parallel to the film, then the central ray need not be angled but is directed perpendicular to the midthoracic spine. The exposure can be taken while suspending respiration or while the patient breathes quietly (the later is done to blur out rib and pulmonary markings). *(Ballinger [Vol. 1], p 231–232; Bontrager and Anthony, p 305)*

109. The answer is A. For questionable hip fractures in the patient who has received trauma, the routine projections usually include an AP without inverting the foot and a cross-table lateral. These two projections will require as little movement of the patient from the supine position as possible, decreasing the possibility of additional injury to bones and soft-tissue structures of the affected side. An AP projection is performed with the patient in a supine position, and the central ray is directed through the hip, perpendicular to the film. A cross-table lateral is performed with the film placed medial to the affected hip for a superoinferior projection or with film placed on the lateral aspect of the affected hip joint for an axiolateral or inferosuperior projection. For either cross-table lateral projection, the unaffected leg is abducted and the central ray is directed through the femoral neck of the injured leg, perpendicular to the film. A frog lateral, oblique, and PA projection require more movement of the patient, therefore increasing the possibility of additional trauma; also, two projections at right angles to one another, as in an AP and cross-table lateral projection, are usually required for accurate evaluation of a part. *(Ballinger [Vol. 1], p 102–106, 108–109; Bontrager and Anthony, p 180–186)*

110. The answer is C. The transthoracic lateral projection of the proximal humerus is easily performed on a traumatized patient whose arm cannot or should not be moved in order to avoid additional trauma to the upper humerus. For the transthoracic lateral projection, patients are placed so that their affected humerus is nearest to the film while they are either standing, seated, or lying supine with the film to their side. The arm of the unaffected side is raised above as much as possible, with the hand resting on the head. The central ray is directed through the thorax and to the surgical neck of the humerus, perpendicular to the film. A transaxillary, Bennett, or any other projection that requires abduction of the affected arm may not only be difficult for the patient to perform but contraindicated as well. *(Ballinger [Vol. 1], p 151; Bontrager and Anthony, p 107)*

111. The answer is D. The joint space between the talus and fibula is well seen by inverting the foot and ankle and directing the central ray perpendicular to the film, through the ankle joint. This AP projection of the ankle joint is performed with the patient's leg extended, dorsal portion of the ankle in contact with film and plantar aspect at right angles to the plane of the film. Besides opening up the talofibular articulation, this projection demonstrates the distal tibia and fibula and the talus. *(Ballinger [Vol. 1], p 61)*

112. The answer is A. The diagram that accompanies the question demonstrates the position of the head and central ray required for an axiolateral projection using the Lysholm method. As demonstrated, the patient's head is adjusted to the true lateral position so that the interpupillary line is perpendicular to the film plane and the midsagittal plane of the face is parallel to the film plane. The central ray is directed at an angle of 30 to 35° caudad, entering the temporal region of the side up and emerging at a point about 1 inch below the external auditory meatus of the side in contact with the film. The Lysholm axiolateral method is useful in projecting an oblique view of the cranial base, mastoid portion of the temporal bones, and carotid canals. Both sides of the head are examined for comparison. *(Ballinger [Vol. 2], p 395, 436)*

113. The answer is D. The Camp-Coventry PA axial projection, Béclère AP axial, and Holmblad PA axial projections are all useful in demonstrating the intercondyloid fossa and tibial eminences. The Camp-Coventry method is performed with the patient in the prone position with the thigh in contact with the film. The knee is flexed so that anterior surface of the lower leg forms a 40 to 50° angle to the plane of the film, and the lower leg and foot are supported. The central ray is angled so that it is perpendicular to the long axis of the lower leg, caudally (40 to 50°) through the depression behind the knee. This method affords a more "opened" view of the intercondyloid fossa than do the Holmblad and Béclère methods. The Holmblad method of examining the intercondyloid fossa is also a PA projection, but the patient is placed in a kneeling position on "all fours" so that the long axes of the lower legs are parallel to the table and film. The long axis of the femora should form a 70° angle to the horizon, and the central ray is directed perpendicular to the long axis of the tibia through the patellar apex. The Holmblad method affords one of the best views of the joint space and bone surfaces. The Béclère method requires the patient to be placed in a supine position with the knee flexed so that the femur forms a 60° angle to the long axis of the tibia. Either a curved cassette or built-up straight cassette and film are placed under the knee, and the central ray is directed perpendicular to the long axis of the tibia through the knee joint. *(Ballinger [Vol. 1], p 73–75; Bontrager and Anthony, p 166)*

114. The answer is C. The cross-table lateral projection is the first and most important projection in examining the cervical vertebrae of an acutely injured patient, as it does not require head and neck movement, which could inflict more injury on the spine or cord. With the patient lying supine with the shoulders depressed, a film in a holder is placed in contact with one of the shoulders. The x-ray beam is directed horizontally through the fourth cervical vertebra, perpendicular to the film. This lateral projection is helpful in establishing the alignment of the vertebrae and in ruling out fractures. After this, the physician determines whether or not the patient can be positioned for additional views of the neck. AP projections of the cervical spine with the mouth open or jaw wagging are taken to demonstrate the upper cervical segments. Pillar projections are useful in demonstrating the posterior elements, articular facets, spinous processes, and laminae of the cervical and upper thoracic vertebrae. *(Ballinger [Vol. 1], p 212, 223–224, 226; Bontrager and Anthony, p 308, 314–315)*

115. The answer is A. In a patient with a high transverse stomach, it is sometimes difficult to visualize the stomach curvatures, pyloric antrum, and duodenal bulb in routine projections. With the patient prone (or in a RAO position) and the central ray directed 35 to 45° cephalad, the stomach appears opened up, allowing visualization of the lesser and greater curvatures, pylorus, and duodenal bulb. The cephalic angulation will make the stomach appear more J-shaped, resembling the average sthenic contour. *(Ballinger [Vol. 3], p 656; Bontrager and Anthony, p 19)*

116. The answer is B. Pneumoencephalography is a radiographic examination of the subarachnoid and ventricular system of the brain following the injection of a gaseous contrast agent into the subarachnoid space of the spinal canal via lumbar puncture. In order to distribute the gaseous contrast agent to various structures of the ventricular system, the patient must be rotated laterally, forward and backward. A specially designed somersault chair is extremely advantageous for this task. Because air is lighter than the CSF within the subarachnoid space and ventricular system, it tends to rise to the highest level in the structure in which it is contained. A brow-up position means that the patient's face or brow is up and the posterior aspect of the head is down. Air would tend to rise to the uppermost (anterior) portion of the ventricular system, this being the frontal and temporal horns of the lateral ventricles and the anterior portion of the third ventricle. The brow-down position, on the other hand, would allow air to rise to the posterior aspects of the ventricular system such as the occipital horns of the lateral ventricles, posterior portion of the third ventricle, and the fourth ventricle. *(Ballinger [Vol. 3], p 773–778; Meschan, p 289–298)*

117. The answer is C. Intraoral projections will demonstrate the maxillae to the best advantage radiographically. For all intraoral projections, the film (usually nonscreen type) is placed in the patient's mouth and secured in place by closing the mouth. The central ray is directed from a point above the head toward the feet. For a superoinferior intraoral projection, the patients are adjusted in the supine position so that their head is straight and the midsagittal plane is perpendicular to the table. The central ray is directed perpendicular to the film through the midsagittal plane, passing through the face. The dental arch, palatine processes, and roof of the mouth (horizontal plates of the maxillae) are demonstrated in this projection. The alveolar processes, anterior portion of the hard palate, and superior incisors are demonstrated with the AP axial intraoral projection with the patient's head positioned as above, but the central ray is directed at an angle of 60 to 65° caudad through the distal portion of the nose. The posterior part of the hard palate, alveolar processes, canines, premolars, and molars can be demonstrated by the AP axial oblique intraoral projection. For this projection, the patient's head is rotated 30° away from the side being radiographed and the central ray is angled 60° caudad, entering a point lateral to the nose through the canine fossa. *(Ballinger [Vol. 2], p 484–486)*

118. The answer is B. The Chassard-Lapiné axial projection requires that the patient be seated at the end of the radiographic table in the knee-to-chest position, with the thighs abducted and hands grasping the ankles. The central ray is directed vertically through the lumbosacral region at the level of the greater trochanters and at right angles to the plane of the film. This projection is useful in demonstrating the hip joints, pelvic bones, opacified urinary bladder, and sigmoid colon. *(Ballinger [Vol. 1], p 101)*

119. The answer is B. In the PA oblique projection of the acetabulum (Teufel method), the patient is oblique so that the unaffected side is elevated and forms an angle of 38° to the plane of the film. The central ray is directed 12° cephalad through the acetabulum of the affected side. This projection is useful in demonstrating the superoposterior acetabular wall. *(Ballinger [Vol. 1], p 111)*

120. The answer is B. The foot and ankle assume a true lateral position when placed so that their medial aspect is in contact with the film. In order to assume this position, the patient is turned from the supine position, away from the affected side. The knee of the affected side is elevated slightly so that the patella is at right angles to the film. The plantar surface of the affected foot should also be perpendicular to the film. The central ray is directed perpendicular to the film and enters the base of the third metatarsal. The bones of the foot and ankle will be demonstrated in a true, exact lateral position (tibia and fibula should be superimposed as well as metatarsals and phalanges). The foot can also be radiographed in the lateral position, with its lateral aspect in contact with the film (mediolateral projection), but the truest lateral is assumed with the medial aspect of the foot down. *(Ballinger [Vol. 1], p 48–49; Bontrager and Anthony, p 143)*

121. The answer is C. AP projections of the knee while the patient stands erect are best for revealing joint space narrowing due to arthritis. This projection and position are helpful in identifying deformities associated with arthritic disease as well as for preoperative and postoperative joint evaluation. The patient stands balanced, with the back of the knee in contact with the film, and the central ray is directed perpendicular to the level of the patellar apices (lower margin of the patellas) between both knees. AP supine projections/positions of the knees may not reveal as much information concerning arthritic joint changes as the AP weight-bearing projections will. *(Ballinger [Vol. 1], p 70)*

122. The answer is C. The radiograph that accompanies the question represents a lateral projection of a selective vertebral arteriogram demonstrating the posterior circulation of the brain. For a selective vertebral arteriogram, a catheter is usually placed into the femoral artery by using the Seldinger technique and is advanced under fluoroscopy to the vertebral artery of interest. Iodinated contrast medium is injected, and serial films are taken. Usually an AP axial projection is performed using a 30° caudal tube angulation, as well as a cross-table lateral projection. The vertebral arteries arise from the subclavian arteries, pass upward through the foramina of the cervical vertebrae, and enter the cranium through the foramen magnum, where they unite to form the basilar artery. The posterior fossa structures of the brain are supplied with blood from branches of the vertebrobasilar system of arteries. The radiograph that accompanies the question can be identified as a vertebral arteriogram as opposed to an internal or external carotid arteriogram because the opacified blood vessels are located in the posterior aspect of the cranium. If an external carotid arteriogram were performed, the vascular structures of the face and extracranial structures would be opacified. An internal carotid arteriogram would demonstrate the anterior circulation of the brain, and a brachiocephalic arteriogram would demonstrate vessels of the right arm and right side of the head and neck. *(Ballinger [Vol. 3], p*

779–781, 804; Bontrager and Anthony, p 374–375, 379–380; Meschan, p 299–309; Tortorici, p 186–188, 200–202)

123–125. The answers are 123-B, 124-A, 125-A. A variety of selective visceral angiographic procedures can be performed by manipulation of a catheter in the aortic lumen. The abdominal aorta gives off numerous branches that supply organs in the abdominal and pelvic cavities. Most of these vessels can be selectively catheterized using the Seldinger technique and injecting water-soluble iodinated contrast medium for angiographic study. For a selective superior mesenteric arteriogram, the catheter is inserted most often by a femoral artery approach and advanced under fluoroscopic control to the abdominal aorta, where it is manipulated by the radiologist into the lumen of the SMA. The SMA arises from the anterior aspect of the aorta at above the level of the first lumbar vertebra and passes downward to the lumbosacral region. For an AP projection of the SMA and its branches, the central ray is directed to the midsagittal plane at the level of the third lumbar vertebra (midway between the origination and termination of the SMA). Blood supply to most of the small intestine and right half of the large intestine can be visualized radiographically.

The celiac axis can also be catheterized selectively, using a femoral approach. The celiac axis is a short trunk that arises from the front of the abdominal aorta just beneath the diaphragm, at about the level of the 12th thoracic vertebra. It gives rises to three major vascular branches: the left gastric, splenic, and hepatic arteries. For radiographic demonstration of the opacified celiac and its branches, the central ray is directed perpendicularly to the level of the first lumbar vertebra and midsagittal plane for the AP projection. Blood supply to the liver, spleen, stomach, and duodenum can be visualized following injection of water-soluble iodinated contrast into the celiac axis.

A selective left renal arteriogram can be performed following catheterization of the left renal artery by way of a femoral approach to the abdominal aorta. A "coned-in" AP projection of the circulation to the left kidney is made by directing the central ray perpendicularly to the left sagittal plane (midway between the midsagittal plane and left side of the patient) at the level of the first lumbar vertebra. Positioning can be ascertained by examining previous urographic studies of the kidney of interest. Oblique projections of the kidney are sometimes required in order to demonstrate various anatomic structures.

Angiography of the visceral branches of the abdominal aorta are often required in order to identify vascular abnormalities associated with stenosis, infarction, hemorrhage, aneurysms, tumors, and congenital anomalies. Rapid serial filming will allow demonstration of arterial, capillary, and venous structures and any possible abnormalities present. *(Ballinger [Vol. 3], p 804, 806–808; Katzen, p 23–32; Snopek, p 197–210; Tortorici, p 223–228, 236–244)*

126. The answer is B. In order to prevent crossing of the radius over the ulna, the hand must be supinated to project the bones of the forearm without superimposition. Pronation causes the radius to cross over the ulna and results in an oblique position of the forearm. Oblique and lateral positioning of the hand will result in some superimposition and will not provide an AP projection of the forearm bones. The AP projection of the forearm requires that the arm be extended at the elbow joint and the hand be supinated; the central ray is directed perpendicularly to the midshaft of the forearm bones. Routine examination of the forearm usually calls for AP and lateral projections. *(Ballinger [Vol. 1], p 138; Bontrager and Anthony, p 99–101)*

127. The answer is D. Arthrography is a radiographic examination of the soft-tissue structures within a joint following the injection of radiopaque and/or radiolucent contrast media into a joint. Aqueous iodinated contrast may be used for an opaque arthrogram, gas may be used for a pneumoarthrogram, or both types of contrast may be used together for a double-contrast arthrogram. Arthrography is useful in evaluating ligaments, cartilage, bursae, and menisci of various joints. The procedure is performed using aseptic technique and a local anesthetic. Arthrography is commonly performed to evaluate athletic injuries to various joints, such as the knee, shoulder, ankle, elbow, and hip. *(Ballinger [Vol. 1], p 88–90; Bontrager and Anthony, p 537)*

128. The answer is D. Bronchography is a radiographic study of the bronchial tree following administration of a positive contrast medium, usually an oily iodinated agent. The contrast medium can be administered in a variety of ways, including supraglottic or intraglottic cannulation, intratracheal intubation, percutaneous cricothyroid or percutaneous transtracheal method, and selective catheterization method. Most methods rely on body positioning for distribution of the contrast medium to various segments of the bronchial tree. However, the selective catheterization method allows for direct filling of the segments under investigation without much body maneuvering. Patient cooperation, mild sedation, and sometimes local anesthesia are required in order to suppress the patient's gag and cough reflexes. This is essential for successful bronchial filling and examination and will keep alveolar filling to a minimum. After the examination has been completed and adequate fluoroscopic spot films and routine radiographs have been obtained, the patient is instructed to gently cough up the contrast medium. Postural drainage may be employed to facilitate movement of the contrast medium from various bronchial segments. The patient is not allowed to have food or drink until the effects of anesthesia have worn off, since aspiration might occur. *(Ballinger [Vol. 3], p 598–600; Bontrager and Anthony, p 530; Snopek, p 241–251)*

129. The answer is D. A herniated or ruptured intervertebral disk may be demonstrated radiographically by a variety of methods. A CT scan will demonstrate the intervertebral space anatomy by cross-sectional tomographic cuts taken through the level of interest, and myelography is useful in demonstrating the structures of the subarachnoid space of the spinal canal following the injection of contrast media. Both radiographic examinations are useful in demonstrating herniation of a disk as well as other spinal abnormalities. Diskography, as its name implies, is the study of individual intervertebral disks. Iodinated contrast is injected directly into the center of the disk (nucleus pulposus), and films are taken of that area. This study is also useful in demonstrating ruptured disks radiographically. *(Ballinger [Vol. 3], p 754–770, 837; Bontrager and Anthony, p 539–540; Meschan, p 155–162)*

130. The answer is B. Because the pelvis of the male and female differ in architectural structure, different angulations of the central ray are required for demonstration of the pubic and ischial rami of the pelvis. For males, the central ray is angled 20 to 35° cephalad; for females, a greater angulation is required, 30 to 45° cephalad. For this projection, the patient assumes a supine position and the central ray passes through a point 2 inches below the superior ridge of the pubic symphysis. *(Ballinger [Vol. 1], p 113)*

131. The answer is A. In most routine examinations of the facial bones, a parietoacanthial projection using the Waters method along with a lateral projection are performed. In the Waters method, the patient is adjusted in the prone or PA erect position so that the head rests on the extended chin, with the nose about ½ inch above the film holder and the orbitomeatal line forming a 37 to 40° angle to the film plane. The midsagittal plane should be perpendicular to the film, and the head should not be rotated. The perpendicularly directed central ray enters the vertex and exits the acanthion (anterior nasal spine). The orbits, zygomatic arches, maxillae, and maxillary sinuses are well seen in the angulated frontal projection of the facial bones. A properly positioned Waters projection should demonstrate the petrous ridges just below the maxillary sinus shadows. An AP axial projection may be performed when the patient cannot lie prone or sit erect. For this projection, the patient's infraorbitomeatal line should be perpendicular to the film plane and the central ray angled 30° cephalad just distal to the lips and midsagittal plane. This projection gives similar results as the PA Waters, except the facial structures are more magnified. A modified Waters projection may also be employed for the radiographic demonstration of blowout fractures of the orbit. The head is adjusted so that the orbitomeatal line forms an angle of 55° instead of 37° to the film plane, as the head is adjusted to rest on the chin and nose. *(Ballinger [Vol. 2], p 466, 468–469; Bontrager and Anthony, p 222, 224)*

132. The answer is D. For examination of the acromioclavicular joints when there is a question of separation or dislocation, it is best to position the patient erect (standing or seated), because the recumbent positions may tend to reduce the acromioclavicular separation. For radiographic examination of the acromioclavicular joints, the patient drops both arms down at the sides and may be instructed to hold equal weights in each hand (if able), as this will pull the shoulders down and show acromioclavicular joint separation. Both joints are usually radiographed on one film or two separate films for comparison. AP, PA, or lateral projections can be used in examination of the acromioclavicular joints, with the AP projection being most common. *(Ballinger [Vol. 1], p 170–171; Bontrager and Anthony, p 124)*

133. The answer is C. For the purpose of demonstrating the superior orbital fissures in a PA axial projection, the central ray is directed 20 to 25° caudad, emerging through the inferior orbital margins. The patient's head is positioned so that the forehead and nose are in contact with the film holder and the midsagittal and orbitomeatal line are perpendicular to the film. The superior orbital fissures are projected between the lesser and greater wings of the sphenoid bone on the medial aspect of the orbits. To demonstrate the inferior orbital fissures medial to the mandibular rami and lateral to the pterygoid processes, the patient is positioned PA erect or recumbent so that the infraorbitomeatal line and midsagittal plane are perpendicular to the film plane. The central ray is directed 20 to 25° cephalad, emerging at the level of the nasion. *(Ballinger [Vol. 2], p 410–411)*

134–135. The answers are 134-D, 135-A. The optic foramina are radiographed exceptionally well with the parieto-orbital oblique projection using the Rhese method, and the foramina rotundum are well seen in the parietoacanthial projection using the Waters method. The rotundum and optic foramina are located in the greater and lesser wings of the sphenoid bone, respectively, at the base of the skull. Because of their different positions, it is necessary to take two different projections, to demonstrate radiographically each pair of foramina. Because these foramina transmit nerves and blood vessels, it is often necessary to examine them radiographically in order to check for erosion associated with neurogenic or angiogenic problems. For the demonstration of the optic foramina, a parieto-orbital oblique projection/Rhese method is most often employed. For this projection, the seated or prone patient is adjusted so that the head rests on the chin, nose, and zygoma; the midsagittal plane of the head forms a 53° angle to the film plane. The acanthiomeatal line is placed at right angles to the film, and the central ray is directed perpendicular to the orbit closest to the film. The final radiograph should demonstrate the optic canal in cross-section, located in the lower outer quadrant of the orbit. Usually both sides are radiographed for comparison. The opposite of this projection, the orbitoparietal/Rhese method, will demonstrate the same anatomy. This projection requires the patient's head to be resting on the vertex and rotated so that the midsagittal plane forms a 53° angle to the film plane and the acanthiomeatal line is perpendicular to the film plane. The central ray is directed perpendicularly to the lower outer quadrant of the uppermost orbit.

For the demonstration of the foramina rotundum, a parietoacanthial projection/Waters method is employed. For the Waters method, the patient is adjusted in the PA erect or prone position. The head is extended, the chin is in contact with the film holder, and the nose is approximately ½ inch above the film holder. The orbitomeatal line should form a 37° angle to the film, and the midsagittal plane should be perpendicular. The central ray is directed perpendicularly through the vertex and midsagittal plane, exiting the acanthion (anterior nasal spine). The foramina rotundum will be located just inferior to the medial aspect of the floor of the orbits and superior to the upper maxillary sinuses, bilaterally. *(Ballinger [Vol. 2], p 402–405, 514–515; Bontrager and Anthony, p 219–220, 222, 232)*

136. The answer is D. Free air (spontaneous pneumoperitoneum) may be the result of an acute abdominal problem such as perforated ulcer, rupture of a hollow organ, or trauma. In addition to an AP projection of the abdomen with the patient supine, other projections (AP erect, lateral and dorsal decubitus), which employ a horizontal x-ray beam, may be necessary in order to demonstrate free air in the peritoneal cavity. When performing an erect projection of the abdomen, it is imperative to include the top of the diaphragm on the film when free air is suspected, as air rises to the highest point. When performing lateral decubitus projections, patients are usually placed in a left lateral recumbent position, with the film in contact with their anterior or posterior aspect. Free air would rise to the side up (in this case, the right side), if present. For a dorsal decubitus projection, patients lie in the supine position with the film in contact with either their left or right side. The beam is directed horizontally at right angles to the film. Free air, if present, would rise to the anterior aspect of the abdomen, which is up. *(Ballinger [Vol. 3], p 610–611; Bontrager and Anthony, p 66, 68–71)*

137. The answer is D. For a lateral projection of the scapula, it is best to place the patient in an oblique position, with the affected side in contact with the film (RAO for the right scapula and LAO for the left scapula). It is usually easiest for patients to be seated or erect, facing the film holder. They are then rotated so that the flat surface of the scapula is perpendicular to the film, or in a true lateral position. The central ray is directed perpendicularly to the midvertebral border of the scapula. Radiographically, the scapula should be demonstrated free of the rib cage. When the anterior oblique position is not possible, posterior obliques may be performed, but a greater amount of patient rotation is needed. *(Ballinger [Vol. 1], p 179; Bontrager and Anthony, p 126)*

138. The answer is D. J-tipped guide wires should be used preferentially during the catheterization process of angiography in order to negotiate the twists and turns of tortuous blood vessels. Difficulty in manipulation could be encountered if a straight-tipped guide wire were used. Atherosclerotic vessels have lipid and plaque deposits on their inner lumen wall, which often necessitates the use of a J-tipped guide wire, which bounces away from the plaque and avoids dislodging it. A straight-tipped guide wire could inadvertently be advanced underneath the plaque, loosen it, and cause distal emoblization. J-tipped guide wires are usually safer to use in tortuous atherosclerotic vessels because they avoid causing injury or embolization. *(Tortorici, p 88–92)*

139–141. The answers are 139-D, 140-A, 141-B. The suprasternal notch is located at the same level as the top of the third thoracic vertebra (or the interspace between T-2 and T-3). The suprasternal notch is easily palpated at the top of the sternum, in the midline. It is a useful landmark for radiographic positioning as it corresponds to a vertebral level that can be identified easily for "coned-down" projections of various structures in this area of the body.

The gonion, or angle of the mandible, can be palpated easily as the prominent angles on the lateral aspects of the jaw. The gonion corresponds to the same level as the third cervical vertebra when the head is in a neutral position. This palpable landmark can also be used in positioning body parts in this area for radiography.

The thyroid cartilage, another easily palpated structure situated in the anterior neck, is often referred to as the Adam's apple as it gives rise to the laryngeal protruberance in the midline. The thyroid cartilage lies at the same level as the fifth cervical vertebra. It too is used to locate anatomic structures topographically for use in radiographic positioning. *(Bontrager and Anthony, p 297–298)*

142. The answer is D. The filling of the renal pelvis and calyces with opaque contrast medium can be enhanced during excretory urography by the application of ureteric compression or by placing the patient in the Trendelenburg and/or prone positions. Ureteric compression involves the application of a specially designed belt and inflatable balloons over the lower abdomen. When the balloons are inflated, pressure is placed on the ureters, allowing the contrast media to stay in the upper collecting systems longer and enhancing their opacity. Ureteric compression may be contraindicated in cases of abdominal masses, surgery, pain, trauma, aortic aneurysms, or ureterolithiasis. The Trendelenburg position may be used for contrast enhancement of the upper collecting systems by making use of gravitational force; when the kidneys are at a lower position than the rest of the collecting system, contrast will stay in them longer. The prone position is useful in enhancing opacification of the renal pelvicalyceal systems by exerting pressure on the abdomen and causing gas in the stomach to move into the fundus, thereby displacing gas shadows out of the way of the kidneys and enhancing visualization of their opacified structures. *(Ballinger [Vol. 3], p 695, 697; Bontrager and Anthony, p 511, 520)*

143. The answer is D. Routine positioning of the sternum usually includes a RAO and a lateral. The RAO position allows the sternum to be projected away from the spine and over the shadow of the heart by rotating the patient 15 to 20° from the prone position. The central ray is directed at right angles to the film through the midsternum, just left of the midsagittal plane. Shallow breathing technique is often used in an effort to blur pulmonary and rib shadows. The lateral projection of the sternum may be performed in either the lateral erect or recumbent positions or as a cross-table lateral projection. The patient's arms should be positioned out of the way of the anterior chest wall and sternum. The central ray is directed perpendicularly through the midsternum and anterior chest wall. Respiration is usually suspended for the lateral projection. A LAO may be performed as an alternative to a RAO when necessary. *(Ballinger [Vol. 1], p 188–189; Bontrager and Anthony, p 325–326)*

144. The answer is D. The foramen magnum is best demonstrated in its entirety with the patient positioned for an AP axial projection and the central ray directed 50 to 60° caudad. For this axial projection, patients are adjusted in the supine or AP erect position so that their midsagittal plane and orbitomeatal line are perpendicular to the film plane. The central ray will enter the cranial vertex at an angle of 50 to 60° caudad, emerging at the foramen magnum. This will demonstrate the occipital region, jugular foramina, and entire foramen magnum. A 0° angulation with the patient positioned as described above would not provide adequate visualization of the foramen magnum. AP axial projections with the central ray angled 30° caudally and the orbitomeatal line perpendicular to the film or with the central ray angled 37° caudally and the infraorbitomeatal line perpendicular to the film are useful in demonstrating the occipital bone, petrous pyramids, and the posterior portion of the foramen magnum with the posterior parts of the sella projected within its shadow. *(Ballinger [Vol. 2], p 386–388, 437)*

RADIOGRAPHIC EXPOSURE AND PROCESSING

145. It is frequently necessary in radiography to change the exposure parameters without changing the resulting radiographic density. A shoot-through lateral hip taken in the x-ray department is exposed at 40-inch focus-film distance (FFD) with 38 mAs. When a follow-up examination is requested after surgery, a FFD of 48 inches has to be used. What mAs will provide the same radiographic density as the original examination?

A. 26 mAs
B. 42 mAs
C. 46 mAs
D. 55 mAs

146. The x-ray tube has been designed to produce a beam of desired quantity and quality in a way that will optimize the geometry of image formation. What effect does the line-focus principle have on image formation?

1. Image sharpness will vary from the anode to cathode end of a 14 × 17-inch radiograph
2. Magnification will be reduced
3. Distortion will be increased

A. 1 only
B. 2 only
C. 3 only
D. 1, 2, and 3

147. In the diagnostic energy range, most x-ray photons are either photoelectrically absorbed, Compton scattered, or transmitted. Which of the following photons contribute most to the formation of the x-ray image?

A. Transmitted
B. Compton scattered
C. Absorbed
D. Thompson scattered

148. The image-intensifier tube creates an amplified fluoroscopic image several thousand times brighter than the direct fluoroscopic image. This is accomplished partly by reducing the size of the output image to 1 to 2 inches across, while the input image size varies between 4 and 14 inches across. What is the other component of the overall brightness improvement?

A. Minification
B. Magnification mode
C. The output phosphor conversion efficiency
D. Flux gain

149. If the image is found to be 2.5 times as large as the anatomic object radiographed, where was that anatomic object positioned in relation to the film plane, if a FFD of 40 inches was used?

A. 16 inches from the film plane
B. 19 inches from the film plane
C. 21 inches from the film plane
D. 24 inches from the film plane

150–153. For each numbered term listed below, select the imaging technique with which it is most closely associated. Each heading may be used once, more than once, or not at all.

    A. CT scan
    B. Magnetic resonance
    C. Xeroradiography
    D. Ultrasonography

150. Window width and level

151. Translate and rotate

152. Predetector collimation

153. Toner cloud

154. A high-speed rotating anode, rather than the average 3,000-rpm anode, has some great advantages. Faster rotational speed helps to improve image quality because

    A. the penumbra is reduced
    B. more mA can be delivered in a shorter time
    C. the anode's electrical conduction function is improved
    D. image density is increased

155. All factors that affect the amount of geometric unsharpness in any image have been summarized into an equation called the penumbra formula. Where FID stands for focus-image distance, FOD stands for focus-object distance, and OID stands for object-image distance, the penumbra formula is represented by

    A. $\text{FID} \times \dfrac{\text{FOD}}{\text{width of effective focal spot}}$

    B. $\text{width of effective focal spot} \times \dfrac{\text{OID}}{\text{FOD}}$

    C. $\text{FOD} \times \dfrac{\text{width of actual focal spot}}{\text{FID}}$

    D. $\text{width of actual focal spot} \times \dfrac{\text{OID}}{\text{FID}^2}$

156. Of the factors listed below, which affect both radiographic density and the sharpness with which anatomic details are recorded?

    1. FID
    2. Volume of tissue irradiated
    3. mAs selected

    A. 1 and 2
    B. 1 and 3
    C. 2 and 3
    D. 1, 2, and 3

157. Patient dose for a tomographic exposure is generally slightly larger than for a plain radiographic exposure of exactly the same anatomy. What are the differences between the two that contribute to increased dose to the patient?

    1. The mAs is increased because kVp must be kept low to maintain contrast
    2. The angled tube produces a slightly larger field size at each end of the excursion
    3. Higher mAs is required because the angled central ray traverses greater tissue volume

  A. 1 and 2
  B. 1 and 3
  C. 2 and 3
  D. 1, 2, and 3

158. Humans are not evenly dense, thick blocks of tissue that image in a uniform way. The technologist does, however, have a variety of methods and techniques that help in obtaining the optimally exposed radiograph. Which of the following diagrams illustrates a compensating filter that will show all the structures in the chest to best advantage?

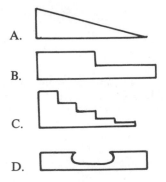

A.

B.

C.

D.

Questions 159 and 160 consist of four lettered headings followed by a list of numbered words or phrases. For each numbered word or phrase, select the one heading with which it is most closely related. Each heading may be used once, more than once, or not at all.

  A. Luminescence
  B. Photomultiplier tube
  C. Conversion efficiency
  D. X-ray tube output

159. Roentgen

160. Automatic exposure control

161. Which of the following groups of exposure factors would produce the greatest optical density in the finished radiograph (where SID stands for source-image distance)?

A. 150 mA, 4/5 seconds, 63 kVp, 40 inches FFD/SID
B. 175 mA, 4/10 seconds, 85 kVp, 48 inches FFD/SID
C. 225 mA, 3/5 seconds, 72 kVp, 54 inches FFD/SID
D. 300 mA, 3/10 seconds, 100 kVp, 84 inches FFD/SID

162. Which of the following are generalized changes that sooner or later occur as the body ages and that affect x-ray transmission and absorption?

1. Bone volume and density decrease
2. Fat replaces some muscle tissue
3. Fluid content of tissues is increased

A. 1 and 2
B. 1 and 3
C. 2 and 3
D. 1, 2, and 3

163. It is sometimes difficult to obtain a radiograph of excellent quality for an obese patient who is having a survey abdominal examination. Which of the following will improve contrast in this situation?

1. Collimation ¼ inch smaller than cassette size
2. Rare earth intensifying screens
3. A 16:1 grid

A. 1 and 2
B. 1 and 3
C. 2 and 3
D. 1, 2, and 3

164. Tomographic x-ray units that maintain fixed FFD and fixed focus-object:object-film ratios throughout the exposure produce a superior image. Which specific aspects of this Grossman method image are improved?

1. Radiographic density is uniform throughout the image
2. Magnification is uniform at a known percentage
3. Contrast is markedly higher

A. 1 and 2
B. 1 and 3
C. 2 and 3
D. 1, 2, and 3

165. Which of the following statements are true regarding the anode cooling curve below?

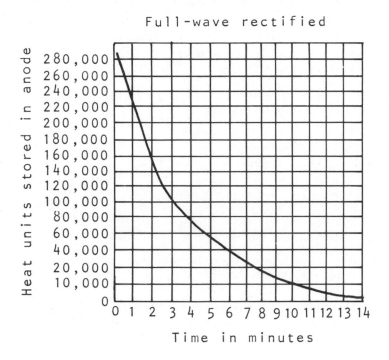

1. It takes 12 minutes to cool completely from four exposures of 85 kV, 600 mA, 0.7 second
2. It takes 7 minutes to cool completely from three exposures of 95 kV, 400 mA, 0.8 second
3. It takes 13 minutes to cool completely from eight exposures of 70 kV, 200 mA, 2 seconds

A. 1 and 2
B. 1 and 3
C. 2 and 3
D. 1, 2, and 3

166. Distortion in the image is usually recognized as such, but only infrequently can it be remedied. Which of the following affects the shape of the image?

A. OID
B. Object thickness
C. Distance of the object from the central ray
D. Size of the effective focal spot

167. Radiographic density is very important to the x-ray image, but without "contrast" there would be no image. Image contrast results from

A. photoelectric absorption
B. the transmitted photon
C. differential absorption
D. the scattered photon

168. X-ray units sometimes behave in ways that produce easily recognizable signs of their incorrect functioning. What has probably occurred if the tube output suddenly drops to 50% of its original level?

A. The target is cracked
B. The anode is emitting electrons
C. Two vacuum tube rectifiers have failed
D. The glass insert is punctured

169. The formation of radiographic contrast relies heavily on photoelectric interactions. Photoelectric interactions are correctly described as

A. more likely to occur in fat than in muscle
B. unrelated to photon energy
C. occurring equally often in soft tissues and in bone
D. more frequent in tissues with a higher atomic number

170. Numerous changes can be made in the construction of an intensifying screen in order to change its speed. These changes are not under the technologist's control. Which of the construction characteristics listed below will reduce the speed of an intensifying screen?

A. A thicker active layer
B. Larger phosphor crystal size
C. The presence of reflective material
D. Dye added to the binder of the active layer

171. Because silver is expensive, recovery units are often used with automatic processors in order to reclaim the silver in fixing solutions. All of the following methods are used for recovering silver EXCEPT

A. silver straining
B. electrolytic recovery
C. chemical precipitation
D. metallic replacement

172. Film contrast is most commonly defined numerically by the

A. average gradient
B. ratio of absorbed to transmitted photons
C. densitometer
D. kVp of the primary beam

173. Which of the following imaging systems would be expected to give the highest resolution?

A. Par-speed intensifying screen with screen-type film
B. High-speed intensifying screen with screen-type film
C. Slow-speed intensifying screen with screen-type film
D. Direct-exposure film used without an intensifying screen

174. The CT image is different from any other in the field of radiology. Which of the following statements best describes how the CT image is formed?

A. The remnant x-ray beam strikes the image-intensifier tube, and the image is transmitted to the console monitor
B. The remnant beam strikes a gas or scintillation detector, which measures beam intensity and transmits the information to the computer and then to the console monitor
C. The remnant beam strikes the film and is photographed, and that image is displayed on the console monitor
D. The remnant beam strikes the image-intensifier tube, which transmits the image to the computer, where it is stored for later recall or display on the console monitor

175. Some of the factors affecting image sharpness are within the technologist's control, whereas others are inherent in the equipment available in any x-ray department. Which of the following will give the sharpest image?

A. Par-speed screens, 1-mm focal spot, 400 mA
B. Par-speed screens, 1-mm focal spot, 100 mA
C. High-speed screens, 2-mm focal spot, 100 mA
D. High-speed screens, 2-mm focal spot, 100 mA

176. One of the goals of a quality assurance program in a radiology department is to reduce materials waste, mainly film waste, as this is one of the most expensive portions of operating costs. Waste due to "repeats" in large institutions constitutes about 4% of all film used and also represents that same percentage of unnecessary exposure to patients. The vast majority of repeated radiographs are caused by

A. dirty or damaged intensifying screens
B. improper positioning or incorrect choice of exposure factors
C. equipment malfunctioning and processor error
D. cassettes loaded with the wrong film

177. The vast majority of diagnostic x-ray tubes are diode vacuum tubes—that is, they have two electrical terminals, one positive and one negative. There is also a diagnostic x-ray tube with three terminals, a triode. This special-purpose tube is called a

A. reverse emission tube
B. Coolidge tube
C. grid-biased tube
D. trifocus tube

178. Tomography is a radiographic method of "removing" superimposed structures through motion in order to image an unobstructed view of a specific anatomic plane. Uniform radiographic density is produced in the image when the tube

    A. and cassette travel parallel to the table

    B. and cassette travel in an arc

    C. travels parallel to the table and the cassette travels in an arc

    D. travels in an arc and the cassette travels parallel to the table

179. The spectrum of recording and viewing methods available with intensified fluoroscopy offers something for every individual clinical occasion. Which recording system is most appropriate when a dynamic study must be evaluated in the shortest period of time?

    A. Cassette spot films

    B. Video disk

    C. Videotape

    D. Cinefluorography

180. It is not always possible in radiography to use the standard 40-inch (100-cm) FFD, although technique charts are usually established on that basis. An emergency room patient has cervical spine radiographs taken at a FFD of 35 inches with 14 mAs. When the patient is later taken to the x-ray department, his radiographs can then be made at the standard 40-inch FFD. What mAs will provide the same radiographic density as the emergency room examination?

    A. 11 mAs

    B. 16 mAs

    C. 18 mAs

    D. 24 mAs

181. Tube failure is brought about when one important component actually fails or when tube output becomes so erratic that it is unusable, the result of continued or sudden thermal stresses. If only tube life were being considered, which of the following would definitely increase its length?

    A. Warming the tube with a maximum kVp/mAs combination

    B. Choosing high kVp and low mAs combinations of exposure factors

    C. Running the rotor at least 30 seconds so that the exposure can be made instantaneously

    D. Selecting low mA stations and using very long exposure times so that low kVp can be selected for high-contrast radiographs

182. The image characteristic that has an ambivalent or dual nature in that at different times its presence can either make interpretation very difficult or actually serve to clarify a diagnosis is

    A. density

    B. contrast

    C. distortion

    D. detail sharpness

183. The production of scattered radiation, the great reducer of image contrast, will increase in volume with an increase in

A. photon wavelength
B. tissue thickness irradiated
C. object-film distance (OFD)
D. size of air gap used

184. Equally diagnostic film quality can result when an air gap is used instead of a grid in

A. cerebral angiography
B. plain abdominal radiography of adults
C. pediatric radiography
D. barium studies

185. Separate radiographic grids, which can be fastened to the front of a cassette as needed to make a grid cassette, are still in use in many radiology departments. Should the focused grid be attached upside down with the "tube side" against the cassette, the resulting radiograph will not be useful. How can such a grid-use error be immediately recognized?

A. Grid lines completely obscure the image
B. A strip of adequate density appears lengthwise at the center of the radiograph only
C. Only the left and right sides of the radiograph are correctly exposed
D. Only the upper and lower edges of the radiograph appear normally exposed

186. Digital fluorography can improve conventional imaging in a number of ways, by making use of current computer technology. Which of the following is NOT an advantage of digital imaging?

A. Scattered radiation noise in the image is reduced
B. Processing time is reduced
C. Subtracted images are available for viewing immediately
D. Incorrect exposure factors are readily correctable

187. One of the advantages of CT is the ability to modify the image electronically without exposing the patient to additional radiation. All of the following are methods of electronic image manipulation EXCEPT

A. back-projection
B. window width and level selection
C. magnification
D. subtraction

188. The technique chart for each individual radiographic room should indicate kVp and/or mAs values required to accommodate grid use. This permits a wider range of techniques to be used, based on the requirements of each clinical situation. The extra amount of radiation required for grid use over nongrid use is called

A. the Bucky factor
B. K
C. selectivity
D. modulation transfer function

189. The exposure rate of a diagnostic x-ray beam can be measured and expressed in roentgens or milliroentgens. The exposure rate of any diagnostic beam will be increased by

    A. an increase in distance from the source
    B. a decrease in tube potential
    C. an increase in tube current
    D. an increase in primary-beam filtration

190. Radiographic contrast consists of subject contrast (anatomic plus beam variables) and the contrast inherent in the materials used in the imaging process. Which of the following would demonstrate the greatest radiographic contrast if all other conditions of the imaging process were the same?

    A. Soft-tissue mass in the abdomen
    B. Osteolytic metastasis
    C. Liver cirrhosis
    D. Pneumothorax

191. Radiographic contrast is a most central component of the image because it permits the perception of anatomic detail. High radiographic contrast requires the use of low kVp. Which of the following is a disadvantage of high contrast?

    A. Decreased differential absorption
    B. Reduced exposure latitude
    C. A longer gray scale
    D. Reduced patient dose

192. Which of the following groups of exposure variables would produce the greatest optical density in a processed radiograph?

    A.   75 mA, 3/10 second, 100 kVp, 72 inches FFD/SID, high-speed screens
    B. 200 mA, 4/5 second, 74 kVp, 40 inches FFD/SID, par-speed screens
    C. 250 mA, 3/5 second, 118 kVp, 36 inches FFD/SID, detail/fine-speed screens
    D. 600 mA, 3/20 second, 85 kVp, 60 inches FFD/SID, par-speed screens

193. Many factors that affect the x-ray emission spectrum, although not under the control of the technologist, have a significant effect on radiographic density. Their presence or absence may explain why no two x-ray units perform in exactly the same way. Radiographic density would be increased by

    A. adding filtration beyond the required minimum
    B. using three-phase voltage waveform
    C. having a target material of a low atomic number
    D. increasing photon wavelength

194. For the purpose of computer reconstruction of the CT image, the "slice" of tissue irradiated is usually represented as an array of square cells or elements arranged in rows or columns. What is the name given to each square cell or element as shown on the monitor?

    A. CT number
    B. Pixel
    C. Matrix
    D. Voxel

195. Radiographic density is defined by a numeric value that indicates the relationship beween the light striking one side of a radiograph (from a standard illuminator) and the light transmitted through the radiograph. What percentage of light is transmitted when radiographic or optical density is 1?

    A.   0.1%
    B.   1%
    C.   10%
    D. 100%

196. Sharpness in the radiographic image is mainly the result of limiting inherent unsharpness in beam geometry and imaging equipment. Which of the following would give the sharpest image?

    A. High-speed screens, 1-mm focal spot, 38-inch FOD, 48-inch FFD
    B. Detail/fine screens, 2-mm focal spot, 28-inch FOD, 42-inch FFD
    C. Detail/fine screens, 1-mm focal spot, 36-inch FOD, 46-inch FFD
    D. Detail/fine screens, 1-mm focal spot, 38-inch FOD, 40-inch FFD

Questions 197–200 consist of four lettered headings followed by a list of numbered words or phrases. For each numbered word or phrase, select the heading with which it is most closely related. Each heading may be used once, more than once, or not at all.

    A. Line-focus principle
    B. Kilovoltage
    C. Focal spot selection
    D. Angle of anode

197. Scatter production

198. Primary-beam wavelength

199. Radiographic contrast

200. Exposure rate

201. Tomography of the internal auditory canal requires very thin "slices," or in-focus sections, to visualize all the details of the anatomy well. What changes occur in the image characteristics as section or "cut" thickness is decreased in the multidirectional tomographic unit?

    1. Radiographic density decreases
    2. Radiographic contrast decreases
    3. Sharpness increases

    A. 1 and 2
    B. 1 and 3
    C. 2 and 3
    D. 1, 2, and 3

202. Quality assurance testing of diagnostic x-ray equipment can be viewed from two perspectives: image quality and patient/personnel exposure. Which of the following tests are primarily directed at restricting day-to-day nonproductive patient/personnel exposure?

      1. Spinning top test
      2. Half-value layer (HVL) measurement
      3. X-ray field/light field congruency test

  A. 1 and 2
  B. 1 and 3
  C. 2 and 3
  D. 1, 2, and 3

203. To keep tube use within safe limits, charts are provided to indicate maximum and minimum values for exposure factors. Which of the following statements referring to the tube rating chart below are correct?

      1. The shortest exposure time for 90 kVp, 200 mAs is 0.4 second
      2. The shortest exposure time for 60 kVp, 50 mAs is 0.02 second
      3. The shortest exposure time for 70 kVp, 240 mAs is 0.4 second

  A. 1 and 2
  B. 1 and 3
  C. 2 and 3
  D. 1, 2, and 3

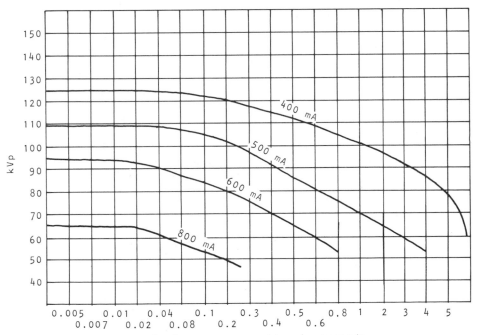

204 The term "gassy tube" is one that all technologists have heard from the equipment service man when erratic tube output has to be explained. This troublesome gas may result from

      1. vaporized metal of the target
      2. a punctured insert that admits vaporized oil
      3. a vaporized filament

A. 1 and 2
B. 1 and 3
C. 2 and 3
D. 1, 2, and 3

205. Which of the following factors will have some impact on total radiographic density?

      1. The presence of disease processes
      2. Compression of the tissues to be imaged
      3. The atomic number of the target material

A. 1 and 2
B. 1 and 3
C. 2 and 3
D. 1, 2, and 3

206. Several factors referred to as "noise" work to undermine image quality. Some of them are inherent to the x-ray imaging process and some to the imaging equipment. Which of the following would reduce radiographic noise?

      1. Low kVp, high mAs, and slow-speed screens
      2. High kVp, low mAs, and very fast screens
      3. High mAs, low kVp, and a nonscreen system

A. 1 and 2
B. 1 and 3
C. 2 and 3
D. 1, 2, and 3

207. Radiographic contrast is always maximized by the greatest possible restriction of the primary beam. Which beam-limiting device is currently used in addition to a collimator when a high-contrast, high-definition radiograph is required of a small anatomic area?

A. Cone
B. Aperture diaphragm
C. Extension cylinder
D. Tube port

208. X-ray photons are correctly described as all of the following EXCEPT

    A. leaving the x-ray tube in straight lines
    B. producing biologic changes by ionization
    C. electrically neutral
    D. focused by a lens

209. The image-intensifier tube increases the brightness of the fluoroscopic image to a level at which it can be viewed with the improved visual acuity of the retina's cone cells. The x-ray image is converted to an electron image at the

    A. focusing electrodes and the anode
    B. input phosphor
    C. input phosphor and the photocathode
    D. output phosphor

210. Film that is sensitive to all colors or wavelengths of light in the spectrum is called

    A. panchromatic
    B. orthochromatic
    C. monochromatic
    D. direct-exposure

211. Which of the following are recommended for the storage and handling of radiographic film?

    1. Cool and dry conditions
    2. Bright and airy conditions
    3. Lead-lined storage areas

    A. 1 only
    B. 1 and 3
    C. 2 and 3
    D. 1, 2, and 3

212. Which of the following statements are true concerning the characteristic curves of the films depicted in the graph below?

       1. Film A is faster than film B

       2. Film A has greater contrast than film B

       3. The combined base plus fog densities of film A are greater than those of film B

A. 1 and 2

B. 1 and 3

C. 2 and 3

D. 1, 2, and 3

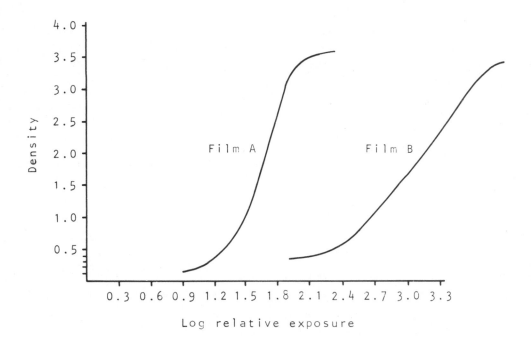

213. If a film-screen combination with a film speed of 1 and a screen speed of 400 is used to expose a part and a technique of 50 mAs and 75 kVp is required for the proper exposure (radiographic density and contrast), how will the exposure factors be changed in order to reproduce a correctly exposed radiograph of the same part, if a film with a speed factor of 0.5 is used in combination with a screen speed of 200?

A. The mAs should be doubled and kVp should be doubled

B. The mAs should be quartered and kVp remains the same

C. The mAs should be quadrupled and kVp remains the same

D. The mAs stays the same and kVp is quadrupled

214. If a certain type of film possesses a base density of 0.05 and a fog density of 0.04, between what two densities will one measure the average gradient or contrast of this film on a characteristic curve?

    A. 0.16 and 1.91
    B. 0.29 and 2.59
    C. 0.30 and 2.04
    D. 0.34 and 2.09

215. If using densities of 0.34 (D_1) and 2.09 (D_2) on the characteristic curve, what is the average gradient or numeric representation of the film's contrast if D_1 and D_2 correspond to Log Relative Exposures of 0.85 and 1.90, respectively?

    A. 0.32
    B. 1.05
    C. 1.66
    D. 3.30

216. The xeroradiographic image differs in a number of respects from the radiographic film-screen image with which we are more familiar. Which of the following statements does NOT accurately describe xeroradiography?

    A. The image is high contrast
    B. Dose is increased over film-screen imaging
    C. Edge effect is a diagnostic aid
    D. Dry processing is automatic

BODY—RADIOGRAPHIC EXPOSURE AND PROCESSING
ANSWERS, EXPLANATIONS, AND REFERENCES

145. The answer is D. The mAs-distance formula is derived from the inverse square law. However, in the situation described in the question it is required to find the beam intensity (mAs) that will keep exposure at the film constant, even as distance (focus-film distance [FFD]) is changed. When FFD is doubled, mAs must be quadrupled to maintain a constant film density. The following calculations yield the answer to the example given in the question *(Bushong, p 63–65; Selman, p 341–344):*

$$\frac{mAs_1}{mAs_2} = \left(\frac{D_1}{D_2}\right)^2 \rightarrow \frac{38}{X} = \left(\frac{40}{48}\right)^2 \rightarrow \frac{38}{X} = \frac{1,600}{2,304} \rightarrow 1,600X = 87,552 \rightarrow X =$$

$54.72 \rightarrow X = 55$ mAs.

146. The answer is A. The target (focal spot) of the anode is angled toward the filament to present both a large area for heat dissipation (actual focal spot) and a small area to provide a sharp image (effective focal spot). However, the size of the effective focal spot varies depending on whether it is viewed from directly beneath it from under the cathode or from under the anode. The effective focal spot appears smallest at the anode and largest at the cathode end, resulting in a variation in sharpness when the entire beam is used to expose the film. Magnification, which is a source of unsharpness in the image, is independent of the line-focus principle and dependent on the position of the object, between the focal spot and image. Distortion or inaccurate representation of the size or shape of an object radiographed is also independent of the line-focus principle; shape distortion depends on the location of the object relative to a central ray that is perpendicular to the image plane. *(Bushong, p 117–118; Selman, p 213–216)*

147. The answer is A. The x-ray image is mainly the result of photons having sufficient energy to penetrate the anatomic part and interact with the intensifying screens to produce radiographic density. It is these transmitted photons that carry information about the differences in atomic density of the materials through which they have passed. Photoelectrically absorbed photons also make a contribution to the image. They do not add to radiographic density because they are absorbed before reaching the image receptor but are notable as a lack of density—they provide contrast. Scattered photons do not contribute useful information because their path has not been direct; they do in fact degrade image quality. *(Bushong, p 165–167; Selman, p 189–190)*

148. The answer is D. Flux gain refers to the increase in image brightness resulting from accelerating the electrons across the vacuum tube, with many more light photons emitted at the output phosphor than were originally required to generate the electron stream at the photocathode. Roughly 25 kV sufficiently increases the kinetic energy of the electrons between the photocathode and the anode to produce a gain in brightness of about 50 times. Minification is the brightness improvement achieved by reducing the size of the output phosphor. Magnification mode is an optical image magnification system available with many image-intensifier tubes. The input and output phosphors are very similar in conversion efficiency. *(Bushong, p 294–295; Selman, p 405–409)*

149. The answer is D. The following equation, derived from geometric relationships between similar triangles, is used to solve problems involving magnification: MF = FFD/FOD.

$$\frac{2.5 = 40 \text{ inches}}{X} \rightarrow 2.5X = 40 \text{ inches} \rightarrow X = 16 \text{ inches.}$$

If the FOD = 16 inches and the FFD = 40 inches, then the anatomic object is 24 inches from the film plane (40 − 16 = 24). *(Bushong, p 272–273; Selman, p 356)*

150–153. The answers are 150-A, 151-A, 152-A, 153-C.   Each pixel displayed on the CT monitor represents a level of brightness that can range from CT numbers −1,000 to +1,000. The CT monitor can represent a gray scale of about 20 to 30 shades. This discrepancy in information display is solved by the selection of a "window," or only a single group of CT numbers to be displayed at any one time, the width indicating the range of the window. The window level is the position of the selected range on the overall scale of CT numbers available.

   Translate and *rotate* are terms that refer to the methods by which the earlier CT units gathered information on the attenuation values for the tissues being imaged. One translation is a single pass of the tube/detector assembly, across the patient from side to side. The tube detector assembly then returns to its initial position, rotates a set number of degrees (from the original path), and makes another translation across the tissue. The computer uses these discrete attenuation values to reconstruct the image.

   Considerably less scattered radiation is produced with the CT pencil or fan beam and prepatient collimation as compared with the larger-area beam used in conventional radiography. The scatter that is produced is again reduced by the use of predetector collimators placed between the patient and the detector.

   In the xeroradiographic development chamber, a fine mist of charged powder particles is blown onto the electrostatically charged plate. The charged powder is the toner cloud, which adheres to the plate, forming a visible image. Depending on the charge of the toner cloud, the finished image may be a positive or a negative. In the transfer station, the powder image is transferred from the Xerox plate to paper. *(Bushong, p 321–322, 366–369, 374; Chesney and Chesney [1984], p 475)*

154. The answer is B.   A high-speed rotating anode, usually 10,000 rpm, increases the rate at which heat is dissipated from the anode disk. This permits larger exposures to be made (that is, the tube rating is increased), or any given magnitude of mA and kVp can be made in a shorter time period. When the patient is unable to cooperate fully with the technologist to suspend respiration or remain motionless for the duration of the exposure, the ability to complete the exposure in half or a quarter of the time can prevent motion in the radiograph and can possibly prevent the need for a second exposure. *(Bushong, p 114–116; Selman, p 215–218)*

155. The answer is B.   The most important aspect of geometric unsharpness is the size of the effective focal spot. (Actual focal spot size is significant only in tube heat-loading capacity.) As the effective focal spot increases in width, the penumbra or geometric unsharpness increases in width. Secondly, the penumbra is affected by the location of the anatomic part between the focal spot and the image plane. As the part is moved farther away from the image plane (or closer to the focal spot), object-image distance (OID) is increasing and so is the penumbra, but when the part is moved closer to the image plane (or farther from the focal spot), the penumbra is decreased. Thus penumbra is defined as being directly proportional to both effective focal spot size and OID and inversely proportional to FOD, or the penumbra (P) = width of effective focal spot OID/FOD. *(Bushong, p 278–281; Selman, p 327–330)*

156. The answer is D.   For any given OID, a change in focus-image distance (FID) will vary magnification in the image, and that will affect sharpness. A variation in FID will also vary density, according to the inverse square law. As tissue volume increases, radiographic density decreases and more anatomic structures are moved farther from the image plane, increasing magnification and unsharpness. The mA varies radiographic density. As mA increases, effective focal spot size also increases, regardless of the focal spot selected. The larger the mA, the more difficult it is for the focusing cup to control the electron stream. *(Bushong, p 288; Selman, p 327–335, 338–345)*

157. The answer is D.   Certain factors contribute to an increase in patient exposure received from a tomographic "cut" as compared with a radiographic exposure of the same area. Radiographic contrast decreases with decreasing cut thickness, and relatively low kVp must be used to counteract this trend. This means that mAs must be increased to achieve correct radiographic density. A square x-ray field from an overhead tube is elongated into a rectangle when that tube is angled, as at the beginning and end of each tomographic excursion. The larger field size increases the dose to the patient. Higher mAs is required (higher kVp would decrease contrast) when the central ray is passing obliquely through a greater tissue volume, as when the tube is angled at the beginning and end of each excursion. *(Bushong, p 306–307; Selman, p 433– 434)*

158. The answer is D.   A compensating filter is an aluminum or plastic device placed in the primary beam, usually on the tracks of the collimator, to absorb some areas of the beam while transmitting others. The primary beam is then nonuniform when it interacts with the patient, producing a more uniform image density. In the figure that accompanies the question, **D** is a double wedge or trough filter, which reduces radiation intensity reaching the lung fields but leaves unchanged that portion of the beam that would expose the mediastinum, resulting in uniform imaging of the whole chest. A wedge filter **(A)** is suitable for lateral views of the spine. A stepped filter **(B)** is suitable for imaging the vasculature of the entire leg. Diagram C is not a compensating filter. *(Bushong, p 179–180; Chesney and Chesney [1984], p 506–507)*

159–160. The answers are 159-D, 160-B.   The quantity or intensity output of the x-ray tube is measured in roentgens (coulombs/kg) or milliroentgens. This is a measurement of the number of ion pairs produced in an air volume by a quantity of x-rays. The roentgen is a unit of radiation exposure or intensity that applies only to x-rays and gamma rays.
   Automatic exposure controls, or "phototimers" (as they are still called), can be of two types, one of which is the fluorescent screen/photomultiplier tube type. Radiation passes through the patient and cassette and strikes a fluorescent screen in a light-tight box. The visible light from the fluorescent screen is "seen" by a photomultiplier tube, which emits proportional electrons. These constitute a current, which terminates the exposure. The acceptable level of radiation reaching the fluorescent screen is predetermined for the density requirements of the examination. *(Bushong, p 12–13, 124–125)*

161. The answer is B.   Of the choices listed in the question, 175 mA, 4/10 seconds, 85 kVp, 48 inches FFD/source-image distance (SID) will produce the greatest optical density in the finished radiograph. This can be shown in the following steps: *Step 1:* Multiply mA × seconds; mAs is directly proportional to optical density, or in choice **A**, 120 mAs; choice **B**, 70 mAs; choice **C**, 135 mAs; and choice **D**, 90 mAs. *Step 2:* kVp is related to optical density, in that increasing kVp by 15% doubles optical density; reducing kVp by 15% halves optical density. Increasing kVp by 15% and halving mAs or decreasing kVp by 15% *and* doubling mAs will keep optical density constant. For **A**, increase the original kVp of 63 by 15%, to 72, and halve the original mAs of 120, to 60. Optical density is unchanged. For **B**, decrease the original kVp of 85 by 15%, to 72, and double the origianl mAs of 70, to 140. Optical density has remained constant. For **D**, decrease the original kVp of 100 by 15%, to 85, and increase original mAs of 90, to 180. Again, decrease kVp by 15%, to 72, and increase mAs to 360. Optical density is unchanged. To summarize, **A:** 60 mAs, 72 kVp; **B:** 140 mAs, 72 kVp; **C:** 135 mAs, 72 kVp; and **D:** 360 mAs, 72 kVp. *Step 3:* Optical density varies inversely with the square of the FFD/SID. Halving the FFD/SID quadruples optical density. The mAs/distance equation will keep optical density proportional when FFD/SID is changed:

For A, $\dfrac{mAs_1}{mAs_2} = \left(\dfrac{D_1}{D_2}\right)^2 \rightarrow \dfrac{60}{X} = \left(\dfrac{40}{48}\right)^2 \rightarrow \dfrac{60}{X} = \dfrac{1,600}{2,304} \rightarrow 1,600X =$

$138,240 \rightarrow X = 86.4$ mAs.

For C, $\dfrac{mAs_1}{mAs_2} = \left(\dfrac{D_1}{D_2}\right)^2 \rightarrow \dfrac{135}{X} = \left(\dfrac{54}{48}\right)^2 \rightarrow \dfrac{135}{X} = \dfrac{2,916}{2,304} \rightarrow 2,916X =$

$311,040 \rightarrow X = 106.66$ mAs.

For **D**, $\dfrac{mAs_1}{mAs_2} = \left(\dfrac{D_1}{D_2}\right)^2 \rightarrow \dfrac{360}{X} = \left(\dfrac{84}{48}\right)^2 \rightarrow \dfrac{360}{X} = \dfrac{7,056}{2,304} \rightarrow 7,056X =$

$829,440 \rightarrow X = 117.55$ mAs.

Final summary:
A. 86 mAs, 72 kVp, 48 inches FFD/SID
B. 140 mAs, 72 kVp, 48 inches FFD/SID
C. 107 mAs, 72 kVp, 48 inches FFD/SID
D. 118 mAs, 72 kVp, 48 inches FFD/SID
In the final comparison, it is clear that **B** has the greatest optical density.

162. The answer is A. Bone density and volume decrease most markedly in women after about age 60, but these changes are encountered in all elderly people as a manifestation of skeletal atrophy. Atrophy occurs in soft tissues, too, where muscle mass diminishes but volume of tissue may remain constant because of increased fat deposition. In general, the fluid content of tissues decreases as the vascular supply decreases, plus adipose tissue replaces muscle and contains less water than muscle does. As tissues atrophy and diminish in volume in elderly persons, they transmit radiation more readily, requiring lower exposure factors. *(Thompson, p 241; Tortora and Anagnostakos, p 72–73)*

163. The answer is D. Collimation is the easiest and most effective method of increasing radiographic contrast through the reduction of scattered radiation. For a large abdominal tissue volume, scattered photons that interfere with the image may account for as much as 50% of radiographic density, and scatter can be dramatically reduced when tissue area irradiated is reduced through tight collimation. Rare earth intensifying screens, because of their increased speed, tend to increase radiographic contrast. Another advantage of their use in this situation is that they allow reduced exposure time. Other aspects of the grid aside, as grid ratio increases, radiographic contrast also increases. A 16:1 grid is the highest grid ratio currently available. *(Bushong, p 182–195; Selman, p 371–374)*

164. The answer is A. During the tomographic exposure, the tube and cassette move in equal and opposite directions across or around the part being imaged. If the FFD is not constant from the beginning to the end of exposure, then radiographic density will not be uniform across the image. When the tube is farther away from the cassette, fewer photons will arrive at the image plane than when the tube is closer. When the focus-object:object-film ratios are constant throughout the exposure, the magnification rate is constant and can easily be measured. When focus-object:object-film ratios vary during the exposure, the structure under examination appears distorted in shape. Contrast is neither increased nor decreased as a function of FFD or focus-object:object-film ratios but depends primarily on kVp selected, characteristics of the imaging system, and the tissues being imaged. *(Bushong, p 306; Selman, p 430)*

165. The answer is B. To determine the cooling time in statement **1** in the question, 85 kV × 600 mA × 0.7 second × 4 = 142,800. Find 143,000 on the vertical axis and follow across to where it intersects with the cooling curve; move straight down and read the time on the horizontal axis: 2 minutes. It takes 14−2 minutes, or 12 minutes, to cool completely. To determine the cooling time in **2**, 95 kV × 400 mA × 0.8 second × = 91,200. Find 91,000 on the vertical axis and follow the line across to the intersection of the cooling curve; move straight down and read the time on the horizontal axis: approximately 3 minutes. It takes 14−3 minutes, or 11 minutes, to cool completely. For statement **3**, 70 kV × 200 mA × 2 seconds × 8 = 224,000. Find 225,000 on the vertical axis and follow the line across to the intersection of the cooling curve; move straight down and read the time on the horizontal axis: approximately 1 minute. To cool completely takes 14−1 minute, or 13 minutes. *(Bushong, p 136–137)*

166. The answer is C. Shape distortion is defined as unequal magnification of different parts of a single object or structure. Objects positioned under the central ray have the advantage of being imaged by photons traveling perpendicular to the image plane, whereas those removed to either the anode or cathode side will be imaged by photons diverging at greater and greater angles relative to the central ray, as the edge of the beam is approached. The most distant parts of any object (from the central ray) will be most distorted. OID and the thickness of the object affect magnification, and the size of the effective focal spot affects geometric unsharpness in the image. *(Bushong, p 276–277; Selman, p 359–361)*

167. The answer is C. Differential absorption refers to the amounts of energy lost by each of the image-forming photons as they pass through the tissue being imaged. Differential absorption results from the energy variations in (1) those photons that lose all their energy in the tissue—the photoelectrically absorbed photons that do not interact with the imaging system at all and (2) those photons that are transmitted and do not interact with the tissue at all but arrive at the imaging system. The photoelectrically absorbed photons are conspicuous by their absence: The "light," or lucent, areas of the radiograph indicate the presence of dense materials, whereas the darker gray tones indicate materials or tissues of less opacity, those in which the transmitted photons lost varying amounts of energy but retained enough to interact with the imaging system. It is the entire range of tones resulting from absorbed and transmitted photons that together provide contrast in the radiograph. *(Bushong, p 164–169; Selman, p 347–349)*

168. The answer is C. Alternating current changes direction 60 times a second and so is not suitable for uniform generation of x-rays. However, when it is rectified (by either four vacuum tubes or solid-state rectifiers) into a pulsating direct current, it can be passed to the x-ray tube. As the alternating current flows in one direction, it is sent through two vacuum tubes and on to the x-ray tube. When the direction of the alternating current changes, it flows through the other two vacuum tubes and then to the x-ray tube. When half of the rectification system's vacuum tubes are not functioning, only half of the alternating current pulses are passed to the x-ray tube, resulting in half of the expected tube output. A cracked target, a punctured insert, and emission of electrons by the anode would all result in variable and reduced output, but not in exactly a 50% reduction. *(Bushong, p 100–103; Selman, p 143–152)*

169. The answer is D. The probability of a photoelectric interaction occurring is directly proportional to the third power of the atomic number of the absorber; photoelectric interactions occur more frequently in tissues with a higher atomic number. Bone has an effective atomic number of almost 14, muscle about 7.5, and fat about 6.0. The probability of photoelectric interactions is also dependent on photon energy. The photon energy must be equal to or greater than the binding energy of the electron ejected, and the probability of this interaction is inversely proportional to the third power of the photon energy. Photoelectric interactions occur most frequently at the lower end of the diagnostic energy range and also occur more frequently in bone than in soft tissue. *(Bushong, p 160–163; Selman, p 189–191)*

170. The answer is D. Adding a dye to the binder of the active phosphor layer will result in absorption of fluorescent light from the phosphors by the dye and, therefore, reduced intensity of fluorescence by the screen or reduced speed. Dyes are usually added in the construction of slow, fine-detail intensifying screens when increased resolution is desired more than speed. Thicker active layers, as well as large crystals, will result in increased light output by the screen or increased speed. The presence of a reflective material behind the phosphor layer will also increase light output or increase speed of the screen, as it helps to redirect the scattered light from the phosphors in the direction of the film. Often, however, as intensifying screen speed is increased, image sharpness is sacrificed because the fluorescent light spreads before reaching the film emulsion. Manufacturers may vary the type of phosphor material used in order to increase or decrease the speed of a screen. Rare earth phosphors, for example, are very efficient in converting x-rays to light; therefore, they are employed in some of the faster screens available today. *(Bushong, p 245–248; Selman, p 286–290)*

171. The answer is A.   The three methods primarily used to recover silver from fixing solutions are electrolytic recovery, chemical precipitation, and metallic replacement. In the chemical precipitation method, sodium sulfide is added to the used fixer solution, causing silver to be precipitated out as silver sulfide. Metallic replacement involves the chemical process of placing a metal such as steel wool into expended fixer solution. Iron ions from the steel wool will go into solution, and the silver from the fixer replaces the iron and plates out on the steel wool. These two methods render the fixer solution unusable; therefore, used fixer is collected from the processor and stored in a container until the silver can be recovered. Then the solution is discarded. Electrolytic recovery (electrolysis) is the process of reclaiming silver after a chemical change produced by electric current passed through an ionized solution. Two electrodes are used for this purpose and are contained in a unit attached to the processor, through which fixer solution passes. Positive silver ions will eventually plate out on the cathode (negative electrode). *(Chesney and Chesney [1981], p 162–175; Thompson, p 274–276)*

172. The answer is A.   Radiographic contrast is usually evaluated by technologists through visual inspection, but when a numeric value is required to compare products, the average graident is generally used. The average gradient is the slope of a straight line on the characteristic, or Hurter and Driffield (H and D), curve joining two points that correspond to density levels 0.25 and 2.0 above the combined base and fog densities. A densitometer is an instrument that measures optical or radiographic density. It is required in the construction of a characteristic curve. The kVp in the primary beam is the variable the technologist uses to control radiographic contrast, but this does not take into account any patient factors. The relationship between percent of absrobed photons to those transmitted is not constant but changes with changing kVp. *(Bushong, p 266–267; Selman, p 350)*

173. The answer is D.   Resolution is the ability of an imaging system to demonstrate sharpness of details in the radiographic image. If an imaging system can reproduce an object's image faithfully, in good focus, then it is said to have good resolution, or resolving power. When using direct-exposure (nonscreen) film to image any body part, the greatest amount of resolution can be obtained. When intensifying screens are used for imaging, resolution decreases, the resolving power being inversely proportional to the speed of the screen used. In other words, high-speed (faster) screens reduce resolution; par-speed screens produce better resolution than high-speed; slow, or fine-detail screens produce even better resolution; and nonscreen technique provides the best resolution of all. Resolution can be measured numerically in order to accurately compare imaging systems; the use of a line-pair test pattern is used for this purpose. The more line pairs/mm that can be imaged, the better the resolution. For example, direct-exposure film can resolve 50 to 100 line pairs/mm, whereas fast screens can resolve between 7 and 15 line pairs/mm. *(Bushong, p 245–248; Chesney and Chesney [1981], p 102–109; Selman, p 293, 334–337; Thompson, p 70–78)*

174. The answer is B.   The CT image is a reconstruction from numeric values generated by the attenuated, or remnant, beam intensities. The remnant beam does not form an image that can be viewed, as in radiography. The remnant beam strikes the detector, which transmits information regarding the intensity of radiation detected to the computer, where it is stored as numeric data. When sufficient discrete "pieces" of information have been received, the computer, by using algorithms, reconstructs the information into the visual format and either stores or displays it on the console monitor. No image receptor, either film or an image-intensifier tube, is required initially because the data gathered are numeric and cannot be represented visually until processed by the computer. *(Bushong, p 363–366, 374–375; Chesney and Chesney [1984], p 458–470)*

175. The answer is B.   The faster the intensifying screen speed, the less the image sharpness. Par-speed screens have an approximate speed of 100, whereas high-speed screens have an approximate speed of 200 to 300. Focal spot size is directly related to geometric unsharpness, or penumbra. Focal spot size also changes from the given size designation as increasing mA is used.

A larger mA, for any given focal spot size, produces a greater space charge in the electron stream and reaches the target area after having spread out considerably. A larger area on the target is bombarded by the electrons, creating a larger focal spot and increasing penumbra. *(Bushong, p 245, 279–281; Selman, p 331–333)*

176. The answer is B.   In studies made at many institutions across the country, almost all repeated radiographs were found to be the result of improper positioning and/or incorrect choice of exposure factors. When automatic exposure controls (phototimers) were used, incorrect positioning generally resulted in a radiograph too underexposed or overexposed to be of any clinical use. Artifacts caused by dirty or damaged intensifying screens, grid malfunctioning, processor error, plus incorrect loading of cassettes and double exposure do not contribute significantly to the retake rate. They constitute only a tiny part of it. *(Bushong, p 547)*

177. The answer is C.   An x-ray tube with three terminals is called a grid-biased, or grid-controlled, tube and is useful in that it acts as its own exposure switch. The "grid" is frequently a wire mesh placed directly in front of, or actually a part of, the cathode focusing cup. A negative charge on the grid can prevent electrons from flowing across the tube, thus starting or stopping the exposure. The reverse emission, or conical focus, tube was a very early x-ray tube in use about 80 years ago. The Coolidge tube is the heated-filament x-ray tube, basically the one in use today. A trifocus tube is an image-amplifier tube that has an ordinary viewing mode plus the choice of two additional magnification modes. *(Chesney and Chesney [1984], p 172–174; Selman, p 270–271)*

178. The answer is B.   In tomography, only when the tube and cassette travel through an arc is FFD constant for the duration of the exposure, producing uniform radiographic density in the image. The parallel motion of the tube or cassette results in longer FFD at the beginning and end of the exposure and shorter FFD at the midpoint of the exposure, when the tube is directly over the part and the film is directly underneath. Many x-ray units that are used for general radiography as well as for tomography use less expensive setups in which FFD varies during the exposure. *(Bushong, p 303–307; Selman, p 417–438)*

179. The answer is C.   When time is the most important consideration, then a videotape recording of a motion study is ideal. The tape can be viewed immediately after recording because it does not require chemical development; in fact, it can be run before the patient is released from the radiographic room to make sure that all necessary information is recorded. Cinefluorography image quality is superior to that of videotape, but a considerable delay is necessary while the film is unloaded, processed, and set up for viewing. Cassette spot films cannot record motion studies. Video disk records individual frames that can be run continuously to approximate a motion study, but the lack of smoothness is so distracting that its main use is in "still" imaging. *(Bushong, p 302; Chesney and Chesney [1984], p 398–402)*

180. The answer is C.   The mAs-distance formula is derived from the inverse square law of radiation relating beam attenuation over distance and mAs required for a specific film density. This equation is solved in the following way *(Bushong, p 63–65; Selman, p 341–344)*:

$$\frac{mAs_1}{mAs_2} = \left(\frac{D_1}{D_2}\right)^2 \rightarrow \frac{14}{X} = \left(\frac{35}{40}\right)^2 \rightarrow \frac{14}{X} = \frac{1,225}{1,600} \rightarrow$$

$1,225X = 22,400 \rightarrow X = 18.28 \rightarrow X = 18$ mAs.

181. The answer is B.   The damage caused by heat eventually renders the x-ray tube useless, and heat production is a by-product of x-ray production. X-ray efficiency increases with increasing kVp—that is, the percentage of x-rays produced increases relative to the percentage of heat produced. Heat units can be calculated simply by multiplying kVp by mAs: 68 kVp and 100 mAs will generate 6,800 heat units, and 78 kVp and 50 mAs will generate only 3,900 heat units, yet both of these exposures will provide the same radiographic density. The anode must be warmed gradually by low-heat exposures to prevent vaporization of the metal or even possible cracking of the anode. Running the rotor longer than is absolutely essential will vaporize the filament, leading to gas in the tube and/or plating out of the tungsten on the inside of the glass insert and contributing to electric failure of the tube. *(Bushong, p 133–135; Selman, p 220–225)*

182. The answer is C. Distortion, or misrepresentation of the true size or shape of an anatomic detail, is caused by the geometry of the beam and the three-dimensionality of the patient. If the anatomic detail is placed as close to the image plane as possible, size distortion will be minimal. If the anatomic detail is imaged as close to the center of the beam as possible and with a central ray perpendicular to the imaging plane, shape distortion will be reduced. Many oblique or tube-angled projections make use of shape distortion to remove superimposed anatomic details from the detail of interest or to visualize an anatomic part that is not presented accurately in the AP or PA projection. The difference in the amount of size distortion of two parts imaged on the same film can identify the spatial relationship of those two parts. However, distortion always decreases sharpness. *(Bushong, p 276–278; Selman, p 355–360)*

183. The answer is B. As the thickness of the tissue irradiated increases, more x-rays scatter more than once, increasing the total production of scattered photons. Scatter production is a function of x-ray beam and patient factors. Photon wavelength or energy is significant in scatter production, but a decrease in photon wavelength (an increase in energy) is required for an increase in scatter production. Object-film distance (OFD) and air gap size are synonomous, and, although they will affect scatter volume reaching the image receptor, neither affects scatter production. *(Bushong, p 183–187; Selman, p 373)*

184. The answer is A. In cerebral angiography (especially biplane), where kVp is relatively low to maintain high contrast, scatter formed in the part will not be traveling in the same direction as the transmitted photons, and simply removing the image receptor 4 to 6 inches from the part will prevent the scatter from reaching the film. Image sharpness can be maintained with use of a small focal spot and short exposure times. In abdominal radiography, the volume of scatter would be much larger, and magnification plus unsharpness could be serious if a large focal spot were required. In pediatric radiography, a grid is rarely required as the body part is usually small. In addition, speed of exposure to exclude motion may be more important than a small loss of contrast from not using a grid. The high kVp and larger body parts in barium studies require a high-ratio grid. An air gap is equivalent to about an 8:1 grid. *(Bushong, p 210–211, 310–311; Selman, p 364)*

185. The answer is B. The focused grid is constructed so that the angled lead strips running lengthwise in relation to the cassette approximate or coincide with the angle of the diverging photons of the primary beam. This permits passage of transmitted photons but absorbs scattered photons that are traveling in a different trajectory or path. The photons in the central part of the x-ray beam are less divergent than those at the edge; consequently, grid strips are less angled at the center than they are at the sides of the grid. When the grid's tube side faces the cassette, the slightly angled center strips will permit passage of the primary beam, resulting in acceptable exposure. However, as grid strips increase in angulation toward the sides, more photons will be absorbed, and little to no radiographic density will be present at the sides. *(Bushong, p 204, 208; Selman, p 386–387)*

186. The answer is B. In fluorography, the image is not received directly by film as in conventional imaging but is converted into a digital signal from the image-intensifier output phosphor. The electronic image is available immediately; it does not require processing. Scattered radiation noise can be reduced with computer enhancement of the image. An image subtraction can be made and viewed while the examination is still in progress. Errors in choice of exposure factors can frequently be overcome by electronic manipulation of the attenuation numbers. This is especially helpful in angiography, when it may not be possible to give additional contrast media for repeat films. *(Bushong, p 345–347; Curry et al., p 420–460)*

187. The answer is A.   Back-projection describes a mathematical computer method for reconstructing the image from the attenuation numbers. The total range of CT numbers available may be as large as 2,000, but the maximum number of shades of gray with which those numbers are represented is slightly above 30. Window selection permits a small group of CT numbers to be visualized over the whole gray scale range. Magnification and subtraction are methods of increasing visual information available by increasing the size of one part of the image or by removing superfluous information from the image that is distracting. *(Bushong, p 348, 354, 378–379; Chesney and Chesney [1984], p 474–476)*

188. The answer is A.   The grid's function is to absorb scatter, but the grid also absorbs a small percentage of primary radiation. This absorbed radiation would contribute to film blackening, or radiographic density. The radiographic density is reduced when a grid is introduced into the imaging system, so control panel factors of kVp and/or mAs must be increased. The precise amount of increase is referred to as the Bucky factor. K is contrast improvement factor. Selectivity is a grid performance function, relating the grid's ability to transmit primary radiation while absorbing scattered radiation. Modulation transfer function is a mathematical representation of the sum of all the factors that alter image quality. *(Selman, p 387–388)*

189. The answer is C.   Tube current is the number of electrons flowing from cathode to anode and is directly related to the number of photons produced at the anode. An increase in tube current will proportionally increase exposure rate or beam intensity. If the exposure rate is measured farther from the anode or source, less intensity will be noted in accordance with the inverse square law of radiation. Either a decrease in tube potential (kVp) or an increase in the aluminum filtration of the primary beam will decrease exposure rate—decreased tube potential by decreasing the number of photons generated, and increased primary-beam filtration by reducing the number of photons through absorption in the aluminum. *(Bushong, p 173; Selman, p 166–169)*

190. The answer is B.   Without reference to the sensitometric curve, radiographic contrast can be defined as the difference in the ratio of photons incident on one small area of film as compared with photons incident on an adjacent equal small area of film. In an osteolytic metastatic process, bone is actually destroyed, leaving radiolucent areas in an otherwise radiodense material and resulting in high contrast. Except for the lumbar spine and pelvis, the abdomen is a low-contrast area, and a soft-tissue mass in an area of similar density will not have good contrast. A relatively small change in the density of a solid organ such as the liver will not change its absorption characteristics sufficiently to give it good contrast. A pneumothorax is still air in a normally air-filled cavity—a low-contrast situation. *(Selman, p 347; Thompson, p 240–247)*

191. The answer is B.   Exposure latitude defines the range of kVp/mAs combinations that will produce a diagnostically acceptable radiograph; it is the range of error permissible that can still result in an acceptable radiograph. A small error in a high-contrast radiograph frequently results in a retake. High-contrast (low kVp) factors enhance small density differences, producing a very short gray scale, or range of tonal differences visible. Reduced patient dose is a major advantage of low-contrast factors, whereas low kVp requires higher mAs (mAs is linearly related to dose) to achieve any given density. *(Selman, p 345–351; Thompson, p 122–125)*

192. The answer is C.   Of the choices given in the question, 250 mA, 3/5 seconds, 118 kVp, 36 inches FFD/SID detail/fine screens will provide the greatest optical density on the processed radiograph. This can be shown in the following steps: *Step 1:* Multiply mA × seconds; mAs is directly proportional to optical density; or in choice A, 22.5 mAs; choice B, 160 mAs; choice C, 150 mAs; and choice D, 90 mAs. *Step 2:* kVp is related to optical density in that increasing kVp by 15% doubles optical density; reducing kVp by 15% halves optical density. Increasing kVp by 15% *and* halving mAs or decreasing kVp by 15% *and* doubling mAs will keep optical density constant. For **A**, decrease the original kVp of 100 by 15%, to 85, and double the original mAs of 22.5 to 45. Optical density has remained unchanged. For **B**, increase the original kVp of 74 by

15%, to 85, and halve the original mAs of 160, to 80. Optical density has not varied. For **C**, decrease the original kVp of 118 by 15%, to 100, and double the original mAs of 150, to 300. Again decrease kVp by 15%, to 85, and double mAs, to 600. Optical density has not changed. To summarize, **A:** 45 mAs, 85 kVp; **B:** 80 mAs, 85 kVp; **C:** 600 mAs, 85 kVp; and **D:** 90 mAs, 85 kVp. *Step 3:* Optical density varies inversely with the square of the FFD/SID. Doubling FFD/SID will reduce optical density to one-quarter of the original density. Use the mAs/distance equation to deep optical density proportional as FFD/SID changes:

For **B**, $\dfrac{mAs_1}{mAs_2} = \left(\dfrac{D_1}{D_2}\right)^2 \rightarrow \dfrac{80}{X} = \left(\dfrac{40}{72}\right)^2 \rightarrow \dfrac{80}{X} = \dfrac{1,600}{5,184} \rightarrow 1,600X = 414,720 \rightarrow$

$X = 259.2$ mAs.

For **C**, $\dfrac{mAs_1}{mAs_2} = \left(\dfrac{D_1}{D_2}\right)^2 \rightarrow \dfrac{600}{X} = \left(\dfrac{36}{72}\right)^2 \rightarrow \dfrac{600}{X} = \dfrac{1,296}{5,184} \rightarrow 1,296X = 3,110,400 \rightarrow$

$X = 2,400$ mAs.

For **D**, $\dfrac{mAs_1}{mAs_2} = \left(\dfrac{D_1}{D_2}\right)^2 \rightarrow \dfrac{90}{X} = \left(\dfrac{60}{72}\right)^2 \rightarrow \dfrac{90}{X} = \dfrac{3,600}{5,184} \rightarrow 3,600X = 466,560 \rightarrow$

$X = 129.6$ mAs.

To summarize, **A:** 45 mAs, 85 kVp, 72 inches FFD/SID; **B:** 259 mAs, 85 kVp, 72 inches FFD/SID; **C:** 2,400 mAs, 85 kVp, 72 inches FFD/SID; and **D:** 130 mAs, 85 kVp, 72 inches FFD/SID. *Step 4:* The speed of intensifying screens used is directly related to optical density. A par-speed screen is considered the "standard," with a speed designation of 100. Detail or fine screens have a speed designation of 50, and their use would reduce optical density by half over a par-speed system. High-speed screens have a speed designation of 200 to 300 and would increase optical density two to three times over a par-speed system. For **A**, high-speed screens will increase optical density two to three times. Multiplying 45 mAs by 2 and 3 results in 90 to 135 mAs. For **C**, detail or fine screens will reduce optical density by half. Multiplying 2,400 mAs by ½ results in 1,200 mAs.

Final summary:
A. 90–135 mAs, 85 kVp, 72 inches FFD/SID, par-speed screens
B. 259 mAs, 85 kVp, 72 inches FFD/SID, par-speed screens
C. 1,200 mAs, 85 kVp, 72 inches FFD/SID, par-speed screens
D. 130 mAs, 85 kVp, 72 inches FFD/SID, par-speed screens

In the final comparison it is clear that **C** has the greatest density, now that all variables are reduced to the same terms.

193. The answer is B.   Three-phase operation is considerably more efficient than single-phase, half, or full-wave rectification. The number of photons produced and the average energy of those photons are increased, thereby increasing radiographic density. Adding excess filtration to the beam decreases the number of photons; target material of a low atomic number reduces both the number of photons and their average energy. Both would result in reduced radiographic density. Photon wavelength is inversely proportional to photon energy. Increasing photon wavelength is a decrease of photon energy, resulting in reduced radiographic density. (*Bushong, p 147–155; Selman, p 263–265*)

194. The answer is B. Each square cell or element of a CT image is a two-dimensional "pixel," or picture element. Each pixel represents the surface of what is really a three-dimensional volume of tissue, the depth of that volume being the thickness of "slice" irradiated. The tissue volume is called a voxel. For each irradiation of a voxel of tissue, the radiation detector receives the beam attenuated by the tissue volume and passes these data electronically to the computer, where a number is generated for that tissue volume representing its attenuation coefficient. This number, called the CT number, can vary with the kVp and filtration of the beam. The matrix, or the array of pixels, has varied from 80×80 (6,400 pixels) to 512×512 (262,144 pixels). The larger the matrix, the smaller is each individual pixel. *(Bushong, p 377–378; Chesney and Chesney [1984], p 462–466)*

195. The answer is C. At a radiographic or optical density of 1, 10% of the light incident on the radiograph from the viewbox illuminator is transmitted. Although the useful range of radiographic densities is about 0.25 to 2.5, the majority of diagnostic radiographs fall within the range of 0.5 to 1.5, or very close to 10% light transmission. All diagnostic radiographs should then have a range of densities that average about 1, regardless of beam generation characteristics, patient variables, and the differences between all the various image-receptor systems. *(Bushong, p 262–266; Selman, p 339)*

196. The answer is D. Sharpness in the image is inversely proportional to screen speed. High-speed screens have an approximate speed of 200 to 300, whereas detail/fine screens have an approximate speed of 50. Focal spot size is directly related to geometric unsharpness, and a smaller focal spot size will contribute to a sharper image. Magnification increases as the object is moved away from the image or film plane, closer to the focal spot. Magnification is a major factor in the production of penumbra, or geometric unsharpness. The OFDs for the examples in the question are **A**, 10 inches; **B**, 4 inches; **C**, 10 inches; and **D**, 2 inches, demonstrating that **D** will produce the sharpest image. *(Bushong, p 245, 272–276; Selman, p 327–333)*

197–200. The answers are 197-B, 198-B, 199-B, 200-B. Scatter production in tissue increases with increasing kV. Scattered radiation frequently reaches the image receptor, especially when kV is high and contributes an overall gray haze, adding to image density and undermining image contrast. When large body parts are to be imaged, a grid is required to remove scatter from the beam and improve image quality.

The wavelength of a primary-beam photon is inversely proportional to its energy and is dependent on the kV applied to the tube. The kV controls the speed at which the electrons travel to the anode (their kinetic energy). This energy is transferred to the photons produced at the target. Increasing kV decreases photon wavelength.

Radiographic contrast exists because x-rays penetrate tissue to different degrees, depending on their energy and the atomic number and density of the tissue. At low kV, many photons are absorbed in the denser body materials, and relatively few have the energy to penetrate all tissues and reach the image receptor. This high-contrast image shows few gray tones and appears mainly black and white. As kV increases, more photons are transmitted through the denser body materials and reach the image receptor and few are absorbed. This image has low contrast, showing many gray tones and very few blacks and whites.

The exposure rate or intensity of the primary beam is considerably influenced by the level of kV selected. As kV is increased, the efficiency of x-ray production increases, with more photons at all energy levels being produced plus more higher-energy photons. Exposure rate is roughly proportional to kV^2. *(Bushong, p 141, 149–151, 160–162, 164–169, 170–171, 195–197)*

201. The answer is C. Radiographic contrast is decreased when (as in a very thin "slice") only a single tissue density is being imaged. (Contrast is defined as the difference in adjacent densities.) This effect can be reduced by using a high-contrast film-screen combination. With the mechanically excellent multidirectional tomographic units, the sharpness of the in-focus plane is maintained even with minimum plane thickness, and the increasing blurring in all structures outside the in-focus plane accentuates the clarity of the structures to be imaged. Radiographic density is not a function of cut thickness but varies with FFD, kVp, mAs, patient factors, and film-screen systems used. *(Bushong, p 306; Curry et al., p 248–249)*

202. The answer is B.   The spinning top test is used to detect inaccuracies in the exposure timer, which can result in the need for repeated patient exposures to obtain an acceptable radiograph. It is extremely important that the light field coincide quite accurately with the invisible x-ray field (x-ray field/light field congruency test), or the patient may receive exposure to anatomic areas not being imaged. In addition, anatomic areas required to be in the image may be collimated off, requiring an additional exposure before an adequate radiograph is obtained. The measurement of the half-value layer (HVL) results in information regarding beam quality or penetrability, and, although patient entrance or skin dose decreases as the HVL increases, image contrast also decreases as HVL increases. Therefore, an acceptable balance between these aspects must be settled on when the tube and collimator are installed. HVL measurement is subsequently used to determine variability in beam quality. *(Chesney and Chesney [1984], p 571–582, 597, 615–616; Gray et al., p 70–71, 84, 95–96)*

203. The answer is B.   To determine the exposure time for statement 1 in the question, find the line on the vertical axis for 90 kVp. Follow that line to the right until it intersects with the first mA station; drop down to the horizontal and read the time, 0.04 second (600 × 0.04 = 24 mAs). Continue along the 90-kVp line until it intersects with the second mA station; drop down to the horizontal and read the time, 0.4 second (500 × 0.4 = mAs). For **3**, find the 70-kVp line on the vertical axis and follow it to the right until it intersects with the first mA station; drop down to the horizontal line and read the time, 0.4 second (600 × 0.4 = 240 mAs). For **2**, follow the 60-kVp line from the vertical axis to the right until it meets the first mA indicator; drop down to the horizontal line and read the time, 0.04 second (800 × 0.04 = 500 mAs). *(Bushong, p 135–136)*

204. The answer is B.   Improper use of the x-ray tube causes the metal atoms of the anode to become vaporized. Using high kVp/mAs combinations may heat up an unwarmed anode unevenly and also too rapidly, beyond the limits suggested in the instantaneous ratings. Continued overheating, keeping the anode at its thermal tolerance for periods of time, will have the same effect and will also cause damage to the anode surface. The filament vaporizes slightly under normal operating conditions: The exposure cannot be made until the rotor is up to speed; the filaments heat throughout this time period, but maintaining this filament heating for longer than absolutely necessary considerably speeds up the vaporization process, and the electric failure of the tube or the filaments will eventually cause breakage. Following puncture of the insert, oil will be drawn into the tube, but it does not vaporize. *(Bushong, p 133–135; Chesney and Chesney [1984], p 627)*

205. The answer is D.   X-ray imaging is valuable primarily because changes in tissue density and volume (disease processes or injury) alter beam absorption and transmission, creating an image that is visibly different from "normal." Normal radiographic density may be either increased or decreased, depending on the type of process at work. Compression bands can decrease tissue volume to be imaged by moving it out of the area of the x-ray field. Radiographic density will be increased when the tissue volume is decreased. As the atomic number of the target material increases, both the number of photons produced and the average energy of those photons increase, resulting in an increase in radiographic density. *(Bushong, p 151–153; Thompson, p 238, 240–247)*

206. The answer is B.   Interference with the transfer of information to the film (noise) is mainly the result of characteristics of the intensifying screen and the unevenness of photon distribution in the beam. When an image is formed using large numbers of photons (high mAs), small variations in photon density from one area to another will not be noticeable as actual variations in radiographic density. However, when a fast-speed imaging system is being used and only a relatively small number of photons are required to produce sufficient radiographic density, the variations become visible and reduce overall image quality. High mAs and slow-speed screens or no screens (a direct-imaging system) would eliminate this "quantum mottle" source of noise, whereas a fast-speed screen system and few photons would exaggerate it. *(Bushong, p 259–260; Selman, p 336– 337)*

207. The answer is C.   An extension cylinder is an effective beam restrictor that, when used in addition to a collimator, can increase contrast and sharpness over the use of the collimator alone. This cylinder can be extended very close to the patient's skin, dramatically limiting scatter formation. Furthermore, the length of the cylinder when extended reduces the penumbra by restricting the beam equally at both the top and bottom opening. Both a cone and an aperture diaphragm restrict the beam only at the upper opening. The tube port restricts the beam before it enters the collimator. *(Bushong, p 188–190; Selman, p 393–395)*

208. The answer is D.   X-ray photons cannot be focused by a lens. They are penetrating, invisible quanta of energy that are associated with both electric and magnetic fields, and they have no mass or charge. They travel from the target of the x-ray tube in straight lines, diverging from the target as they move away. They affect photographic film and cause fluorescence in some crystals. As produced in the diagnostic x-ray tube, they have a wide range of energies. They cause changes in the biologic material with which they interact, mainly by ionization. *(Selman, p 165)*

209. The answer is C.   The input phosphor of the image-intensifier tube is made of cesium iodide, which emits a light image proportional in intensity to the x-ray image that it received. The photocathode is bonded to the input phosphor, and it is here that the light image from the input phosphor causes electrons to be emitted by the photocathode, in the same pattern of intensities as the visible image. The focusing electrodes "compress" the electron stream as it is accelerated toward the anode. The electron stream diverges slightly from the anode and strikes the output phosphor, where light photons are emitted, again forming the original image but one that is 3 to 10,000 times brighter. *(Bushong, p 294–295; Chesney and Chesney [1984], p 383–389)*

210. The answer is A.   Panchromatic film is sensitive to the entire spectrum of visible light. This type of film is generally used in photography and must be processed in darkened conditions to avoid unwanted exposure (fog). Orthochromatic film is sensitive to all regions (colors) in the visible-light spectrum except red. In radiography, this type of film is also referred to as "green-sensitive" film and is used with many rare earth intensifying screens. The use of a red safelight filter is recommended with this type of film in order to avoid fog. Monochromatic film is mainly sensitive to one region in the visible-light spectrum. In radiography, this type of film is called blue-sensitive, as it responds to intensifying screens that give off light in the blue-violet region. Amber or red safelight filters can be used in conjunction with this type of film during its handling and processing. The spectral sensitivity of a film is an essential factor to consider when using intensifying screens, as the color or wavelength of light emitted by the screen should be matched to the spectral sensitivity of the film in order to provide maximum efficiency in speed and in dose reduction. Direct-exposure film is sensitive to the direct action of x-rays and is not used in conjunction with an intensifying screen. *(Bushong, p 218–219; Chesney and Chesney [1981], p 32–33; Thompson, p 23)*

211. The answer is B.   Radiographic film should be stored in a cool, dry area, as elevated temperatures and increased humidity reduce film contrast and increase film fog. Temperature should be less than 70°F, and relative humidity should be between 40 and 60%. Film should also be stored away from sources of light and radiation, as exposure to either can result in unwanted darkening or fog, rendering an unacceptable radiographic image. Film storage bins and darkrooms should be well sealed off from light and constructed of a material such as lead to protect film from radiation sources from within the radiology department. The environment should be clean when storing and handling film, and films should be stored on edge rather than flat to avoid unwanted artifacts and warping. Films with the oldest expiration dates should be used first, as a long storage period can cause decreased film contrast, loss of speed, and increased fog density. *(Bushong, p 223–224; Chesney and Chesney [1981], p 244–248; Selman, p 279–280; Thompson, p 252–256)*

212. The answer is A. The characteristic curve of a film allows one to determine the degree of contrast and speed of a film and also expresses the film's base plus fog, useful and maximum densities, and their relationship to exposure. The curve is generally divided into three parts: the toe, straight-line, and shoulder regions. The toe is the lower-density (underexposure) region, the straight line is the useful density (correct exposure) region, and the shoulder is the higher-density (overexposure) region. The base plus fog density is found in the low-density region, and for film A in the question, 0.1 represents this density. The base plus fog density for film B is 0.4, which is greater than that of film A. Film contrast can be determined by the slope of the straight-line portion of the curve. The steeper the slope, the greater the contrast; therefore, film A has higher contrast than film B because of film A's greater slope steepness. Speed can be determined by the position of the characteristic curves on a graph, the faster films being positioned nearer to the left of the graph than the slower films. Speed is also determined by the amount of exposure needed to produce a certain density; the less exposure needed to produce a certain density (e.g., 1.0), the faster the film. Film A lies closer to the left of the graph than film B and requires less log relative exposure (LRE) to produce a density of 1.0. Film A took a LRE of approximately 1.5 to produce a density of 1.0, whereas film B took a LRE of approximately 2.7 to produce the same film density. The characteristic curve is an important sensitometric tool in evaluating a film's response to exposure and processing. Other names for this curve include sensitometric curve and H and D curve. *(Bushong, p 261–272; Chesney and Chesney [1981], p 56–79; Selman, p 349–351; Thompson, p 37–43)*

213. The answer is C. In order to produce another properly exposed radiograph with similar density and contrast as the first image (of the same part) using a different film-screen combination, one must determine the intensification factor between the two systems used. In the case described in the question, a comparison must be made between the two imaging systems. A film speed of 1 used with a screen speed of 400 equals a total system speed of 400 (1×400). The second system used is a film with a speed of 0.5 in combination with a screen speed of 200. This equals a total system speed of 100 (0.5×200). (The higher the number assigned to a system, the faster or more sensitive it is.) The intensification factor between these two systems is 400/100, or 4. Therefore, the first film-screen combination used with a system speed of 400 is four times faster than the second film-screen combination with a system speed of 100. In order to reproduce a properly exposed radiograph of the same part, technical factors will be adjusted by multiplying the original mAs by a factor of four, as this is the intensification factor between the two systems (mAs must be changed in order to maintain the same average density); kVp will remain the same, in order to maintain a similar level of contrast between films. The faster-speed intensifying screen (400) will produce a slight increase in radiographic contrast compared with the slower-speed intensifying screen (200). The first system used a 400-speed film-screen combination with 50 mAs at 75 kVp. The second system used to radiograph the same part used a 100-speed film-screen combination (only one-quarter as fast as the first), and the new factors required are 200 mAs at 75 kVp. *(Bushong, p 245; Curry et al., p 119; Selman, p 338–340, 345–350)*

214. The answer is D. The average gradient is a numeric way of expressing film contrast. The average gradient is the slope of a straight line drawn between two points at density levels 0.25 and 2.0 above the combined base plus fog densities on a characteristic curve of a film. If the combined base plus fog densities of a film are 0.09, then the two densities points between which the average gradient or film contrast would be evaluated are 0.34 and 2.09 ($0.05 + 0.04 + 0.25 = 0.34$, and $0.05 + 0.04 + 2.0 = 2.09$). *(Bushong, p 266–268; Thompson, p 42–43)*

215. The answer is C.   In the example given in the question, the average gradient is 1.66. The following equation is used to determine the average gradient or numeric representation of film contrast:

$$\text{average gradient} = \frac{D_2 - D_1}{LRE_2 - LRE_1}$$

D_2 is the density point on the characteristic curve 2.0 above the base plus fog densities. D_2 in this case is 2.09. D_1 is the density point on the characteristic curve 0.25 above the base plus fog densities. D_1 in this case is 0.34. LRE_2 is the LRE associated with D_2, or 1.90. LRE_1 is the LRE associated with D_1, or 0.85. Therefore, average gradient is expressed as follows:

$$\frac{2.09 - 0.34}{1.90 - 0.85} = \frac{1.75}{1.05} = 1.66$$

The higher the average gradient number, the higher the film contrast. *(Bushong, p 265–268)*

216. The answer is A.   The xeroradiographic image is one of high latitude and low contrast. One of its advantages is that bone and soft-tissue structures are imaged equally well at the same time. The edge effect, or edge enhancement, that is unique to xeroradiography gives the illusion of high contrast at tissue interfaces. This effect occurs regardless of the difference in tissue densities. Image processing takes place in a closed cabinet and is entirely automatic. The greatest disadvantage of xeroradiography is that the amount of exposure required is larger than for a comparable film-screen image. Xeroradiography is currently limited in use to mammography and examination of the larynx and other small body parts. *(Bushong, p 318–324; Selman, p 438–441)*

PHYSICS AND EQUIPMENT

217. Which of the following does not belong to the group?

A. Direct current
B. Electromotive force
C. Potential difference
D. Voltage

218. X-ray tubes have variable life spans, depending on their construction and the care with which they are operated. Which of the following is the most common reason for very sudden tube failure?

A. The target surface becomes roughened and pitted
B. Vaporized tungsten builds up on the inside of the glass insert
C. The filament vaporizes and finally severs
D. Molecules of gas are present within the glass insert

219. Which of the following statements are true concerning magnets?

1. Unlike poles of two magnets will repel each other
2. Magnetic lines of force travel from the north to the south pole outside a magnet
3. If a magnet is divided into small pieces, each piece becomes a magnet

A. 1 and 2
B. 1 and 3
C. 2 and 3
D. 1, 2, and 3

220. Which of the following are associated with Magnetic Resonance Imaging (MRI)?

1. Acoustic impedance
2. Larmor frequency
3. Spin density

A. 1 and 2
B. 1 and 3
C. 2 and 3
D. 1, 2, and 3

221. Mechanical energy can be converted into electrical energy by a

A. battery
B. generator
C. motor
D. rectifier

222. Which of the following elements remains constant in all parts of a parallel electric circuit?

A. Capacitance
B. Current
C. Resistance
D. Voltage

223. The smallest divisional unit of a compound that is characteristically the same as that compound is called

    A. an element
    B. a molecule
    C. an atom
    D. an ion

224. The apparatus used to provide a quantitative measure of the amount of film blackening on an exposed, processed radiograph is a

    A. densitometer
    B. sensitometer
    C. penetrometer
    D. galvanometer

225. Which of the following is NOT a method of electrification?

    A. Contact
    B. Friction
    C. Induction
    D. Convection

226. In electrodynamics, resistance in an electric circuit is measured in

    A. amperes
    B. farads
    C. ohms
    D. volts

227. Which of the following are fundamental laws of electrostatics?

    1. Unlike charges attract, like charges repel each other
    2. Positive charges move in solid conductors
    3. Electric charges can be found on the external surface of a conductor

    A. 1 only
    B. 1 and 3
    C. 2 and 3
    D. 1, 2, and 3

228. If a respirator machine had a total resistance of 15 ohms (Ω) and was plugged into a 110-V receptacle in an intensive care unit, how much current would it take?

    A. 0.13 A
    B. 7.3 A
    C. 55 A
    D. 1,650 A

229. The autotransformer, frequently located in the control panel or console, is that division of the x-ray machine that receives the power first. The autotransformer serves to

    1. supply variable voltage to the filament circuit
    2. monitor voltage coming to the x-ray unit and adjust it to a constant magnitude
    3. step up the incoming voltage for use by the x-ray tube

A. 1 only
B. 2 only
C. 3 only
D. 1, 2, and 3

230. The mass number of an element that contains 53 protons, 74 neutrons, and 53 electrons is

A.   53
B.   74
C. 127
D. 180

231. The high-voltage section of the x-ray machine is usually located in a large metal oil-filled container, frequently placed in a corner of the x-ray room. The high-voltage section includes components such as the

    1. exposure timer circuit
    2. autotransformer
    3. rectifiers

A. 1 only
B. 2 only
C. 3 only
D. 1, 2, and 3

232. The radiographic image results from interactions between the beam, the subject, and the image receptor. Which of the following is NOT essential to image formation?

A. Transmitted photons
B. Differential absorption
C. Photoelectric absorption
D. Classical, or Thompson, scattering

233. When magnetic flux or force lines in a magnetic field are crossed by a conductor, a flow of current and electromotive force is induced in the conductor. Which of the following factors will increase the electromotive force induced?

    1. Increased magnetic field strength
    2. A straight, uncoiled conductor
    3. A 90° angle between the (moving) conductor and magnetic flux lines

A. 1 and 2
B. 1 and 3
C. 2 and 3
D. 1, 2, and 3

234. Magnification radiography is now quite a common procedure in the angiographic suite, but it still has some disadvantages. Undesirable aspects of radiographic magnification include

      1. increased patient dose
      2. decreased image resolution
      3. increased scatter production

  A. 1 only
  B. 2 only
  C. 3 only
  D. 1, 2, and 3

235. A wide variety of metals and other materials have been used in the construction of x-ray tubes as the technology of tube construction has increased in sophistication. In most modern tubes, molybdenum is generally used in the

  A. filament and the rotor assembly
  B. filament and the focusing cup
  C. anode disk and the focusing cup
  D. anode disk and the rotor assembly

236. The x-ray tube requires direct current for x-ray production, necessitating the rectification of available alternating current. Which of the voltage waveforms illustrated below represents unrectified three-phase power?

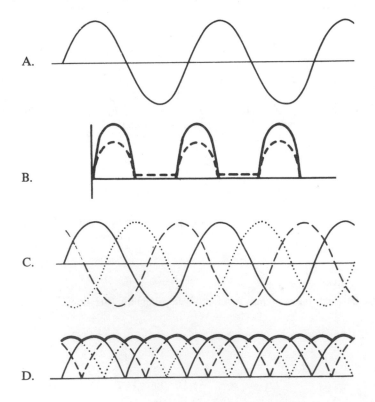

A.

B.

C.

D.

237. In the image-intensifier tube, the path that electrons follow from the photocathode to the output phosphor must be carefully controlled if an accurate image is to be formed. That control is primarily provided by the

    A. anode
    B. electrostatic lenses
    C. photocathode
    D. vacuum

238. Several types of mobile (portable) x-ray units are currently available and are commonly used. Which of these has the advantage of being free from incoming line voltage fluctuations while still being dependent on the institution power supply?

    A. Mains dependent
    B. Battery powered
    C. Condenser (capacitor) discharge
    D. Hand-carried portable

239. Which of the following may be incorporated into an electric circuit to store electric charges?

    A. Capacitor (condenser)
    B. Ammeter
    C. Rheostat
    D. Choke coil

Questions **240–241** consist of four lettered headings followed by a list of numbered words or phrases. For each numbered word or phrase, select the one heading which is most closely related to it. Each heading may be used once, more than once, or not at all.

    A. Image amplifier or intensifier
    B. Objective plane
    C. Ion chamber phototimer (automatic exposure control)
    D. Photofluorographic unit

240. Brightness gain

241. Cesium iodide

242. The following information was obtained during the operation of an x-ray tube. Beam intensity was measured each time 0.5 mm of filter was added. What is the HVL of this x-ray beam?

Millimeters of aluminum	mR
0	100
0.5	89
1.0	79
1.5	68
2.0	60
2.5	50
3.0	43
3.5	37
4.0	32

A. 68 mR
B. 1.5 mm of aluminum
C. 2.5 mm of aluminum
D. 3.5 mm of aluminum

243. Which of the following devices controls voltage in a circuit by varying resistance?

A. Transformer
B. Rectifier
C. Rheostat
D. Autotransformer

244. Increased radiographic density in a film emerging from an automatic processor is NOT likely the result of

A. developer overreplenishment
B. excessive hydroquinone and phenidone in the developer
C. lack of a hardener in the developer
D. increased temperature

245. The primary x-ray beam, as it emerges from the collimator, is made up of photons with a wide range of energies resulting from several aspects of beam generation. Those aspects that affect the range of beam energies produced include the

1. target material
2. tube current
3. filtration

A. 1 and 2
B. 1 and 3
C. 2 and 3
D. 1, 2, and 3

246. The x-ray tube is really a very inefficient converter of energy, considering the percentage of heat production versus the percentage of x-ray production. Furthermore, of the small percentage of x-rays produced, only a fraction are used. It is not possible to use more of the x-rays produced at the target because

A. a monoenergetic beam is required for x-ray imaging
B. most x-rays are emitted from the target in a direction other than toward the patient
C. a very small tube port is required to maintain good detail sharpness
D. 80% of the photons produced are absorbed in the air between the tube and the patient

Questions **247–249** consist of four lettered headings followed by a list of numbered words or phrases. For each numbered word or phrase, select the one heading with which it is most closely related. Each heading may be used once, more than once, or not at all.

A. Radiographic grid
B. Single-phase current
C. Magnification radiography
D. Tomography

247. Selectivity

248. Exposure angle

249. Contrast improvement factor

250. The atomic number of the target material affects both the number and the effective energy of x-rays. Target materials with a higher atomic number are correctly described as

A. having low melting points and requiring long cool-down periods
B. producing a higher-energy beam with low contrast
C. increasing the number of characteristic photons but decreasing the number of bremsstrahlung photons
D. producing higher-energy characteristic radiation

251. Besides its advantage of elemental composition discrimination, another significant advantage of magnetic resonance imaging (MRI) is that it

A. is inexpensive
B. does not use ionizing radiation
C. does not require computer assistance
D. uses short scanning times

252. Many dental units and some portable units are half-wave rectified, but almost all fixed x-ray units have full-wave rectification. What is advantageous about full-wave rectification?

1. The anticipated life of the x-ray tube is longer
2. Radiographic density is increased by 15%
3. Heat-loading efficiency of the x-ray tube is improved

A. 1 only
B. 2 only
C. 3 only
D. 1, 2, and 3

BODY—PHYSICS AND EQUIPMENT
ANSWERS, EXPLANATIONS, AND REFERENCES

217. The answer is A.   Current refers to the amount of charge flowing in an electric circuit and is measured in ampere units. Two types of current are direct and alternating; direct current flows in one direction, whereas alternating current changes directions constantly. Electromotive force, potential difference, and voltage are all terms used to describe the force that drives or moves electrons along an electric circuit. Potential difference refers to the difference in pressure or energy between two points in a circuit carrying electricity. Electromotive force is the the amount of energy needed to move electric charges between two points in a circuit. Voltage is the amount of pressure that moves the current (electric charges) along a conductor. The unit for measuring electromotive force, potential difference, and voltage is the volt. *(Bushong, p 76, 80–82; Selman, p 68–70)*

218. The answer is C.   With continued operation of an x-ray tube, the tungsten filament vaporizes over time as a result of the very high temperature at which this component operates. Finally it can break completely, resulting in no tube current and no x-ray beam production. When a tube is subjected to heavy or prolonged use, always operating at its maximum heat capacity, vaporized metal from both target and filament may be present within the tube as gas molecules; this generally results in variable tube output, as does a roughened and pitted target surface. The vaporized metal can condense on the inside of the glass insert and can cause slightly reduced output due to the filtering effect, or it can interfere with the cathode stream, causing variable output. *(Bushong, p 133–134; Selman, p 220–221)*

219. The answer is C.   The laws of magnetism state that all magnets have a north and a south pole and that unlike poles of two magnets will attract whereas two similar poles will repel each other. This attraction or repulsion increases with increased strength of the magnets and decreases as the distance between the magnets is increased. All magnets are surrounded by a magnetic field consisting of lines of forces (magnetic flux), which travel from the north to the south pole around the outside of a magnet and pass through the inside of that magnet in a direction from the south to the north pole. A unique property of a magnet is that it can be broken down into smaller pieces that behave as individual magnets, each piece possessing a north and south pole. Another interesting characteristic of a magnet is that if it is brought in contact with a material that is highly permeable to magnetism, such as iron and nickel, that material becomes magnetized. The portion of the magnetic material in contact with the magnet will acquire the opposite polarity of that of the magnet pole it touches, reaffirming one of the basic laws of magnetism. *(Bushong, p 82–86; Selman, p 87–95)*

220. The answer is C.   Magnetic resonance imaging is a new modality in diagnostic imaging that uses magnetic fields and radio waves to produce body images in transverse, sagittal, coronal, and oblique planes. Larmor frequency and spin density are associated with the physical principles of MRI. Larmor frequency refers to the frequency of precession or "wobble" of nuclei in an external magnetic field. This physical property can be demonstrated when an atomic nucleus such as that of hydrogen within body tissue is placed in an external magnetic field as used in MRI; each hydrogen nucleus will wobble in a tiny circle or precess about the direction of the external field's magnetic lines. Each hydrogen nucleus has inherent magnetism (north and south poles, charge, and spin) called a magnetic moment and is randomly oriented in tissue. When these randomly oriented magnetic moments are placed in a strong field, most of the nuclei will align themselves in the same direction of the magnetic field and precess. The speed of precession, or Larmor frequency, is determined by the type of nucleus involved and the strength of the magnetic field; this is called the Larmor relationship.
This property of Larmor precession frequency can be used to analyze various materials and body tissues, as in diagnostic MRI. If an unknown material were put into a magnetic field of known strength and the frequencies of precession are determined, then the magnetogyric ratio

(characteristic which is unique for a particular nucleus) for the nuclei in the unknown material can be determined by using the Larmor relationship. Since magnetogyric ratio is unique for each type of nucleus, the type and abundance of nuclei present can be determined, and an image produced of the interior of the material being evaluated (body tissue).

MRI consists of a scanner that contains a primary magnet to create the magnetic field that will cause the alignment and precession of nuclei. The type of nuclei being evaluated is that of hydrogen. A radio transmitter sends pulsed radio-frequency waves to precessing nuclei in the material being examined. Resonance then occurs, causing the nuclei to flip in the external magnetic field by absorbing radio-frequency waves. Removal of the radio-frequency waves will cause the nuclei to oscillate back to their normal state, called "relaxation." During this period of "free induction decay," a radio-frequency signal is emitted; it is from this signal that the nuclear magnetic resonance image is constructed. The number of precessing nuclei within the MRI scanner is directly proportional to the strength of the signal.

Spin density refers to the quantity of nuclei in tissue precessing at the Larmor frequency and comprising the nuclear magnetic resonance signal. The number of precessing nuclei within the MRI scanner is directly proportional to the strength of the signal emitted by the precessing nuclei. Spin density indicates the concentration of nuclei; the type of nuclei being evaluated is that of hydrogen.

Acoustic impedance refers to the reflection of sound at the interface of tissues. This property is important in the area of ultrasound imaging, and it represents the product of the velocity of sound in a medium and the density of the medium. As the density of the medium and/or velocity of sound increases, so does acoustic impedance. *(Ballinger, [Vol 3], p 841, 872–876; Bushong, p 387–398, 564–565)*

221. The answer is B.   A generator is a device that changes mechanical energy into electric energy. A simple electric generator consists of a coil of wire (armature) and a magnetic field. As a coil of wire is moved in a rotating manner within a magnetic field, a current is induced in the wire (electromagnetic induction), thereby generating electric energy from a mechanical source. A battery or cell is a device that converts chemical energy into electric energy, and a rectifier is a device that converts alternating current into direct current. A motor is somewhat the opposite of a generator. It converts electric energy into mechanical energy, thus allowing various pieces of machinery to do work through some form of movement such as rotation. *(Bushong, p 95–97; Selman, p 68, 106–122)*

222. The answer is D.   In a parallel electric circuit (shown below), component parts (resistors or appliances) are arranged as bridges or connectors between the conductor of the circuit. In a series circuit, component parts are lined up in a row, and the voltage drop is the same in all the component parts of the circuit and is equal to the total voltage in the circuit. Current is divided among each individual circuit element, and the total circuit current is equal to the sum of the individual elements' current. The total resistance (R) is inversely proportional to the sum of the reciprocals of each one of the resistors employed in the circuit. Parallel circuits are most often incorporated in homes, because this arrangement provides equal voltage to each individual appliance throughout the circuit and also allows other appliances to keep working if one of the appliances should fail, since all are on different conductors of the main circuit. *(Bushong, p 78–80; Selman, p 78–82)*

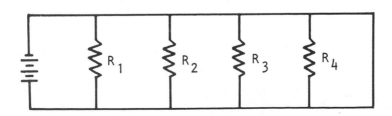

223. The answer is B.   A molecule is the smallest divisional unit of a substance or compound that has the same properties as that compound. A compound is a complex substance that is made chemically by joining together two or more different elements. Compounds have definite compositions; smaller units of the same definite composition are called molecules. Elements are simple substances that cannot be easily broken down; they too have a definite composition. Examples of elements can be found in a periodic table. The smallest divisional unit of an element that is characteristically the same as that element is called an atom. A compound such as sodium chloride is composed of one atom of the element sodium and one atom of the element chloride. A molecule of sodium chloride will always consist of one atom of each of these elements in a definite composition. An ion is an atom that has either lost or gained an electron. *(Bushong, p 30–34; Selman, p 38–40, 52)*

224. The answer is A.   A *densitometer* is a device that measures (quantitates) film blackening, or density. It is constructed with a light source that is directed through a tiny hole. The film being analyzed is slid over the top of this light and pinhole and between a light-sensing device. The amount of light transmitted through each part of the radiograph can be measured by the light sensor and is assigned a numeric value. A *penetrometer* is a device commonly referred to as an aluminum step wedge, as its construction is that of several successively higher steps forming a single aluminum wedge-like structure. When a step wedge is radiographed, successively increasing densities corresponding to the decreasing thicknesses or steps of the penetrometer above will be produced on the film. A *sensitometer* is a device that produces consistent exposures on radiographic film, simulating those produced by x-rays. These exposures can be accurately measured, making the sensitometer a useful tool for measurement of a film's response to exposure and processing (sensitometry). A *galvanometer* is a device used to measure current or voltage in an electric circuit. *(Bushong, p 261; Curry et al., p 220; Selman, p 120–122, 339; Thompson, p 37–39)*

225. The answer is D.   Convection is not a method of electrification but is a mechanical method by which heat is transferred from one area to another. Contact, friction, and induction are the three major methods of electrification. Friction refers to the rubbing off of electrons from one object to another object that is of a different structure or material. Contact is a method of electrification in which a charge is conveyed from a charged object to an uncharged object after they make contact with each other. If an object that has an excess of electrons (negatively charged) touches a neutral object, then the electrons will move from the negatively charged object to the neutral object, causing it to acquire a negative charge. The object being electrified will acquire the same charge as the charged object that it makes contact with in contact electrification. Electrification by induction refers to the transfer of an opposite charge from a charged object to a conductor that is brought into the charged object's electric field. If the negative end of a charged object is near but is not touching a conductive material such as metal, the negative electric field of the charged object will repel electrons in the end of the conductor nearest to the charged object. This will cause the induction of a positive charge in that end of the conductor. When the conductor is removed from the electric field of the charged object, it goes back to its original state. *(Bushong, p 28; Selman, p 56–59)*

226. The answer is C.   Resistance, or the opposition of the flow of current through an electric circuit, is measured in units called ohms. Resistance is dependent on several structural elements of a circuit, including the type of material from which the circuit is made (the conductivity or nonconductivity of the material), the length of the circuit (the longer the distance the current has to travel, the more resistance to its flow), the cross-sectional area of the circuit (if large, it decreases resistance to flow), and temperature (increased temperature puts more resistance on the flow of current through the circuit). Current is measured in amperes, or the flow of electrons per second through a circuit. The greater the current, the higher the amperage. The volt is the unit of measurement of potential difference or the force that moves the electrons through a circuit (voltage). Farads are the units of measurement of capacitance (the quantity of stored electric energy). *(Bushong, p 76–78; Selman, p 68–72, 82–84)*

227. The answer is B.   There are several fundamental laws of electrostatics, including one that states that unlike charges attract each other and like charges repel each other. For example, if a positively charged object is brought in contact with another positively charged object, they will actually repel each other; but if one of the objects were negatively charged, then they would attract each other. Electric charges are found on the outside surface of a conductor; if a metal tube were charged, its charges would reside on the outside and the lumen of the tube would be uncharged. Only electron (negatively charged particle) movement can produce electrification; positive charges stay still. Charges are most abundant on the greatest curvature of a curved conductor. The electrostatic force between two charges varies directly with the product of their strength and inversely to the square of the distance between them. These fundamental laws of electrostatics are elementary to the understanding of charged particles and electricity. *(Bushong, p 70–75; Selman, p 59–64)*

228. The answer is B.   In order to solve the problem presented in the question, Ohm's law should be employed: the voltage of a circuit is equal to the current times the resistance ($V = IR$). If the voltage (V) = 110 and the resistance (R) = 15 ohms (Ω), then one can manipulate the equation to find the unknown current (I):

$$I = \frac{V}{R} \rightarrow I = \frac{110}{15} \, I = 7.3 \text{ A.}$$

A simple way to remember Ohm's law is to learn how the formula can be used to determine an unknown. The figure that follows not only represents Ohm's law, but, by the position of the units in the circle, it permits finding the unknown if two of the elementary factors of the circuit are given.

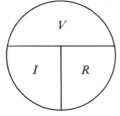

In the figure, $V = IR$, $I = \dfrac{V}{R}$, and $R = \dfrac{V}{I}$ *(Bushong, p 77–78; Selman, p 68–78)*

229. The answer is A.   The autotransformer supplies voltage to both the high-voltage and filament circuits at the magnitude required. This transformer has one core and one winding with variable taps or connections that can enclose a variable number of turns of the transformer, thus permitting it to supply a range of voltages from about half to twice the incoming line voltage. The line voltage compensator monitors and regulates voltage to the x-ray unit. The high-voltage, or step-up, transformer is the device that brings the voltage to a level suitable for use by the x-ray tube. *(Bushong, p 119–122)*

230. The answer is C.   The mass number of an atom equals the number of protons and neutrons contained in its nucleus. In the example given in the question, 53 protons plus 74 neutrons equals a mass of 127, or the atomic mass of the element iodine (used as the basis for many radiopaque contrast agents in radiology). The mass number should not be confused with the atomic number (Z) of an element, which is equal to the number of protons (positively charged particles) in the nucleus. The number of protons is equal to the number of orbital electrons (negatively charged particles) for any particular electrically neutral element. The atomic number is important because it differentiates one element from another. The mass number represents the weight of a specific element, which also varies between one element and another. Elements and their associated mass and atomic numbers can be identified in the periodic table of elements. *(Bushong, p 42–43; Selman, p 43–47)*

231. The answer is C.   The high-voltage section of an x-ray mahcine contains the step-up transformer, the step-down filament transformer, and the rectifiers. This section of the x-ray unit converts the incoming voltage to kilovoltage and then rectifies the waveform to satisfy the requirements of the x-ray tube. The exposure timer circuit is usually located in the operator's console, as is the exposure timer selector. The autotransformer is similarly located in the control panel or operator's console. *(Bushong, p 127; Selman, p 232–233)*

232. The answer is D.   Low-energy x-rays interact with matter by classical, or Thompson, scattering. In some circumstances that scattered photon may contribute to the noise that degrades the image. The image is formed primarily by photons that have enough energy to pass through tissues and reach the image receptor, forming the darker areas of the image. The lighter image areas result from photons photoelectrically absorbed in tissue, not reaching the image receptor at all. Differential absorption describes the variation in image densities (or contrast) that results from the effects of the transmitted and photoelectrically absorbed photons. *(Bushong, p 156–166; Selman, p 189–190)*

233. The answer is B.   As magnetic field strength is increased, more electromotive force is induced in the conductor because of the greater concentration of flux lines in a stronger magnetic field. The steeper the angle with which a conductor cuts through magnetic flux lines, the greater electromotive force induced, because more lines can be cut per unit of time with an angle of 90° than with angles less than 90°. A straight conductor would not be as efficient as a coiled conductor in inducing current or increasing electromotive force, because each turn of a coil cuts across the magnetic flux lines, producing a larger sum of lines cut per second than a single straight conductor. The amount of electromotive force and current induced in any conductor as it moves through a magnetic field (or as a magnetic field moves across a conductor) is dependent on the number of magnetic flux lines crossed per second; the more crossed, the greater the current and electromotive force induced. This law of electromagnetic induction was discovered by Michael Faraday. *(Bushong, p 89, 92–93; Selman, p 99–102)*

234. The answer is A.   To achieve a radiographic magnification factor of two, the anatomic part is positioned halfway between the focal spot and the film, resulting in almost four times the dose as compared with conventional positioning of the part on or close to the film. Image resolution is increased in magnification radiography, because the focal spot is extremely small and each part of the image is spread over a much larger area of the intensifying screen. Scatter production is slightly decreased as a result of lower tube energies, but it does not have the energy or correct trajectory to reach the film. *(Bushong, p 310–311; Selman, p 361–366)*

235. The answer is C.   The anode disk is now generally made of molybdenum, a material that is more stable than tungsten when heated and has a surface coating that resists abrasion. The focusing cup is also constructed of molybdenum. The filament was traditionally constructed of tungsten, but currently the addition of thorium has been found to increase its life span. The body of the rotor assembly consists of copper, for its thermal characteristics. The ball bearings are steel, and either silver or lead is used as the lubricant. *(Chesney and Chesney [1984], p 237–248, 275; Selman, p 209–210, 215–217)*

236. The answer is C.   Alternating current switches direction 60 times a second, as shown by current above the line (the positive half-cycle), and below the line (the negative half-cycle). When this waveform is rectified, the current flows in the same direction to the x-ray tube all the time, as in **d** in the question. A single-phase unrectified voltage waveform is illustrated in **a,** and **b** shows half-wave rectification in which the inverse, or negative, half-cycle is not used. *(Bushong, p 100–105; Selman, p 143–152)*

237. The answer is B. The input phosphor pattern of light and dark areas that represents the anatomy through which the x-ray beam has passed is transformed at the photocathode into an electron pattern that is conveyed to the output phosphor. The electrostatic lenses maintain the integrity of the electron image while reducing its size during the passage from the photocathode to the output phosphor. The anode is the positive terminal in the image-intensifier tube. The photocathode emits proportional electrons in response to light stimulation. The vacuum prevents interference from gas molecules. *(Bushong, p 293–296; Selman, p 407–410)*

238. The answer is C. A condenser discharge type of portable x-ray unit can store charge or mAs in a capacitor and then discharge it through the x-ray tube as exposure is required. The unit is plugged into a power supply in order to charge the capacitor, but it then becomes independent of its power source. A line voltage fluctuation will not interfere with the actual exposure. A battery-powered mobile unit is never dependent on in-house power supply, except during the time that it requires recharging of its batteries. Mains-dependent units and the very small, truly portable hand-carried units both require a plug-in power source and are dependent on that incoming line voltage to control the exposure, regardless of possible variations in it. *(Selman, p 267–269)*

239. The answer is A. A capacitor or condenser is a device that can store electric charges when incorporated into a circuit. A type of condenser known as a parallel plate capacitor is constructed of two plates separated by an insulator such as air. When placed in a circuit where current is supplied, the capacitor can store charges up to a certain amount. This quantity of stored charges is called capacitance, which is measured in units called farads. Capacitance increases with the area of the plates and the closer the plates are to one another, along with the use of better insulating material between the plates. An ammeter is a device that measures the amount of charge flowing per second in an electric circuit. A rheostat is a device that can control voltage and current in a circuit while varying resistance. A choke coil is an electromagnetic device that requires alternating current in order to control current in a circuit. *(Selman, p 82–84, 137–139)*

240–241. The answers are 240-A, 241-A. The image amplifier or intensifier increases the light level of the fluoroscopic image several thousand times to bring it into a range where it can be viewed with the cone cells of the retina, which provide excellent visual acuity. The number of times that the amplified image is improved over the ordinary fluoroscopic image is called the brightness gain. Brightness gain is the product of the increase in the energy of the electrons moving across the tube (flux gain) and minification gain, or an increase in the number of light photons per unit area on the output phosphor as compared with the input phosphor.

Cesium iodide is the phosphor used in all contemporary image-intensifier tubes; it may be used on both the input and output phosphors of the tube. Zinc cadmium sulphide was used in the early image-intensifier tubes. When an x-ray photon or an electron interacts with the phosphor, a burst of visible light is given off, which in total produces a light image identical to the phosphor or electron image. Cesium iodide has a resolving capability of between 4 and 6 line pairs/mm. *(Bushong, p 294–295; Selman, p 405–410)*

242. The answer is C. HVL is used in diagnostic radiology as a measure of the quality or penetrability of an x-ray beam and is defined as that thickness of absorbing material that reduces beam intensity to one-half its original value. In the example given in the question, the x-ray beam is measured initially as 100 mR before any absorber is added. To determine the HVl, it is necessary to know how much absorber, in this case millimeters of aluminum, must be placed in the beam to reduce the original intensity of 100 mR to half, or 50 mR. The beam was reduced to 50 mR by 2.5 mm of the aluminum absorber. *(Bushong, p 177, 210; Selman, p 176, 200)*

243. The answer is C. A *rheostat* is a device that can be employed in a circuit to control the voltage applied to the primary side of a transformer. Its ability to control voltage is related to its ability to vary resistance. Constructed of wire coils and a movable contactor, a rheostat acts as a resistor, producing voltage drop in a circuit. If more of the wire coils of the rheostat are tapped off within the circuit by adjusting the contactor, then resistance increases, causing voltage to decrease. The fewer coils in the rheostat that are tapped off within the circuit, the less the resistance and the greater the voltage to the primary side of a transformer. Excess electric energy is converted into heat by the rheostat. A *transformer* is a device that functions to "step up" or "step down" voltage from a primary (input) to a secondary (output) coil, allowing input voltage to be increased or decreased as necessary. An *autotransformer* is a device similar to a transformer except that it has only one coil around an iron core, which serves as both the primary and secondary coil by use of a contactor. This contactor adjusts the ratio of secondary to primary turns of the coil, and the applied voltage can be varied to the primary coil of the high-voltage transformer in an x-ray machine. When technologists vary kVp on the control panel, they are actually adjusting the autotransformer, which varies input voltage to the transformer. Transformers operate only with alternating current, whereas rheostats can operate on either alternating or direct current. A *rectifier* is a device (valve tube or solid state), that changes alternating current into direct current. All of the devices mentioned are employed in some part of an x-ray machine, each serving its own purpose within the circuitry. The rheostat, transformer, and autotransformer can vary current as well as voltage. *(Bushong, p 79, 97–101, 121–122; Selman, p 132–137)*

244. The answer is C.   Lack of a hardener such as glutaraldehyde in the developer will not cause increased radiographic density. Instead, it is likely to cause the film to emerge from the processor wet or to stick to the transport rollers because of insufficient hardening of the emulsion. Developer overreplenishment, increased developer temperature or time, and too active a developer will cause increased radiographic density or chemical fog. Hydroquinone and phenidone are potent reducing agents that change exposed silver halide to black metallic silver; in excess, they will increase the activity of the developer, producing increased film density. *(Chesney and Chesney [1981], p 183; Thompson, p 278–279)*

245. The answer is B.   The material of which the target is made affects the range, or spectrum, of beam energies; target material of a higher atomic number produces higher-energy photons. Aluminum filtration is placed in the primary beam as a protective measure to remove the lowest-energy photons, which would otherwise be absorbed by the patient. The spectrum of beam energies is thereby increased at the high-energy end and decreased at the low-energy end, resulting in increased average energy of the beam as a whole. A change in tube current or mA causes a proportional increase in the quantity of photons in the beam, but the increase in numbers is equal for all energies, and the range of energies is unchanged by a variation in tube current. *(Bushong, p 114, 149–154; Selman, p 172)*

246. The answer is B.   When x-rays are produced at the target, they are emitted in all directions, isotropically. Those emitted through the tube port in the direction of the patient are referred to as the useful beam, and these are used in the imaging process. The remainder, more than half of all photons produced, pass out of the tube in all direction unless absorbed by the protective, lead-lined metal housing. These unused photons are called "leakage" radiation. Some attenuation of the polyenergetic x-ray beam does occur between the target and the patient, in accordance with the inverse square law, but it is very small because the distance is small. The tube port is designed to pass the entire useful beam, the size and sharpness of which is governed by the anode angle. *(Bushong, p 109, 140–142; Selman, p 160–161)*

247–249. The answers are 247-A, 248-D, 249-A.   Selectivity, is defined as follows:

$$\Sigma = \frac{\text{Primary radiation transmitted through the grid}}{\text{Scatter radiation transmitted through the grid}}$$

The higher the selectivity of a grid, the more efficient it is in performing its job of absorbing scattered photons while transmitting primary photons. Both ratio and frequency (lead lines per unit length) affect the total amount of lead in any grid, and the more lead a grid contains, the greater its selectivity will be.

Exposure angle (tomographic angle) is the angle that the central ray moves through at the fulcrum point during the tomographic sweep of the x-ray tube. It is not the angle described at the fulcrum by the entire motion of the tube because the tube moves before the exposure begins and continues to move after the exposure ends. The significance of exposure angle is that it controls the thickness of the in-focus slice: The larger the angle described, the thinner the in-focus slice (or section) will be.

Contrast improvement factor (K) is defined as follows:

$$k = \frac{\text{Radiographic contrast with a grid}}{\text{Radiographic contrast without a grid}}$$

K is always greater than 1 (1 would represent no contrast improvement whatsoever), and usually is about 2. The function of the grid is to improve radiographic contrast by removing scattered photons from the remnant beam, but its function is circumscribed by all factors that affect the production of scatter: area irradiated, beam energy, and irradiated tissue thickness. *(Bushong, p 200–201, 303–307; Selman, p 379–380, 417–427)*

250. The answer is D.   The energy level of characteristic radiation is equal to the difference in binding energies of the two shell levels of the electrons involved, and higher atomic number materials have higher binding energies. Higher-atomic-number materials do produce a beam with slightly higher effective energy, but peak energy of any beam is set by the technologist, and this is the prime control over contrast. Higher atomic-number targets produce higher-energy characteristic photons and also more bremsstrahlung photons, especially at the higher energy levels. Target materials are selected for their high atomic number plus high melting points, important aspects of everyday function and overall tube life. *(Bushong, p 151–153; Selman, p 163–164)*

251. The answer is B.   A significant advantage of magnetic resonance imaging (MRI) is that it does not require the use of ionizing radiation, therefore eliminating the risk of radiation-induced biologic effects. MRI is a complex imaging modality centered on the activity of atomic nuclei within the body (chiefly hydrogen nuclei). It uses magnetic fields and radio frequency to obtain slices or images of body tissues electronically in many planes (sagittal, coronal, and oblique planes); these can be manipulated by the operator through computer assistance. MRI scanning times, which are usually several minutes long, can present a problem in eliminating motion unsharpness due to involuntary and voluntary patient movement. The cost of MRI is higher than that of most other imaging modalities available at this time. *(Ballinger [Vol. 3], p 872–876; Bushong, p 387–412)*

252. The answer is C.   Half-wave rectification uses only the positive half-cycle of the alternating waveform, which for 60-cycle current means that only 60 pulses pass through the x-ray tube per second. With full-wave rectification, the negative, or inverse, half-cycle is also used by the x-ray tube, resulting in twice as many pulses of current passing through the x-ray tube and twice as many x-ray photons produced in the same time period. The heat-loading efficiency of the tube is thus doubled, as any radiographic density can be achieved in half the exposure time. In any x-ray unit that is functioning normally and is accurately calibrated, radiographic density is primarily the result of mAs, kVp, FFD, and tissue variations. *(Bushong, p 129–132; Selman, p 151–152)*

RADIATION PROTECTION AND RADIOBIOLOGY

253. Because the number of people employed as radiation workers is only a small percentage of the population, radiation workers are permitted a higher maximum permissible dose (MPD) than the general public. How many times greater is the MPD for radiation workers than for the general public?

    A. 50
    B. 20
    C. 10
    D. 5

254. The late or delayed effects of radiation exposure can result not only from quickly delivered acute doses but also from chronic low-level exposures received over quite long periods of time. The most common late effect experienced by the radium watch dial painters of the early 1900s was

    A. liver cancer
    B. skin cancer
    C. cataracts
    D. bone cancer

255. When humans are exposed to levels of whole-body radiation greater than approximately 100 rem, the acute radiation syndrome will probably follow. The latent period of the acute radiation syndrome, which follows the prodromal phase, is a predictor of future events. Which of the following statements correctly describes the predicting aspect of the latent period?

    A. Nausea during the latent period indicates that the gastrointestinal syndrome will follow
    B. The duration of the latent period is an indicator of the severity of effects to come
    C. A very short latent period indicates that no damage occurred
    D. Coma during the latent period indicates that death will follow within 2 weeks

256. Which of the following are currently believed to be a source of unnecessary exposure because of the low yield of diagnostic information?

    1. Annual chest radiography
    2. Routine fluoroscopy in persons older than 40 years
    3. Mammographic examinations in high-risk females

    A. 1 and 2
    B. 1 and 3
    C. 2 and 3
    D. 1, 2, and 3

257. The National Council on Radiation Protection (NCRP) recommends that the dose level in fluoroscopy not exceed a specific rate, measured in air at the point at which the beam enters the patient. What is that specified maximum?

    A. 0.5 R/minute
    B. 10 R/minute
    C. 50 R/hour
    D. 100 R/hour

258. When body parts of nonuniform thickness are being radiographed, either a gradient screen cassette or a wedge compensating filter may be used to produce an image of uniform density. The gradient screen, however, has a distinct disadvantage compared with the wedge filter, in that

A. it is very uncomfortable for the patient
B. patient dose is increased
C. a lower-energy beam must be used
D. image contrast is markedly decreased

Questions 259–262 consist of four lettered headings followed by a list of numbered words or phrases. For each of the following quantities of radiation exposure choose the dose with which it is most closely associated. Each heading may be used once, more than once, or not at all.

A. Less than 18 mrem
B. 35 to 45 mrem
C. 100 mrem
D. 350 mrem

259. Weekly MPD for occupationally exposed persons

260. Medical uses of ionizing radiation when averaged over the United States population

261. Cosmic radiation received per person per year, averaged for the United States

262. Internal sources of ionizing radiation per person per year, averaged for the United States

263. As a patient-protection measure, a sheet of aluminum or aluminum-equivalent material is required by federal guidelines to be present in the primary beam of all general-purpose radiographic/fluorographic units. This aluminum filtration reduces patient dose by

A. emitting characteristic radiation
B. removing the bremsstrahlung photons from the beam
C. removing the shorter-wavelength photons from the beam
D. removing the longer-wavelength photons from the beam

264. Within a few months after x-rays were discovered, they were being used for medical diagnosis and treatment, resulting in the first visible biologic effects of radiation on humans. Which of the following is an immediate or early effect of radiation exposure?

A. Genetic mutation
B. Skin erythema
C. Leukemia
D. Bone cancer

265. Because it is necessary in radiation protection to equate the various degrees of biologic effectiveness of different types of ionizing radiation, the quantity "dose equivalent" has been introduced. The unit of dose equivalent is the

A. MPD
B. rad (or gray)
C. curie
D. rem (or sievert)

266. The property of an x-ray photon that is made use of in all gas-filled detectors is its ability to

A. remain electrically neutral
B. ionize air
C. cause fluorescence of some crystals
D. liberate heat when passing through matter

267. Radiation dose-response relationships, derived from clinical trials, are important in planning treatment schedules for patients with malignant disease. A nonthreshold dose-response relationship is associated with radiation-induced

A. epilation
B. leukemia
C. sterility
D. organ necrosis

268. There are no NCRP recommendations on MPD for the general public for

　　1. medical diagnostic exposure
　　2. background or environmental exposure
　　3. medical therapeutic exposure

A. 1 and 2
B. 1 and 3
C. 2 and 3
D. 1, 2, and 3

269. Many of the effects that follow irradiation of the human body occur in water, because the human body is composed of about 80% water molecules. When water is irradiated, radiolysis occurs, resulting in the breakdown of the water molecules into other products. Some of these products are free radicals, which

A. can exist for substantial periods of time and are very stable
B. can form hydrogen peroxide
C. are molecules containing a total of eight electrons in their outer shell
D. are charged molecules that remain in one location

270. The NCRP has recommended that a minimum amount of aluminum filtration be added to the primary beam of every medical diagnostic x-ray unit. The minimum recommended amount of total filtration for x-ray units with operating kVp below 50 is

A. 0.25 mm
B. 0.5 mm
C. 1.5 mm
D. 2.0 mm

271. Both physical and biologic factors affect the magnitude of the damage from an exposure to ionizing radiation. The response to ionizing radiation is determined by

    1. the total dose in rad

    2. protraction and fractionation in delivery

    3. the sensitivity of the irradiated tissue

  A. 1 and 2

  B. 1 and 3

  C. 2 and 3

  D. 1, 2, and 3

272. Time, distance, and shielding can all be used to reduce dose when appropriate. With the use of shielding, it is important to determine whether primary photons or scattered photons will be incident on the barrier. Which of the following materials is rarely used as a structural secondary barrier?

  A. Lead

  B. Gypsum board

  C. Plate glass

  D. Lead acrylic

273. During fluoroscopy, if technologists are 18 inches from the radiation source they receive a dose of 10 mR/minute. When they can move away from the table, they should do so, to a point that is 7 feet from the source. In using distance for protection, the accumulated dose is reduced to

  A. 0.055 mR/minute

  B. 0.450 mR/minute

  C. 2.142 mR/minute

  D. 2.177 mR/minute

274. The image-intensifier or fluoroscopic carriage assembly must be coupled to the fluoroscopic tube and must not be capable of being energized except when centered to the fluoroscopic tube. This is because the

  A. fluoroscopic grid would image with off-center cutoff

  B. image-intensifier/fluoroscopic assembly is the primary barrier

  C. fluoroscopic timer would not record the time accurately

  D. phototimer pickup would receive unattenuated beam and terminate the exposure too quickly

275. The International Commission on Radiation Protection has recommended application of the "10-day rule" as a simple method of reducing exposure to a specific group of persons. This rule requires that a

  A. patient wait 10 days before a fluoroscopic examination is repeated

  B. reproductive female have elective abdominal/pelvic radiography only in the 10 days after the onset of menstruation

  C. radiation worker exposed to more than 1 rem avoid all exposure in the following 10 days

  D. radiologist perform fluoroscopy daily for no more than 10 consecutive days

276. If only one personnel monitor (probably a film badge) is used by the diagnostic technologist, why is it essential to wear it outside the apron during fluoroscopy and procedures using portable units?

       1. The MPD for hands is 75 rem in any one year
       2. The occupational MPD refers to head and neck exposure
       3. The MPD applies to whole-body exposure

A. 1 and 2
B. 1 and 3
C. 2 and 3
D. 1, 2, and 3

277. The biologic effects of x-ray exposure occur as a result of alterations in atomic structure. By what process is the energy transferred to the tissue atoms from x-ray photons?

A. Bremsstrahlung
B. Ionization
C. Disintegrations per second
D. Relative biologic effectiveness

278. As soon as it was known that x-rays caused biologic damage, it became important to be able to detect and measure their presence. The first radiation detector used was

A. barium tungstate
B. the scintillation counter
C. the thermoluminescent dosimeter
D. photographic emulsion

279. Humans are constantly exposed to ionizing radiation from a variety of sources. Which of the following sources of radiation has varied very little in magnitude in the past half century and also constitutes the largest source of exposure, when compared with others on an annual basis?

A. Natural background radiation
B. Radiopharmaceuticals
C. Fallout from weapons testing
D. Diagnostic uses of x-rays

280. There is a large body of information relating to the effects of various doses of ionizing radiation on the skin. Which of the following effects would be anticipated from a dose of 200 to 600 rad?

       1. Erythema
       2. Epilation
       3. Basal cell death

A. 1 and 2
B. 1 and 3
C. 2 and 3
D. 1, 2, and 3

281. Special MPD guidelines have been established for persons younger than 18 years who may be exposed to ionizing radiation, as student radiographers or in the course of other educational activities. The specific annual dose-limiting recommendation for this group is

    A. 10 mrem/year (0.1 mSv/year)
    B. 100 mrem/year (1 mSv/year)
    C. 1,000 mrem/year (10 mSv/year)
    D. 10,000 mrem/year (100 mSv/year)

282. The dose-limiting recommendation used in designing a nuclear reactor is the entire population-averaged MPD of

    A. 170 mrem/year
    B. 300 mrem/year
    C. 500 mrem/year
    D. 4,000 mrem/year

283. There are four separately named organized systems of units representing the base quantities in physics. Which of the following systems have basic units in common?

    1. Systeme Internationale d'Unités (SI)
    2. Meter-kilogram-second (MKS)
    3. British

    A. 1 and 2
    B. 1 and 3
    C. 2 and 3
    D. 1, 2, and 3

284. Human death resulting from damage to the hematopoietic system would most likely be associated with clinically observable effects such as

    A. motor incoordination and ataxia
    B. the absence of phagocytosis and antibody formation
    C. massive bloody diarrhea and electrolyte imbalance
    D. breathing difficulty and lethargy

285. Radiation-induced breast cancer has been observed in at least one human population, creating much controversy and concern about x-ray detection of breast cancer. Which of the following represent skin or entrance doses received per projection for current mammographic examinations?

    1. 10 to 50 mrad
    2. 0.2 to 1.0 rad
    3. 8 to 15 R

    A. 1 and 2
    B. 1 and 3
    C. 2 and 3
    D. 1, 2, and 3

286. It has been known for some time that x-rays are harmful, but the precise effect that will result from diagnostic levels of x-rays cannot yet be predicted. What is known, however, is that following irradiation, a molecule can

    A. never function normally again
    B. recover from the radiation damage
    C. be unable to neutralize its ionized atoms
    D. continue to function with altered chemical-binding properties

287. The type of interaction that an x-ray photon will have with the material through which it is passing depends partly on the energy of that photon. In the diagnostic x-ray beam, the energy of any photon is controlled by the technologist, who can decrease the possibility of photoelectric absorption by increasing

    A. photon wavelength
    B. imaging system speed
    C. kVp
    D. FFD

288. When humans are exposed to very high doses of whole-body radiation, approximately 5,000 rem and above, death can be expected to follow in about

    A. 2 to 72 hours
    B. 4 to 8 days
    C. 1 to 2 weeks
    D. 1 month

289. Human cells reproduce by two slightly different processes, meiosis and mitosis. What differentiates meiosis from mitosis is that meiosis

    A. is a process of reduction division
    B. occurs only in somatic cells
    C. begins its process with 23 chromosomes
    D. consists of one division resulting in two daughter cells

290. At present, there are many types of gonadal shields. They are usually designed for specific examinations or situations. For a young man having a complete lumbar spine examination, which of the following types would be most effective?

    A. Shaped contact shield
    B. Lead apron
    C. Shadow shield
    D. Lead glove

291. DNA is a complex macromolecule that is found primarily in the cell nucleus and is composed of deoxyribose and phosphate segments, plus nitrogenous bases. Which of the following are base-bonding combinations?

    1. Adenine/thymine
    2. Cytosine/guanine
    3. Thymine/cytosine

    A. 1 and 2
    B. 1 and 3
    C. 2 and 3
    D. 1, 2, and 3

292. For the purpose of personnel protection during fluoroscopic procedures, a drape and/or a hinged shield can be used to reduce scattered radiation in the immediate vicinity of the x-ray table. The minimum value of lead equivalency for these shields as required by federal guidelines is

    A. 0.25 mm
    B. 0.50 mm
    C. 1.50 mm
    D. 2.00 mm

293. Technologists who work mainly in special procedures (angiography) often have their hands quite close to the primary beam and may use a second personnel dosimeter on the wrist or hand to monitor extremity exposure. The annual MPD for the hands is

    A. 25 rem
    B. 50 rem
    C. 75 rem
    D. 100 rem

294. Many factors affect the survival of a cell following a dose of radiation. Some of these factors relate to the dose rate at which the radiation is delivered. The reduction of total biologic effect by extending the time period in which the dose is delivered is called

    A. protraction
    B. tissue oxygenation
    C. fractionation
    D. linear energy transfer

295. When performing a diagnostic radiographic examination, gonad shielding should NOT be provided for the patient with reproductive potential if the situation is such that

    A. only scattered radiation will reach the gonads
    B. only partial exposure of the gonads by the primary beam will occur
    C. use of a higher-speed imaging system would reduce the dose just as effectively
    D. use of gonad shielding would interfere with the goal of the examination

296. Radiation workers are monitored for personal exposure as a check on the safety of the working environment, and they require a personal monitor if they

   1. are occupationally exposed
   2. are potentially reproductive
   3. might receive one-quarter of the MPD annually

   A. 1 and 2
   B. 1 and 3
   C. 2 and 3
   D. 1, 2, and 3

Questions 297–300 consist of four lettered headings followed by a list of numbered words or phrases. For each of the situations described below, choose the radiation dose with which it is most likely to be associated. Each lettered item may be used once, more than once, or not at all.

   A. Less than 50 mR
   B. 500 to 2,000 mR
   C. 50 to 100 R
   D. Greater than 100 rem

297. Lateral lumbar spine projection on a 14 × 17-inch film

298. Acute radiation syndrome

299. AP or PA projection of the chest

300. 10 minutes of fluoroscopy

BODY—RADIATION PROTECTION AND RADIOBIOLOGY
ANSWERS, EXPLANATIONS, AND REFERENCES

253. The answer is C. The general public is permitted 0.5 rem, or one-tenth, the annual exposure that a radiation worker may receive. This low exposure level is intended to reduce exposure to reproductive organs, thereby lessening the possibility of genetic effects. This maximum permissible dose (MPD) for the general public does not include medically essential radiation exposure and is not usually measured. It is used, however, in the design of radiation barriers for the public in hospitals and clinics. *(National Council on Radiation Protection [NCRP, No. 39], p 94; Bushong, p 511)*

254. The answer is D. The young women who painted watch dials with radium-based paint in the 1920s ingested significant amounts of the paint by making the brush into a fine point with the lips or tongue. Radium, chemically similar to calcium, was deposited in bony structures and delivered high doses to bone, as it has a half-life of almost 2,000 years. Many of these people died of the acute effects, and many that initially survived developed bone cancers in later years. *(Bushong, p 494-495; Frankel, p 30-31)*

255. The answer is B. The duration of the latent period is inversely proportional to both the dose received and the severity of effects. The longest latent period occurs in the hematopoietic syndrome, which results from the lowest doses. The shortest latent period occurs when the central nervous system has been damaged, and death will certainly result. The latent period is that time span, following a large radiation dose to the whole body, when the prodromal symptoms have subsided, the individual feels well, and there are no visible signs of radiation-induced illness. *(Bushong, p 466-467; NCRP [No. 33], p 46)*

256. The answer is A. In the very recent past, many types of x-ray examinations were performed on a "routine" basis or as part of annual physical checkups and revealed almost no diagnostic information. Only very rarely was a completely unsuspected disease discovered in an asymptomatic individual. X-ray examinations are recommended only when physical history and/or clinical findings and symptoms suggest the presence of disease. Annual chest radiography and routine fluoroscopy in persons older than 40 years are therefore believed to be a source of unnecessary exposure because they so seldom yield any useful information. The mammographic examination is the best available diagnostic tool for the early detection of breast cancer and is recommended for high-risk women of any age and for all women during and after menopause. *(Bushong, p 312-313, 325, 546-547)*

257. The answer is B. Most modern fluoroscopic equipment has many built-in devices that either keep the patient and operator exposure within certain limits or indicate to the operator the extent of beam-on time used. The maximum exposure rate permitted at the tabletop is 10 R/minute, and many units indicate this level of exposure rate with a continuous visible signal on the operator's control panel. Most fluoroscopic examinations can be performed at lower beam intensity, frequently between 4 and 7 R/minute. *(Bushong, p 514; NCRP [No. 33], p 10)*

258. The answer is B. When body parts of nonuniform thickness are being radiographed, a compensating filter may be placed in the rails of the collimator to absorb excess radiation that would overexpose thinner body parts. A gradient screen simply converts the remnant radiation in the slower end of the screen to less light, which results in less exposure to the film. The compensating filter reduces dose by absorbing the excess radiation before it reaches the patient. *(Bushong, p 179)*

259–262. The answers are 259-C, 260-C, 261-B, 262-A. The weekly MPD for occupationally exposed individuals is 100 mrem. This is derived from the NCRP recommended MPD of 5,000 mrem per year. Radiology technologists receive very little exposure in the course of their occupations, and none of that is whole-body exposure. In many large institutions (where protection is stressed), most working technologists have been found to receive annually less than one-tenth of the MPD.

Medical uses of ionizing radiation when averaged over the United States population annually constitute close to 100 mrem per person. This includes dental uses, diagnostic and therapeutic sources, and all radiopharmaceuticals. This amount does not represent whole-body exposure or even total exposure to any one site, but is simply the sum of all doses incurred.

The amount of cosmic radiation received per person per year for the entire United States is 35 to 45 mrem. Cosmic radiation, mainly charged particles from extraterrestrial sources, interacts with the earth's atmosphere to produce secondary particles that reach us all. This dose is lowest at sea level and almost doubles at an elevation of 1 mile. Those individuals who spend a lot of time at high elevations may receive a considerably larger dose of cosmic radiation than does the average person.

From internal sources of ionizing radiation, the amount of radiation received per person per year averaged for the United States is less than 18 mrem. Very small amounts of radioactive nuclides are contained within the body, either temporarily or on a consistent basis, depending on diet and metabolism. These radionuclides are ingested in foods or water or may be inhaled with air. They reach us through our food chains from the terrestrial presence of uranium, thorium, radiopotassium, and radiocarbon. *(Bushong, p 4, 530; NCRP [No. 39], p 10-14)*

263. The answer is D. Aluminum filtration in the primary beam removes lower-energy (longer-wavelength) photons by photoelectric absorption. These lower-energy photons would otherwise reach the patient but do not have sufficient energy to be transmitted through the patient to the image receptor, adding only to patient dose but not to image formation. The characteristic radiation of the aluminum filtration does not affect the patient dose. Bremsstrahlung photons have a wide energy range, the lowest portion of which would be absorbed by the filtration, but the majority of bremsstrahlung photons are energetic enough to make up the image. *(Frankel, p 108; Bushong, p 177-178)*

264. The answer is B. High doses of relatively low-energy x-rays, such as those produced in the years immediately after their discovery, produced skin erythema or reddening in many of the pioneer workers who frequently exposed their hands to the beam to check its intensity. Leukemia and bone cancer are long-term effects that would not be expected to become apparent until at least several years after exposure. Radiation-induced genetic mutations would not be observed for at least one generation (a very long-term effect). *(Bushong, p 9-10, 465)*

265. The answer is D. The rem (or sievert), the product of absorbed dose multiplied by the relative biologic effectiveness of that dose, is the unit of dose equivalent used to measure occupational exposure. Radiation workers may be exposed to various types of ionizing radiations, which may have different biologic effectiveness. Measuring these exposures in rads alone would not give a clear estimate of the biologic changes produced. *(Bushong, p 13-14, 337; Noz and Maguire, p 60, 63)*

266. The answer is B. The x-ray photon property that is made practical use of in the gas-filled detector is its ability to ionize air. A voltage is established between a central electrode and the air-filled chamber wall so that the electrons and the positive ions produced from the ionizations can be collected and measured. The ability of the x-ray photon to cause fluorescence of some crystals is used in phototube phototimers. *(Selman, p 165; Bushong, p 517-518)*

267. The answer is B. Radiation-induced leukemia is associated with a nonthreshold dose-response relationship, indicating that there is no dose that does not carry some risk of inducing leukemia. This type of dose-response relationship is thought to be quite real, according to all the information collected from both animal research and human results after the atomic bombing of Japan. Epilation, sterility, and organ necrosis are somatic effects, represented most accurately by a threshold dose-response relationship. *(Bushong, p 490-491; Frankel, p 21-22)*

268. The answer is D.   All medical radiation exposure, whether diagnostic or therapeutic, is assumed to be necessary for maintaining an individual's health. Risk inherent in exposure to ionizing radiation must be balanced against a reasonable expectation of benefit gained from that exposure and so cannot be limited arbitrarily. Background or natural environmental radiation exposure varies in intensity relative to elevation and location, but it has always been a factor in human existence and is not believed to be deleterious to health. The NCRP has no recommendations on MPD for any of these exposures. *(Bushong, p 4-5; NCRP [No. 39], p 11-12, 95-97, 106)*

269. The answer is B.   Free radicals are formed as a result of radiolysis of water. These uncharged atoms or groups of atoms act together and are highly unstable molecules with life spans of less than a few milliseconds. They are reactive and can disrupt chemical bonds of other molecules at some distance from the site at which they were generated. When oxygen reacts with the aqueous free hydrogen radical, hydrogen peroxide, a toxic substance, can be formed. *(Bushong, p 452-453; Frankel, p 17-18)*

270. The answer is B.   For an x-ray unit with potential that cannot exceed 50 kVp, a minimum of 0.5 mm of total filtration is required in the primary beam. This amount includes the inherent filtration (that provided by the glass window of the x-ray tube through which the beam emerges and the mirror in the light-beam collimator) plus any added aluminum placed in the primary beam, usually between the tube and collimator or in the collimator itself. Radiographic equipment designed for veterinary use may fall into this category, as may some dental radiographic units. *(Bushong, p 178, 512; NCRP [No. 33], p 13)*

271. The answer is D.   The total absorbed dose of ionizing radiation is probably the most important determiner of response; increasing dose results in increasing response. Fractionation is a method of dose delivery in which periods of time separate the periods of exposure, reducing the overall effect. Protraction is a continuous delivery of a radiation dose, but at a reduced dose rate, again resulting in less response. The greater the inherent sensitivity of the tissue irradiated, the greater will be the response. *(Bushong, p 439-441; NCRP [No. 39], p 24-31)*

272. The answer is A.   A secondary barrier is designed to shield against scattered radiation and leakage radiation, which are always less intense than primary radiation. The amount of lead required to shield against secondary radiation would be so tiny that manufacture of such a shield would be very difficult. Gypsum board 2 to 3 inches thick is commonly used in walls, and plate glass up to 2 inches thick or a lesser thickness of lead acrylic is used for the control booth window. *(Bushong, p 515)*

273. The answer is B.   Beam intensity or exposure rate varies inversely as the square of the distance from the source. This can be stated as follows:

$$\left(\frac{\text{Intensity}_1}{\text{Intensity}_2}\right) = \left(\frac{\text{Distance}_2}{\text{Distance}_1}\right)^2.$$

In the example given in the question, Intensity$_1$ is 10 mR/minute, the initial exposure rate. Intensity$_2$ is the unknown new exposure rate. Distance$_2$ is 7 feet, the new distance from the source. Distance$_1$ is 1.5 feet, the original distance from the source. The following calculations may be used to find the new exposure rate *(Selman, p 343):*

$$\frac{10}{X} = \left(\frac{7}{1.5}\right)^2 \rightarrow \frac{10}{X} = \frac{49}{2.25} \rightarrow 49X = 22.5 \rightarrow X = 0.459 \text{ mR/minute.}$$

274. The answer is B.   The image-intensifier/fluoroscopic assembly is the primary protective barrier for the fluoroscopic tube. If the fluoroscopic tube were not coupled to the carriage and if it could be energized independently of the location of the carriage, primary radiation would be incident on barriers designed only for protection against secondary radiation. The patient could also receive exposure that would not contribute to any useful image. This is a protective measure only and is not related to the operation of any equipment. *(Bushong, p 513; NCRP [No. 33], p 7)*

275. The answer is B.   If all elective abdominal and pelvic radiography were performed on potentially reproductive women only during the first 10 days after the onset of menstruation, the chances of unknowingly exposing an embryo to x-radiation would be greatly diminished. The patient can be assisted in implementing the 10-day rule by either direct questions or a questionnaire. Of course, this rule would only be applicable when no medical urgency existed. *(Bushong, p 550)*

276. The answer is C.   The MPD recommendation of 5 rem/year refers not only to whole-body exposure but also to specific body parts or organs, the lens of the eye, gonads, and red bone marrow. All exposure received should be recorded on the monitor, so the monitor should be placed outside the apron to record dose to the head and neck area accurately. If the monitor were placed beneath the apron, a falsely low dose would be recorded. If any specific body area (such as the hands) receives extensive exposure, an additional monitor should be used to record that dose. *(Bushong, p 542-543; NCRP [No. 39], p 89)*

277. The answer is B.   It is in the process of ionization, through which an electron is removed from or added to an atom, that the energy is transferred to the tissue atoms from x-ray photons. This can cause a change in the ability of an atom to combine chemically and so can cause important molecules to break up. Serious effects can occur if important molecules become unable to function normally or unable to function at all. *(Bushong, p 425; Noz and Maguire, p 3)*

278. The answer is D.   Photographic emulsion was the first radiation detector used. The principle that optical density is directly proportional to the logarithm of relative dose received is still applied today in film badge monitoring of personnel exposure. The thermoluminescent dosimeter is becoming more widely used in personnel monitoring; the scintillation counter is used in both imaging and photon spectroscopy; and barium tungstate is found in phototube phototimer devices. *(Bushong, p 517; Selman, p 191)*

279. The answer is A.   Natural background radiation, the sum of cosmic, terrestrial, and internal sources of exposure to humans, represents roughly 100 mrad/person/year. The largest dose received from a non-natural source is that from diagnostic x-rays, currently averaged to be about 70 mrad/person/year. It should be noted that natural background radiation is relatively constant through time, whereas exposure from diagnostic x-rays, radiopharmaceuticals, and fallout may vary among individuals or regions. *(NCRP [No. 39], p 4; Bushong, p 4)*

280. The answer is A.   At a dose level of 200 to 600 rad to the skin, skin reddening (erythema) and hair loss (epilation) would be anticipated. Both responses would be expected to be transitory, and repair would include regrowth of hair. Only at very much higher dose levels would the basal cells (the germinal layer) be killed. Late effects could occur at these dose levels, but they would probably not be of a malignant nature. *(Bushong, p 470-472, 484; NCRP [No. 39], p 49)*

281. The answer is B.   The annual MPD for students younger than 18 years is 100 mrem/year (1 mSv/year). Persons who become student radiographers before the age of 18 are generally not scheduled to fluoroscopy or portable (mobile unit) radiography clinical rotation until after their 18th birthday. Students younger than 18 years do use a personal dosimeter, even though no exposure is expected to be recorded. *(Bushong, p 510)*

282. The answer is A.   A MPD of 170 mrem/year averaged over the entire population is the acceptable limit considered when designing a nuclear reactor. This whole-body dose-limiting recommendation is based on the genetic risk to the population as a whole and represents one-third of the exposure permitted any individual. This MPD includes radiation from all sources other than natural background and medically necessary radiation. *(Bushong, p 511; NCRP [No. 39], p 57, 97)*

283. The answer is A.   Both the Systeme Internationale d'Unités (SI) and the meter-kilogram-second (MKS) system use the same base units, whereas the British system uses the foot-pound-second units. The SI system has special units for specific radiological quantities, which will be used worldwide before the end of the decade. The SI unit for activity is the becquerel, for dose equivalent is the sievert, and for absorbed dose is the gray. *(Bushong, p 21-22)*

284. The answer is B.   Radiation exposure of a magnitude sufficient to cause death due to damage to the hematopoietic system will reduce the number of cells in the circulating blood. The lymphocytes, which are prominent in antibody formation and in cell-mediated immunity, and also the granular WBCs, which are primarily responsible for phagocytosis. Difficulty in breathing, lethargy, motor incoordination, and ataxia are responses to very high doses of radiation, the effects of which are so rapidly felt in the central nervous system that other systems do not have time to respond. Massive bloody diarrhea and electrolyte imbalance follow radiation doses large enough to be lethal to the intestinal lining cells. Ulceration of the bowel follows, with bleeding and uncontrollable loss of fluids resulting in electrolyte imbalance. *(Bushong, p 467-468; Frankel, p 26)*

285. The answer is C.   Imaging techniques in mammography have evolved very rapidly over the past 10 years in response to the demand for lower-dose systems. Twenty years ago, all mammographic examinations used a nonscreen system and a general radiographic tube with added filtration removed. This system resulted in a skin or entrance dose in the range of 8 to 15 R per projection. Subsequently, xeroradiographic images were obtained at much lower doses and with further adjustments to equipment and filtration, single-projection doses were reduced to a range of 0.2 to 1.0 rad per projection, roughly the same range as produced by the film-screen systems that are much used currently. *(Bushong, p 496, 535-537; Selman, p 440)*

286. The answer is B.   It is possible for irradiated molecules to recover with the help of repair enzymes. Exposure to radiation ionizes atoms of the molecules, thereby changing that atom's ability to combine chemically, but the atoms can become neutral again by attracting free electrons. It is believed, however, that repair is never 100%, that there is a component that is not repairable. *(Bushong, p 425; Frankel, p 19)*

287. The answer is C.   Increasing the kVp of the x-ray beam will give more photons sufficient energy to be transmitted through the body part to the image receptor. These higher-energy photons are less likely to be absorbed in the body, thus decreasing the energy transferred to tissue. Changing imaging system speed or FFD will have no effect on beam energy. Increasing photon wavelength results in a decrease of photon energy. *(Selman, p 340; Frankel, p 3)*

288. The answer is A.   When more than 5,000 rem is delivered to the whole body at one time, the central nervous system, which is the most radiation-resistant body system, is affected and death cannot be avoided. The greater the radiation dose, the more severe the damage, and in the central nervous system syndrome death can occur within hours or up to a few days later. No amount of clinical support can alter the outcome at doses this high. The initial symptoms of nausea and vomiting, sometimes accompanied by mental confusion, are followed by a latent period of a few hours and finally the period of manifest illness, disorientation, seizures, coma, and death. *(Bushong, p 468-469; Frankel, p 26)*

289. The answer is A. Meiosis is a process of reduction division, starting with a cell having 46 chromosomes. This cell then divides into two cells having 46 chromosomes; then these two cells each divide again without replicating the DNA, resulting in four cells having 23 chromosomes each. This occurs only in the body's germ, or genetic, cells, the oogonia and spermatogonia. These genetic cells, as a result of the reduction division, now have half the chromosomes needed. The other half is supplied at conception. *(Bushong, p 436-437)*

290. The answer is A. The shaped contact shield, which totally encloses the scrotum, is the most effective gonadal shield for reducing dose from both primary and scattered radiation. Flat contact shields are quite effective in reducing primary-beam exposure in the AP position but are difficult to apply for a lateral view, and they cannot protect against scatter in any projection. Although a lead glove generally has twice the lead content of a lead apron, if it is placed on top of patient it can still only reduce exposure from the primary beam, and not from scatter generated in the patient's tissues. *(Frankel, p 106; Bushong, p 10, 548-549)*

291. The answer is A. The DNA molecule has a central structure of alternating deoxyribose (sugar) and phosphate molecules. Attached at each sugar molecule is one of the four nitrogenous organic bases, either one of the purines (adenine or guanine), or one of the pyrimidines (thymine or cytosine). The only possible way for the bases to combine is adenine with thymine and cytosine with guanine. The bases attached to the sugar molecules are analagous to ladder rungs, with the alternating sugar and phosphate molecules likened to the ladder sides. The base, sugar, and phosphate group is called a nucleotide. *(Bushong, p 430-432; Frankel, p 40-44)*

292. The answer is A. The fluoroscopist and technologist, when working at the side of the table, would be receiving scattered radiation were it not for protective shielding. The drape shield is an overlapping lead shield suspended from the fluoroscopy carriage. It may be used together with hinged or sliding panels that snap into place between the patient and others at the table. The minimum lead content is required to be 0.25 mm of lead equivalency. The drape shield is in place at all times during fluoroscopy; however, it may not be possible to use the hinged shield when the patient requires much assistance in moving and turning. *(NCRP [No. 33], p 8; Bushong, p 513)*

293. The answer is C. The MPD for the hands is 75 rem, although this amount of exposure would never be anticipated in diagnostic radiography. Special-procedures technologists may not be able to use protective measures such as shielding for the hands, because the field in which they are working is sterile. From handling radionuclides, nuclear medicine technologists may also receive an appreciable dose to their hands. *(Bushong, p 511; NCRP [No. 39], p 91)*

294. The answer is C. Fractionation, a central factor in the delivery of radiaton therapy, is the reduction of biologic effect by delivery of a radiation dose over a period of time instead of all at once. Alternatively, total doses that might prove lethal can be tolerated if given in increments over time. Protraction is the continuous delivery of a total dose, but at a lower dose rate per unit time. Linear energy transfer, the rate at which energy is transferred from ionizing radiation to soft tissue, depends on the physical aspects of the radiation itself. *(Bushong, p 439; NCRP [No. 39], p 25)*

295. The answer is D. Gonad shielding cannot be used when its use would prevent imaging clinically significant anatomy. This is frequently the case in radiography of females when shielding over the ovaries would prevent visualization of parts of the pelvis in abdominal or pelvic examinations. Shielding of the reproductive organs should, however, be performed on all persons with reproductive potential when the gonads are close to or within the primary field, except as stated above. The use of a faster imaging system would reduce overall dose, if correctly used, but would not reduce dose as much as would actual shielding. *(Bushong, p 549; Frankel, p 107)*

296. The answer is B.   Only occupational or work-related radiation exposure is intended to be monitored, and only when the exposure could reach the magnitude of one-quarter of the MPD, or 1.25 rem/year. Medical or dental exposure of the radiation worker must not be included in occupational dose. In the diagnostic x-ray department, all technologists who perform fluoroscopic, portable radiographic, or angiographic examinations use some form of personal monitoring, regardless of their reproductive potential. Personnel involved in file room, transportation, and secretarial work do not require monitoring. *(Bushong, p 539; NCRP [No. 39], p 84-86)*

297–300. The answers are 297-B, 298-D, 299-A, 300-C.   A lateral lumbar spine projection on a 14 × 17-inch film generates a relatively high dose (500 to 2,000 mR). This dose can be moderated by using the fastest screen system available (probably a 400-speed rare earth system), which has the added advantage of a shorter contrast scale when compared with the 200-speed system. The gonads must be shielded for this projection or they will receive substantial unnecessary exposure from both primary and scattered photons.

An AP or PA projection of the chest is associated with an exposure dose of less than 50 mR. The dose received for a single AP or PA projection of the chest varies over a wide range, because there are many different ways that this examination can be performed. The higher dose results from using 6 feet or greater FFD, with high kVp and a high-ratio grid. The PA or AP projection of the chest can also be performed at 6 feet or 40 inches FFD without any grid, using low to medium kVp for a relatively high-contrast radiograph. There are also occasions when an AP or PA chest must be exposed at 40 inches FFD with the reciprocating grid in the x-ray table.

A dose of 100 rem is assumed to be the threshold level of whole-body radiation delivered at once that precipitates a group of signs, symptoms, and effects known as the acute radiation syndrome. At the threshold level, the most sensitive individuals would experience effects in the hematopoietic system. As the dose increases, more individuals would respond, with effects in the gastrointestinal system being the first to occur. At even higher doses, the relatively resistant cells of the central nervous system would be affected.

Most recently made x-ray units have a fluoroscopic output between roughly 5 R/minute and the recommended maximum of 10 R/minute, resulting in a maximum of 100 R for 10 minutes of fluoroscopy. It must be understood that this total amount of exposure is not received by any one area but is divided over all the anatomic areas visualized during the fluoroscopic examination. For 10 minutes of fluoroscopy, the radiation intensity should not exceed 100 R. *(Bushong, p 438, 514, 532; Bushong [1973], p 59-60)*

POSTTEST

ANATOMY AND PHYSIOLOGY
(including Medical Terminology and Pathology)

1. The kidneys are correctly described by which of the following statements?

    1. The kidneys are retroperitoneal, lying between the level of the last thoracic vertebra and third lumbar vertebra
    2. The kidneys are composed of an outer medullary substance and inner fascia
    3. Glomerular filtration occurs within the microscopic units of the kidneys

    A. 1 only
    B. 1 and 3
    C. 2 and 3
    D. 1, 2, and 3

2. If an opaque contrast medium is injected into the inferior vena cava, the sequence of opacified vascular structures that would normally be visualized fluoroscopically would be

    A. right atrium → right ventricle → left atrium → pulmonary artery → pulmonary veins → left ventricle → aorta
    B. right ventricle → pulmonary artery → pulmonary veins → left ventricle → left atrium → aorta
    C. right atrium → right ventricle → pulmonary artery → pulmonary veins → left atrium → left ventricle → aorta
    D. left atrium → left ventricle → pulmonary artery → pulmonary veins → right atrium → right ventricle → aorta

3. A joint that does not allow movement is functionally classified as being

    A. diarthrodial
    B. synarthrodial
    C. amphiarthrodial
    D. synovial

Questions 4–5 consist of four lettered headings followed by a list of numbered words or phrases. For each of the papillae listed below, choose the body part with which it is most closely associated. Each lettered body part may be used once, more than once, or not at all.

    A. Heart
    B. Tongue
    C. Duodenum
    D. Kidney

4. Circumvallate papilla

5. Papilla of Vater

6. The brain is supplied with blood by

       1. internal carotid arteries
       2. external carotid arteries
       3. vertebral arteries

A. 1 and 2
B. 1 and 3
C. 2 and 3
D. 1, 2, and 3

7. The true layer of skin containing blood vessels, glands, nerves, connective tissue, and muscle is the

A. dermis
B. epidermis
C. subcutaneous
D. synovial membrane

8. The region of the pelvis below the pelvic brim is called the

A. true (lesser) pelvis
B. intermediate pelvis
C. false (greater) pelvis
D. ala of the pelvis

9. The innermost bone of the middle ear, which attaches to the oval window, is the

A. incus
B. malleus
C. stapes
D. cochlea

10. Based on structure and function, principal types of body tissues include

       1. epithelial
       2. nervous
       3. muscular

A. 1 and 2
B. 1 and 3
C. 2 and 3
D. 1, 2, and 3

11. The lateral border of the stomach is called the

A. greater curvature
B. pyloric antrum
C. lesser curvature
D. fundus

12. All of the following are part of the temporal bone EXCEPT the

    A. external auditory canal
    B. mastoid process
    C. greater cornu
    D. pars petrosa

13. Numerous outpouchings in the intestine characterize the condition known as

    A. diverticulosis
    B. multiple polyposis
    C. aneurysms
    D. Crohn's disease

14. A stationary blood clot that has formed within a blood vessel is known as

    A. an embolus
    B. a hematoma
    C. a thrombus
    D. a hemangioma

15. The natural anastomosis located at the base of the brain is the

    A. azygos system
    B. circle of Willis
    C. palmar arch
    D. carotid sinus

16. The knee is correctly described as

    1. a hinge joint
    2. formed by the femur, tibia, fibula, and patella
    3. a synovial joint

    A. 1 and 2
    B. 1 and 3
    C. 2 and 3
    D. 1, 2, and 3

17. Neurons can be classified according to their function. Which of the following types of neurons conduct impulses from the brain and spinal cord to muscles?

    A. Afferent
    B. Efferent
    C. Association
    D. Sensory

18. A condition in which the lungs are partially or entirely airless or functionless is known as

    A. pneumothorax
    B. atelectasis
    C. apnea
    D. emphysema

19. Which of the following statements concerning the digestive tract is NOT true?

    A. The ileum is the longest segment of the alimentary canal
    B. The innermost layer of the wall of the digestive tract is the mucosa
    C. Peristalsis inhibits movement of gastrointestinal contents
    D. Rugae are longitudinal folds prominent in the stomach

20. The first cervical vertebra is known as the

    A. atlas
    B. dens
    C. prominens
    D. axis

21. The movement of water through a cell membrane from an area of higher to lower concentration is called

    A. active transport
    B. absorption
    C. osmosis
    D. facilitated diffusion

22. Which of the following are classified as irregular bones?

    1. Sphenoid
    2. Patellae
    3. Lumbar vertebrae

    A. 1 and 2
    B. 1 and 3
    C. 2 and 3
    D. 1, 2, and 3

23. The obturator foramen is bounded by which of the following bones?

    1. Pubis
    2. Ischium
    3. Ilium

    A. 1 and 2
    B. 1 and 3
    C. 2 and 3
    D. 1, 2, and 3

24. Which of the following may cause intestinal obstruction?

    1. Adhesions
    2. Strangulated hernia
    3. Intussusception

    A. 1 and 2
    B. 1 and 3
    C. 2 and 3
    D. 1, 2, and 3

25. The mitral valve of the heart is correctly described as

      1. located between the left atrium and ventricle
      2. having three cusps, which prevent backward flow
      3. closed during ventricular diastole

  A. 1 only
  B. 2 only
  C. 3 only
  D. 1, 2, and 3

26. Arthritis characterized by inflammation and thickening of the synovial membrane, pain, swelling, joint dysfunction, and bilateral joint involvement is known as

      1. osteoarthritis
      2. rheumatoid arthritis
      3. gout

  A. 1 only
  B. 2 only
  C. 3 only
  D. 1, 2, and 3

27. The abdominopelvic cavity can be thought of as divided into nine regions by two imaginary horizontal and two sagittal planes. The region that contains the cecum and part of the small intestine is the

  A. right hypochondriac
  B. umbilical
  C. right inguinal
  D. right lumbar

Questions 28–32 consist of four lettered headings followed by a list of numbered words. For each hormone listed below, select the name of the endocrine gland that secretes it. Each heading may be used once, more than once, or not at all.

  A. Pituitary
  B. Pancreas
  C. Adrenals
  D. Thyroid

28. Growth hormone

29. Epinephrine

30. Prolactin

31. Insulin

32. Mineralocorticoids

Questions 33–38 refer to the following anatomical sketch of a foot, which certain parts have been labeled with numbers. Each of the following questions is followed by four suggested labels or answers. For each question, select the one best answer.

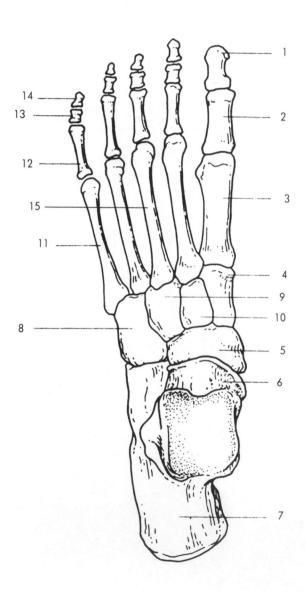

33. The cuboid is the structure labeled with the number

    A. 4
    B. 5
    C. 7
    D. 8

34. The calcaneus is the structure labeled with the number

    A. 5
    B. 6
    C. 7
    D. 9

35. The lateral cuneiform is labeled with the number

    A. 4
    B. 9
    C. 10
    D. 15

36. The navicular bone is the structure labeled with the number

    A. 5
    B. 9
    C. 10
    D. 11

37. The talus, or astragalus, is the structure labeled with the number

    A. 3
    B. 6
    C. 9
    D. 10

38. The first metatarsal is labeled with the number

    A. 1
    B. 3
    C. 4
    D. 11

Questions 39–44 refer to the following figure, which is an AP projection of an abdomen taken after intravenous injection of radiopaque contrast medium. Certain parts of the radiograph have been labeled with numbers. Each of the following questions is followed by four suggested labels or answers. For each question, select the one best answer.

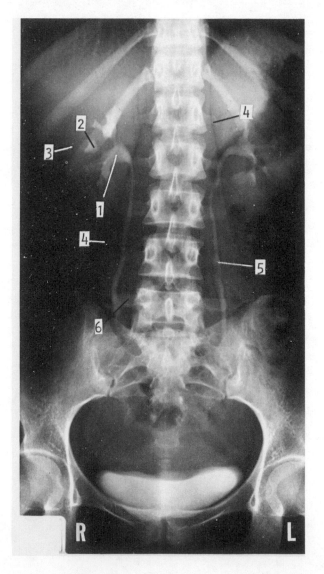

39. The structure labeled with the number 1 is the

    A. ureter
    B. calyx
    C. renal pelvis
    D. nephron

40. The structure labeled with the number 2 is the

    A. calyx
    B. trigone
    C. papilla
    D. pyramid

41. The structure labeled with the number 3 is the

    A. medulla
    B. pelvis
    C. cortex
    D. capsule

42. The structure labeled with the number 4 is the

    A. psoas muscle
    B. latissimus dorsi
    C. renal fascia
    D. rectus abdominis

43. The structure labeled with the number 5 is the

    A. urethra
    B. ureter
    C. collecting tubule
    D. convoluted tubule

44. The structure labeled with the number 6 is the

    A. spinous process
    B. lamina
    C. pedicle
    D. transverse process

Questions 45–48 refer to the radiograph that follows, which is a CT scan taken through the abdomen after oral ingestion of contrast medium. Certain parts of the scan have been labeled with numbers. Each of the following questions is followed by four suggested labels or answers. For each question, select the one best answer.

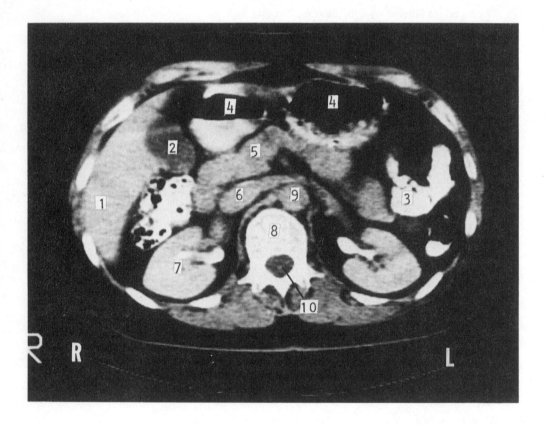

45. The kidney is the structure labeled with the number

    A. 1
    B. 2
    C. 5
    D. 7

46. The pancreas is the structure labeled with the number

    A. 3
    B. 4
    C. 5
    D. 6

47. The aorta is the structure labeled with the number

    A. 4
    B. 6
    C. 9
    D. 10

48. The liver is the structure labeled with the number

    A. 1
    B. 2
    C. 3
    D. 4

POSTTEST—ANATOMY AND PHYSIOLOGY
ANSWERS, EXPLANATIONS, AND REFERENCES

1. The answer is B.   The kidneys are located in the abdomen, behind the peritoneum, lying obliquely between the levels of the last thoracic and third lumbar vertebrae in the typical (sthenic) person. The kidneys are composed of an inner medullary substance containing renal pyramids and collecting tubules, through which urine passes. The outer, compact substance of the kidneys is the cortex, which is between the medulla and the renal capsule. The renal capsule is surrounded by an adipose capsule and is enclosed by fibrous connective tissue called renal fascia. The capsules of the kidneys have a protective function, helping to guard against trauma and spread of infection. The parenchyma of the kidneys consists of microscopic units called nephrons, which function to filter blood, remove wastes, and produce glomerular filtrate. The majority of nephrons are situated in the cortex, and the remainder are found in the medullary substance. *(Ballinger [Vol. 3], p 688-689; Hole, p 750-755; Tortora and Anagnostakos, p 658-663, 667)*

2. The answer is C.   If an opaque contrast agent is injected into the inferior vena cava (the large vein that brings deoxygenated blood back to the heart), a sequence of opacified anatomic structures can be visualized fluoroscopically or recorded on cine film or videotape. According to normal anatomic structure, the contrast agent would pass from the right atrium of the heart to the right ventricle, into the pulmonary arteries of the lungs, into the pulmonary veins, left atrium of the heart, left ventricle, and then into the large artery emerging from the heart, called the aorta. It should be noted that the contrast medium will follow the passage of blood and will normally flow through a series of valves within the heart. *(Hole, p 657-658; Tortora and Anagnostakos, p 458)*

3. The answer is B.   Synarthrodial joints are immovable (synarthrosis) and include such joints as the sutures of the skull and the roots of the teeth. Diarthrodial joints are freely movable (diathrosis); examples of this type of joint include the elbow and knee. Amphiarthrodial joints are only slightly movable (amphiarthrosis); the symphysis pubis and intervertebral joints are classified as such. A synovial joint is a type of diarthrodial or freely movable joint that has a specific fluid-filled structure (bursa) between the articulating bones. The hip and shoulder joints are classified as synovial, diarthrodial joints. *(Chaffee et al., p 116-119; Hole, p 226-227; Tortora and Anagnostakos, p 180-181)*

4–5. The answers are 4-B, 5-C.   Papillae are small nipple-like projections or elevations found on or within certain body parts. The circumvallate papillae are arranged in an inverted V configuration on the posterior portion of the tongue. These papillae, along with most of the fungiform papillae, contain taste buds that perceive sweet, sour, salty, and bitter flavors. Papillae of the tongue also provide a roughened surface and, together with muscles, help maneuver food. The papilla of Vater, or duodenal papilla, is located in the descending segment of the duodenum and can be visualized (endoscopically) within the duodenal lumen at the point where the common bile and pancreatic ducts enter. Liver and pancreatic secretions enter into the duodenum at this area. If this area should become pathologically obstructed by a stone or tumor, secretions may back up into the organs and produce various symptoms such as pain and jaundice. The papilla of Vater is important to locate during endoscopic retrograde cholangiopancreatography, a procedure performed in radiology to demonstrate the bile and pancreatic ducts. Cannulation of the papilla of Vater is necessary in order to inject contrast medium into the ductal system during E.R.C.P. *(Bontrager, p 484; Meschan, p 455-456; Tortora and Anagnostakos, p 375, 587-589, 604-605)*

6. The answer is B.   The internal carotid arteries and vertebral arteries are responsible for supplying blood to the brain. The internal carotid arteries are bilateral branches of the common carotid arteries in the neck. The internal carotid arteries ascend through the cervical region and enter the cranial cavity, where they send off numerous branches that supply the anterior and medial portions of the brain, as well as the eyeballs. The vertebral arteries are branches off the left and right subclavian arteries. They ascend through the foramina of the cervical vertebrae and then enter the cranium through the foramen magnum, where they unite to form a single, basilar artery. The vertebral-basilar system of arteries gives off branches that supply structures of the neck and posterior portions of the brain. Both the internal carotid and vertebral-basilar arteries enter a common arterial anastomosis at the base of the brain, called the circle of Willis. The external carotid arteries also arise from the common carotid arteries in the neck, but they are responsible for supplying blood to structures outside the brain—the face, the scalp, and the neck. All of the arteries listed above carry richly oxygenated blood to structures within the head and neck, but the internal carotid and vertebral arteries are the ones responsible for transporting oxygen to the brain. *(Hole, p 692-693; Tortora and Anagnostakos, p 496-497)*

7. The answer is A.   The dermis is the true layer of skin, or cutaneous membrane, containing blood vessels, glands, nerves, connective tissue, and muscular tissue. It is the thick part of the integumentary system that lies between the thinner epidermis (outermost layer of skin) and the subcutaneous layer (deep layer containing adipose tissue). The skin serves important functions in providing protection for the body against pathogenic organisms, preventing the loss of internal materials, helping to maintain body temperature, receiving external stimuli, and excreting water and wastes. Synovial membranes do not contain epithelium; they function as linings for certain joint cavities. Synovial membranes secrete a lubricating fluid called synovia, which promotes movement at joints and provides nourishmment to the articular cartilage. *(Hole, p 126; Tortora and Anagnostakos, p 99, 106-113)*

8. The answer is A.   The true, or lesser, pelvis is that part of the pelvis situated below the pelvic brim. The pelvic brim is an imaginary boundary line extending from the upper anterior border of the sacrum to the upper border of the symphysis pubis, separating the false (greater) pelvis above from the true (lesser) pelvis below. The pelvic brim is measured in all directions during pelvimetry examinations in order to evaluate its size in relation to the fetus, as the fetus must pass through openings in the pelvis during birth. The upper opening into the true pelvis formed by the pelvic brim is called the pelvic inlet, and the lower opening is the pelvic outlet; between these lies the pelvic cavity. *(Ballinger [Vol. 1], p 95; Tortora and Anagnostakos, p 170)*

9. The answer is C.   The stapes (stirrup), one of three small middle ear bones (auditory ossicles), attaches to the oval window portion of the inner ear. As the stapes vibrates against the oval window, inner ear fluids are set into motion, stimulating hearing receptors. The malleus (hammer) is another ossicle of the middle ear and is attached to the tympanic membrane (eardrum) of the outer ear area, which vibrates synchronously as the eardrum receives sound waves. The vibrations of the malleus are conducted to the incus (anvil), another ossicle of the middle ear, which finally passes the vibrations on to the innermost ossicle, the stapes. The cochlea is part of the labyrinth in the inner ear. *(Chaffee et al., p 277-279; Hole, p 401-404; Tortora and Anagnostakos, p 389-392)*

10. The answer is D.   Epithelial, nervous, and muscular tissue, along with connective tissue, are considered to be the four primary types of body tissues, based on their function and composition. Each primary tissue type can be further categorized into subtypes. Epithelial tissue is further divided into glandular epithelium (forms the secretory portion of glands) and covering and lining epithelium (forms the outer covering of external body surfaces as well as the covering for some internal organs). Glandular epithelium and covering and lining epithelium can be further classified according to specific structure or function. Nervous tissue coordinates body activities through generation and transmission of impulses. Nervous tissue comprises two principle types of cells, neurons and neuroglia. Neurons are the specialized cells that allow conduction of impulses, regulation of glands, activity of muscles, and the process of thinking. Neuroglia form the supportive and protective portion of nervous tissue. Muscular tissue enables movement of the body and is further categorized into muscle subtypes: skeletal (forms the major portion of the muscular system that enables body movement through individual muscle group activity), cardiac (specialized muscle tissue of the heart), and smooth or visceral muscle (forming the wall of various internal organs such as bladder and intestines). Connective tissue, the most abundant primary tissue, helps to protect and support the body and its organs. Connective tissue is classified into two major types, embryonic (exists in the fetus before birth) and adult connective tissue (exists in the newborn and does not change after birth); each of these can be further subdivided into subtypes according to their specific function or structure. Subtypes of adult connective tissue include connective tissue proper, cartilage, bone tissue, and vascular tissue. *(Chaffee et al., p 67; Hole, p 104; Tortora and Anagnostakos, p 82-98, 204, 268-269)*

11. The answer is A. The greater curvature forms the convex lateral wall of the stomach nearest the left side. The pyloric antrum is the lowermost portion of the stomach, which eventually communicates with the duodenum (first portion of the small intestine); the opening between these parts is surrounded by a muscle called the pyloric sphincter. The lesser curvature forms the concave medial border of the stomach, and the fundus is the superior portion of the stomach located above and to the left of the gastroesophageal junction. The body of the stomach constitutes the largest portion and is that part between the fundus and the pylorus. *(Tortora and Anagnostakos, p 597-598; Chaffee et al., p 438)*

12. The answer is C. The greater cornu (horns) are not part of the temporal bones of the skull but form the lateral margins of the hyoid bone, which is situated at the base of the tongue, in the superior portion of the neck. The temporal bones are located bilateral to the sphenoid bone and in front of the occipital bone. Each contains many important parts, including a mastoid portion, squamous portion, tympanic portion, pars petrosa, and styloid process. The pars petrosa, or petrous portion, contains the organ of hearing. This consists of numerous small bones, membranes, and canals, along with sensory and auditory apparatus, which allow for hearing and maintenance of equilibrium. *(Ballinger [Vol. 2], p 370-373; Meschan, p 222, 225, 241, 419)*

13. The answer is A. Diverticulosis is the presence of numerous saclike outpouchings, whereas multiple polyposis is a condition in which numerous new growths of mucous membrane have occurred. Diverticulosis usually occurs in the colon (large intestine) when the muscular layer of the wall becomes weak. This condition may lead to inflammation of one or more diverticula, producing a condition called diverticulitis. An aneurysm is an outpouching or dilatation of a weakened blood vessel wall; there are several types, including berry, fusiform, sacculated, and dissecting. Crohn's disease has an unknown cause and is characterized by severe inflammatory changes, fibrosis, and thickening of the intestinal wall, most often involving the terminal ileum. *(Cawson et al., p 205, 342, 349, 358; Austrin, p 139, 187, 188; Tortora and Anagnostakos, p 513, 624)*

14. The answer is C. A thrombus is an aggregation of blood elements that has formed within and attaches to the inner wall of an artery or vein; this process of clotting in an unbroken vessel is called thrombosis. A thrombus may dissolve spontaneously or may require medical treatment including a variety of anticoagulant and fibrinolytic drugs. If a thrombus remains within the vessel lumen, it may occlude the vessel, cutting off oxygen supply and damaging tissues. A piece of thrombus that breaks away and circulates through the bloodstream is referred to as an embolus, which may eventually occlude smaller vessels. Embolism is the lodgment of an embolus in a vessel, with subsequent curtailment of circulation. An embolus may be composed of other substances besides blood, such as fat, tumor cells, bacteria, air, or foreign material, differentiating it from a thrombus or hematoma, which consists primarily of blood elements. Severe damage or death may result when a thrombus or embolus occludes vessels leading to vital organs such as the brain, heart, and lungs. A hematoma is a collection of extravasated blood and is caused by injury to the skin tissue or an organ; it may become hardened, palpable, swollen, and painful. A hemangioma is a benign tumor of dilated blood vessels. *(Tortora and Anagnostakos, p 446; Gylys and Wedding, p 140; Frenay and Mahoney, p 135; Wroble, p 255)*

15. The answer is B. The circle of Willis is the normal arterial anastomosis at the base of the brain that connects the vertebral artery and the internal carotid artery systems. This union is important because it provides alternate pathways through which blood can reach the brain in the event of a blocked artery. The azygos system is the collection of veins in the thorax that receive venous tributaries from organs in the chest; it also provides a connection between the superior and inferior vena cavae. The palmar arch is a network of arteries in the hand area where branches of the radial and ulnar arteries come together. The carotid sinus is the expanded portion near the base of the internal carotid artery where pressoreceptors are located. *(Hole, p 693-695; Tortora and Anagnostakos, p 496-497, 506-507; Chaffee et al., p 338-339)*

16. The answer is B. The knee is the largest joint in the body, comprising three bones and three different articulations. The three bones of the knee joint are the femur, tibia, and patella. The patella, or kneecap, articulates with the patellar surface of the distal femur, and the medial and lateral condyles of the tibia articulate with the medial and lateral condyles of the femur. The knee joint is a freely movable synovial joint consisting of numerous ligaments, a medial and lateral meniscus (fibrocartilage disks), and bursae. The knee joint allows for flexion and extension at the tibiofemoral articulations and is therefore classified, according to its movement, as a hinge joint. The patellofemoral articulation is classified as a gliding joint, according to its movement. The fibula does not enter into the knee joint but does articulate with the lateral condyle of the tibia proximally. The knee joint is often subject to athletic injuries and arthritis and is therefore radiographed quite often. *(Hole, p 221-224, 227, 233-234; Tortora and Anagnostakos, p 171, 181-182, 194-195)*

17. The answer is B. Efferent, or motor, neurons are responsible for conducting impulses from the brain and spinal cord (central nervous system) to muscle or gland effectors. These impulses may stimulate muscles to contract and glands to secrete. Afferent, or sensory, neurons conduct impulses toward the brain and spinal cord from receptors located in sense organs, internal organs, skin, and skeletal muscles. Association neurons, or interneurons, found within the brain and spinal cord, are responsible for conducting impulses between various parts of the brain or spinal cord as they connect afferent (sensory) to efferent (motor) neurons. Neurons not only differ in their function but vary in structure as well; unipolar neurons have one process extending from their cell bodies, bipolar neurons give rise to two processes, and multipolar neurons give rise to numerous processes. Neurons are the important functional and structural units of nerve tissue; they play an integral part in the body's muscular and glandular activities, as well as in the thinking process. *(Hole, p 308, 325-326; Tortora and Anagnostakos, p 273)*

18. The answer is B. Atelectasis is a condition in which a lung or part of a lung is airless or collapsed. It may be caused by bronchial obstruction (air is absorbed distal to obstruction) or may result from extrinsic pressure exerted on the lung (abnormal fluid or air in the pleural cavity may do this). Atelectasis may also occur in neonates whose lungs fail to expand because of lack of surfactant. Pneumothorax is the abnormal entrance of air into the pleural cavity, outside the lungs. A pneumothorax may be caused by trauma or disease, which can compress the lungs and produce atelectasis. Apnea is a temporary absence of respirations. Emphysema is overaeration of tissues, as seen in pulmonary emphysema when alveoli become abnormally distended with air because of obstruction of distal or proximal air passageways. Emphysema is a serious, chronic lung disease in which the alveoli lose their elasticity and remain filled with air during expiration; this may result in alveolar damage, hyperinflation of the lungs, and reduced expiratory volume. *(Austrin, p 167-169; Cawson et al., p 270-271; Hole, p 582-583, 588, 603-604; Tortora and Anagnostakos, p 559, 575)*

19. The answer is C. Peristalsis does not inhibit gastrointestinal movement but produces movement by alternating waves of contraction and dilatation of the muscular wall. Peristalsis is involuntary and is under the control of the medulla oblongata. Peristalsis begins in the upper esophagus and continues throughout the gastrointestinal tract, moving its contents along toward the end of the canal. The alimentary, or digestive, canal extends from the mouth to the anus and consists of many parts. The longest segment of the canal is the ileum, the last portion of the small intestine, measuring approximately 12 feet in length. The digestive tract is composed of four major layers; from the inside out, they are the mucosa, submucosa, muscularis, and serosa. The outer layer of the esophageal wall, however, does not consist of serosa but a loose connective tissue layer called adventitia. Rugae are longitudinal folds of the mucosa, which are prominent in the stomach. They are best demonstrated when the stomach is empty, as the folds collapse and become more pronounced. When the stomach is full, the rugae stretch out. *(Hole, p 482, 492-493, 507-508; Tortora and Anagnostakos, p 584-585, 595-599, 610)*

20. The answer is A.   The first cervical vertebra, or atlas, is a ringlike structure that has no body or spinous process, making it unique in structure compared with the other vertebrae. Its function is to support and balance the head. The second cervical vertebra, or axis, has a large conical process called the odontoid, or dens, arising from the superior aspect of its body. The dens articulates above with the ring of the atlas serving as a pivot. The prominens is the long, protruding spinous process of the seventh cervical vertebra, which can be palpated at the base of the neck through the skin. *(Ballinger [Vol. 1], p 204-205; Hole, p 206-207; Tortora and Anagnostakos, p 154-155)*

21. The answer is C.   Osmosis is the movement of water through a selectively permeable membrane, from an area of higher to lower concentration of water. Cell membranes provide a means by which various substances can pass into and out of the cell. These movements that allow for passage include osmosis, diffusion, filtration, facilitated diffusion, phagocytosis, pinocytosis, and active transport. Active transport involves the passage of substances through a membrane, from an area of low concentration to higher concentration. In order to move substances across this concentration gradient, adenosine triphosphate provides energy to the cell membrane. Facilitated diffusion involves the passage of certain substances by carriers at the membrane's surface through the membrane. Before combining with the carrier, the substance would not normally be soluble in the phospholipid portion of the membrane; however, once it combines with a soluble carrier, it can be passed through the selectively permeable membrane into the cell. Absorption refers to intake of various substances and fluids by skin or mucous membrane cells. An example of this can be found in the small intestine, where numerous villi in the mucous membrane absorb digestive products from the lumen of the intestine into blood and lymph capillaries. *(Hole, p 10, 54-62; Tortora and Anagnostakos, p 53-57, 87)*

22. The answer is B.   Irregular bones are classified as such because their unusual shape prevents them from fitting into the other categories of bone types. The sphenoid bone and vertebrae fall into the category of irregular bones, as their configurations are unusual and prevent their being classified as long, short, flat, or sesamoid. Lumbar vertebrae consist of a drumlike body with processes extending laterally and posteriorly; their superior and inferior processes articulate with vertebrae above and below. The sphenoid resembles a wedge with winglike extensions, lying in the skull's floor and articulating with all the other bones of the cranium. The patellae are located anteriorly to the knee joint, bilaterally. They are classified as a separate bone type called sesamoid, or round, bones. Sesamoid bones usually develop in tendons near a joint. Small sesamoids are often found in the joints of the digits where the tendons receive compression. *(Ballinger [Vol. 2], p 366; Hole, p 176-177, 196-197, 205-208; Tortora and Anagnostakos, p 138, 145, 151-155)*

23. The answer is C.   The obturator foramen is a large opening in the lower portion of the innominate bone, below the hip joint. The obturator foramen is bounded and formed by the rami of the pubis (anteriorly) and ischium (posteriorly). Its construction should not be confused with that of the acetabulum (the cuplike socket in the innominate bone that receives the femoral head, constituting the hip joint), as it is formed by the union of parts of the ilium, ischium, and pubis. *(Ballinger [Vol. 1], p 92; Tortora and Anagnostakos, p 170-171)*

24. The answer is D.   Intestinal (bowel) obstruction results from a mechanical blockage or peristaltic dysfunction that does not allow for the normal passage of bowel contents. Causes of obstruction include adhesions, strangulated hernia, volvulus, intussusception, tumor, and stricture. Adhesions, or fibrous bands that may form in the abdomen as a result of infection or surgical trauma, may cause parts that are normally separate to fuse together. A strangulated hernia results when blood supply is curtailed from a protruding loop of intestine, causing infarction and possibly gangrene and thereby producing obstruction. Intussusception is the slipping of one segment of intestine into another, or invagination; this may cause obstruction or infarction. Surgical treatment of the problems listed above is usually necessary to reduce the obstruction and any further consequence. *(Cawson et al., p 65, 351-353)*

25. The answer is A.   The mitral, or biscupid, valve is the left atrioventricular valve in the heart. It contains two leaflets, which prevent blood from flowing back to the atrium from the ventricle on the left side. The mitral valve opens during ventricular diastole, allowing freshly oxygenated blood from the left atrium to flow into the left ventricle. The mitral valve may become diseased as a result of rheumatic fever, producing a murmur; it may also be pushed too far back during contraction, causing mitral valve prolapse. *(Tortora and Anagnostakos, p 461, 470; Hole, p 655, 661)*

26. The answer is B.   Rheumatoid arthritis is the most common form of inflammatory arthritis, involving synovial membrane thickening and accumulation of fluid in the joint, resulting in pain and tenderness. The articular cartilages at the ends of the bones may become damaged, fibrous tissue may invade the involved joints, and fusion of the bones of the joint may develop, thereby preventing normal movement. Osteoarthritis is a degenerative joint disease resulting from a combination of wear and tear on joints, irritation, and the aging process. Osteoarthritis is charac- terized by breakdown of the articular cartilage, decreased mobility of the joint, and pain on movement. Gout is a form of arthritis that results from an accumulation of uric acid in the blood, followed by the formation of urate crystals and their deposition in joints and soft tissues, with subsequent inflammation. *(Cawson et al., p 426-434; Hole, p 235, 768; Tortora and Anagnostakos, p 199-200)*

27. The answer is C.   The cecum, appendix, and terminal ileum are located in the right inguinal (iliac) region of the abdomen. The nine divisions include the two upper lateral regions, or left and right hypochondriac; between these lie the epigastric region. Below the epigastric region is the umbilical region, with the left and right lumbar regions on either side. The region below the umbilicus is the hypogastric, surrounded laterally by the left and right inguinal (iliac) regions. (Refer to the figure that accompanies the explanation to question 66 in the body of the text for a diagrammatic representation of these regions.) *(Tortora and Anagnostakos, p 19-20; Ballinger [Vol. 3], p 569)*

28. The answer is A.   Growth hormone (somatotropin) is secreted by the anterior pituitary (adenohypophysis). By increasing the rate at which amino acids enter cells and their ability to convert molecules into proteins, growth hormone stimulates the growth and multiplication of body cells, especially those of the bones and skeletal muscles. An oversecretion of growth hormone may result in developmental diseases such as acromegaly (overgrowth of bone width of hands, feet, and face) and gigantism (overgrowth of bone length resulting in excess height). An undersecretion of growth hormone may produce dwarfism, a condition in which bones do not grow to their expected length. *(Tortora and Anagnostakos, p 407; Hole, p 446-447; Austrin, p 240)*

29. The answer is C.   The adrenal medulla secretes epinephrine (adrenalin) and its related hormone, norepinephrine (noradrenalin). Epinephrine makes up approximately 80% of the total secretion of this gland and is considered more potent than norepinephrine. The effects of these medullary hormones include increasing blood pressure, heart rate, blood sugar concentration, respiratory rate, and airway size. Epinephrine is important in helping the body meet stressful situations by stimulating the sympathetic nervous system. *(Tortora and Anagnostakos, p 421; Hole, p 457-459; Austrin, p 243)*

30. The answer is A.   Prolactin, secreted by the anterior pituitary, functions to stimulate milk production in females. It is responsible for maintaining milk production after the birth of an infant. The actual ejection of milk from the mammary glands is controlled by another hormone, oxytocin, which is stored in the posterior pituitary. Both hormones function together during lactation. *(Tortora and Anagnostakos, p 409; Hole, p 447; Austrin, p 241)*

31. The answer is B.   Insulin, along with glucagon, is secreted by the islets of Langerhans in the pancreas. Insulin is important in storing and using carbohydrates and plays a role in reducing the amount of glucose in the blood by accelerating its transport into body cells. A deficiency of this hormone may result in a common disease, diabetes mellitus. Glucagon's action is opposite to that of insulin; it raises the blood sugar level by accelerating the conversion of glycogen into glucose. *(Tortora and Anagnostakos, p 421-424; Hole, p 462-465; Austrin, p 243)*

32. The answer is C.   Mineralocorticoids are secreted by the adrenal cortex; their chief function is to control the concentrations of extracellular electrolytes. One of the most important mineralocorticoids is aldosterone, which acts on the kidneys to maintain the homeostasis of potassium and sodium ions, conserve water, and reduce urine output. Besides mineralocorticoids, the adrenal cortex secretes glucocorticoids, which help regulate the metabolism of proteins, carbohydrates, and fats. Gonadocorticoids, or sex hormones, affect sexual characteristics of both males and females. *(Tortora and Anagnostakos, p 417-421; Hole, p 459-460; Austrin, p 243)*

33–38. The answers are 33-D, 34-C, 35-B, 36-A, 37-B, 38-B.   In the anatomical sketch of the foot that accompanies the question, the following bones are identified: (1) distal phalanx of first toe, (2) proximal phalanx of first toe, (3) first metatarsal, (4) medial, or first, cuneiform, (5) navicular, (6) talus, (7) calcaneus, (8) cuboid, (9) lateral, or third, cuneiform, (10) intermediate, or second, cuneiform (11) fifth metatarsal, (12) proximal phalanx of fifth toe, (13) middle phalanx of fifth toe, (14) distal phalanx of fifth toe, and (15) third metatarsal. The foot is similar to the hand in structure and consists of 7 tarsal bones, 5 metatarsals, and 14 phalanges. The calcaneus is the largest tarsal bone and is located on the posterior part of the foot, forming the base of the heel. The calcaneus helps to bear the weight of the body and serves as an attachment site for muscles that move the foot. The talus is the uppermost tarsal bone and is located on the posterior part of the foot, medially and on top of the calcaneus. It articulates with the tibia and fibula, forming the ankle joint, and anteriorly with the navicular bone. Unlike the other tarsal bones, which are firmly bound together, the talus moves freely where it meets the tibia and fibula. During walking, the talus first supports the entire weight of the lower extremity then transmits half the weight to the calcaneus, and the remainder of weight is shifted to the other tarsal bones. The navicular articulates with the talus posteriorly and joins the three cuneiform bones anteriorly. It is located on the medial aspect of the foot. The cuboid lies in front of the calcaneus and behind the fourth and fifth metatarsal bones. The three cuneiform bones, composing the tarsus of the foot, lie on its medial aspect. The medial cuneiform lies in front of the navicular and behind the first metatarsal. The intermediate cuneiform lies next to the medial cuneiform, anterior to the navicular and posterior to the second metatarsal. The lateral cuneiform lies between the intermediate cuneiform and cuboid bone, in front of the navicular and behind the third metatarsal bones. The metatarsals are numbered one through five, beginning on the medial aspect of the foot. Each metatarsal bone consists of a head (distally), shaft, and base (proximally). The five metatarsal bones articulate with the three cuneiform bones and the cuboid proximally and with the proximal row of the phalanges distally. The heads, or distal ends, of the metatarsals form the ball of the foot. The phalanges form the toes; each phalanx consists of a base (proximally), a shaft, and a head (distally). The first, or great, toe has only two phalanges, called proximal and distal phalanges. Each of the other four toes (digits) consists of three phalanges— proximal, middle (intermediate), and distal. The proximal row of phalanges in the foot articulates with the five metatarsal bones. *(Tortora and Anagnostakos, p 171-175; Hole, p 224-226; Ballinger [Vol. 1], p 33-38; Meschan, p 92-93; McInnes, p 79)*

39–44. The answers are 39-C, 40-A, 41-C, 42-A, 43-B, 44-D. The radiograph that accompanies the questions is an excretory urogram taken after intravenous injection of radiopaque contrast medium in an effort to demonstrate some of the functional and structural components of the urinary system. This AP projection of the abdomen demonstrates the collecting system of the kidneys, ureters, and bladder, as well as the soft tissues and bones of the abdominopelvic cavities. The following structures are identified: (1) renal pelvis, (2) calyx, (3) cortex, (4) psoas muscle, (5) ureter, and (6) transverse process. The kidneys are located bilateral to the spine, behind the peritoneum, in an oblique plane between the last thoracic vertebra and the first three lumbar vertebrae; position may vary between individuals of different body builds. The kidney substance is composed of an outer cortex and an inner medulla and is surrounded by an adipose capsule and embedded in a sheath of fascia. The cortex lies between the medullary substance and the capsule. It contains millions of microscopic units (nephrons) that filter blood and form urine. The nephron gives rise to renal tubules, which empty urine into collecting tubules. The medullary substance of the kidneys lies between the cortex and calyces and contains numerous collecting tubules arranged in clusters called renal pyramids. The apices of the renal pyramids convey urine into the minor calyces, then into major calyces. The calyces are the cup-shaped portions of the collecting system that convey urine into the funnel-shaped renal pelvis. The calyces and renal pelvis can usually be seen quite well on an intravenous urogram, as the contrast agent follows the same course as the urine, opacifying structures of the collecting system. From the renal pelvis, urine passes into the ureter, a tube approximately 10 to 12 inches long (one from each kidney). The ureters descend behind the peritoneum, in front of the psoas muscle and transverse processes of the lumbar spine and inferiorly curve anteriorly and medially to enter the posterolateral walls of the urinary bladder. The urinary bladder lies in the pelvic cavity and serves as a reservoir for urine. The trigone is the smooth area located at the base of the bladder. It is bounded by two ureteral orifices to the sides and one internal urethral orifice at its apex below. The urethral orifice opens into the urethra, the tube that conveys urine from the bladder to the exterior. The urinary bladder, along with the ureters, can be seen opacified with contrast medium on the radiograph that accompanies the question. Usually, however, the urethra can only be visualized if the patient expels the contrast-laden urine from the bladder during radiography. *(Ballinger [Vol. 3], p 688-697; Meschan, p 356-373; Tortora and Anagnostakos, p 658-663, 677-679; Hole, p 750-758, 770-773)*

45–48. The answers are 45-D, 46-C, 47-C, 48-A. The CT scan that accompanies the question is taken through the abdomen and is a cross-sectional look at the abdominal viscera after oral ingestion of contrast medium. The following structures are identified: (1) liver, (2) gallbladder, (3) small intestine, (4) stomach, (5) pancreas, (6) inferior vena cava, (7) right kidney, (8) vertebral body, (9) aorta, and (10) spinal cord. The hollow organs of the ailmentary canal can be seen filled with air and fluid contrast. The liver is a large, solid organ that occupies a considerable portion of the right side of the upper to mid abdomen. Situated within a fossa on the inferior border of the liver is the gallbladder. The gastrointestinal tract lies within the peritoneum in the anterior portion of the abdomen. Due to the ingestion of opaque contrast medium, this scan reveals air-fluid levels in parts of the gastrointestinal tract. The pancreas is located behind the peritoneum, its head lying close to the duodenal sweep and its tail extending toward the spleen, on the left. The aorta is visualized as a round density just anterior and slightly to the left of the vertebral body. The kidneys lie bilateral to the vertebral body, behind the peritoneum. The inferior vena cava is located anterior to and to the right of the vertebral body, adjacent to the liver. The renal veins can be visualized coming from the hilum of the kidneys and joining the inferior vena cava. The vertebral body is easily seen in the midline posteriorly, with a round lucent area in its posterior section representing the vertebral foramen and spinal cord. The spleen is located adjacent to the left kidney on the left side of the upper abdomen, behind the stomach. It is not easily seen on this scan, as this slice was taken just below the level of the spleen. *(Chiu and Schapiro, p 40, 42, 140-143; Meschan, p 542-543)*

RADIOGRAPHIC POSITIONING AND PROCEDURES

49. Medial and lateral oblique projections of the ankle require that the ankle be positioned at an angle of

A. 25°
B. 35°
C. 45°
D. 55°

50. Which of the following projections or positions are useful in visually "unraveling" the coiled loops of sigmoid colon during a barium enema examination?

1. PA with caudal central ray angulation of 35°
2. AP with Trendelenburg table
3. LPO with a cephalic central ray angulation of 35°

A. 1 and 2
B. 1 and 3
C. 2 and 3
D. 1, 2, and 3

51. An axiolateral (transaxillary) projection of the shoulder joint is obtained by

1. abducting the affected arm and placing the film under the axilla
2. abducting the affected arm and placing the film superior to the shoulder joint
3. abducting the unaffected arm and placing the hand above the head with the film in contact with the humerus of the affected side

A. 1 and 2
B. 1 and 3
C. 2 and 3
D. 1, 2, and 3

52. In which of the following projections and methods are the maxillary sinuses projected to their best advantage?

A. PA axial/Caldwell
B. PA oblique/Rhese
C. Verticosubmental/Schüller
D. Parietoacanthial/Waters

53. The position during an upper gastrointestinal series that will best demonstrate the duodenal cap and pylorus in most body builds resembling the sthenic type is

A. supine
B. right lateral
C. RAO
D. prone

54. The right sacroiliac joint is best demonstrated with the patient in which of the following positions?

    A. 25° LAO

    B. 30° RPO

    C. 30° RAO

    D. 45° LPO

55. Stratification of gallstones can be visualized radiographically by obtaining which of the following positions?

    A. Anterior oblique

    B. Posterior oblique

    C. Erect and decubitus

    D. Lateral

56. Chest radiographs taken during expiration are useful in demonstrating

    A. pneumothorax

    B. empyema

    C. effusion

    D. rib fractures

57. The difference between the angulation of the central ray in the Lysholm, Schüller, and Henschen methods of an axiolateral cranial projection is

    A. 5°

    B. 7°

    C. 10°

    D. 15°

58. Patient rotation can be quickly evaluated in a frontal view of the chest by

    A. the curvature of the thoracic spine

    B. the presence of scapulae in the lung fields

    C. sternoclavicular joint asymmetry

    D. the height of the clavicles

59. In the lateral projection of the wrist, the patient should be positioned so that the

    A. elbow is flexed 90°

    B. entire arm is extended

    C. wrist is in ulnar flexion

    D. wrist is in radial flexion

60. The major difference between excretory, or descending, urography (intravenous pyelography) and retrograde, or ascending, urography (retrograde pyelography) is that

    A. they each require a different type of contrast medium

    B. retrograde studies do not demonstrate renal function

    C. intravenous studies require more films

    D. more contrast media-induced adverse reactions occur with retrograde urography

61. The diagram below is representative of which of the following projections/methods?

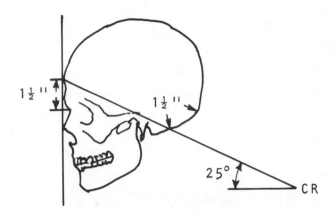

Upright radiography

A. PA/Caldwell method
B. PA axial/Valdini method
C. PA axial/Haas method
D. PA tangential

62. Which of the following positions will best "open up" the aortic arch following opacification with contrast medium?

A. Supine
B. RPO
C. LPO
D. RAO

63. For an AP projection of the sacrum, the central ray is directed

A. perpendicular to the film
B. 10° caudad
C. 15° cephalad
D. 30° cephalad

64. Which of the following are methods of localizing foreign bodies in the eye?

1. Pfeiffer-Comberg
2. Parallax motion
3. Sweet

A. 1 and 2
B. 1 and 3
C. 2 and 3
D. 1, 2, and 3

65. Vertical fractures of the patella are best demonstrated by performing a tangential or axial projection. How is the patient positioned and the central ray directed for this examination?

    A. Knee extended, central ray directed perpendicular to the femoral-tibial joint space

    B. Knee extended, central ray angled 5° cephalad through the patella-femoral joint space

    C. Knee flexed, central ray directed perpendicular to the patella-femoral joint space

    D. Knee flexed, central ray directed perpendicular to the femoral-tibial joint space

66. The position of the patient and x-ray beam in the following radiograph is

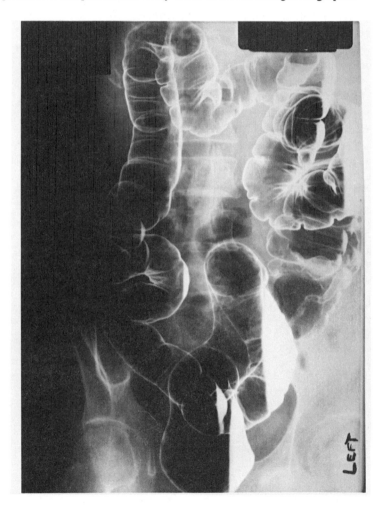

    A. supine/vertical

    B. left lateral recumbent/horizontal

    C. left lateral recumbent/vertical

    D. supine/horizontal

67. In an AP projection of the shoulder, which of the following positions will best demonstrate the greater tuberosity of the humerus in profile?

A. Internal rotation of the entire arm
B. External rotation of the entire arm
C. Neutral position of the arm, palm against the thigh
D. Neutral position of the arm, central ray directed 15° caudad

68. Which of the following is NOT true of lymphography?

A. Indicator dye is used to identify the lymphatic vessels
B. Iodinated contrast is injected using an automatic injector
C. The lymph nodes are opacified immediately when using an oil-based contrast
D. A cutdown is required for cannulation of a lymphatic vessel

69. The intervertebral foramina of the cervical spine open anteriorly at an angle of

A. 45° to the midsagittal plane and at an angle of 15° superiorly to the transverse plane
B. 70° to the midsagittal plane and at an angle of 45° inferiorly to the transverse plane
C. 45° to the midsagittal plane and at an angle of 15° inferiorly to the transverse plane
D. 90° to the midsagittal plane and at an angle of 45° superiorly to the transverse plane

70. For the AP supraorbital projection during internal carotid arteriography, the central ray must

1. be directed caudally in an attempt to superimpose the supraorbital margins on the petrous ridges
2. be directed caudally so as to form a 30° angle to the orbitomeatal line
3. pass through a line about 2 cm above and parallel to the line that passes from the upper margin of the orbit to a point 2 cm above the external auditory meatus

A. 1 and 2
B. 1 and 3
C. 2 and 3
D. 1, 2, and 3

Questions 71–73. For each of the following radiographic presentations, choose the position that would best demonstrate it. Each lettered heading may be used once, more than once, or not at all.

A. Supine
B. Prone
C. RAO
D. RPO

71. Esophagus projected free of the spine

72. Barium in the fundus of the stomach

73. Right colic (hepatic) flexure

74. The glenoid fossa can be best demonstrated in profile by

    A. rotating the patient from an AP position, approximately 45° toward the affected side
    B. an AP projection of the shoulder with the central ray angled 15° cephalad
    C. an AP projection of the shoulder, with the arm internally rotated
    D. rotating the patient from a PA position toward the affected side so that the scapula is perpendicular to the film and the arm is extended above the head

75. The submentovertical projection is useful in demonstrating the

    1. sphenoid sinuses
    2. base of the skull
    3. mastoid process

    A. 1 and 2
    B. 1 and 3
    C. 2 and 3
    D. 1, 2, and 3

76. Which of the following is true concerning mammography?

    1. The fatty breast of a postmenopausal woman requires less exposure than the fibroglandular breast of a young woman
    2. The nipple must be projected in profile for both the craniocaudal and mediolateral projections
    3. Compression of the breast improves definition

    A. 1 and 2
    B. 1 and 3
    C. 2 and 3
    D. 1, 2, and 3

77. In the AP projection of the pelvis, the feet are

    A. pointed upright
    B. inverted 15°
    C. everted 15°
    D. everted 45°

78. The Twining method (sometimes referred to as the Swimmer's view) is taken to demonstrate the

    A. atlas and axis articulation
    B. cervicothoracic region of the spine
    C. lumbosacral region of the spine
    D. dorsolumbar junction

79. An opaque contrast study of the uterus and fallopian tubes is obtained by performing

    A. vaginography
    B. pelvic pneumography
    C. hysterosalpingography
    D. amniography

80. When performing medial and lateral oblique projections of the foot, the angle between the sole of the foot and the film is

    A. 15°
    B. 20°
    C. 30°
    D. 60°

81. The skull radiograph below represents which of the following projections and methods?

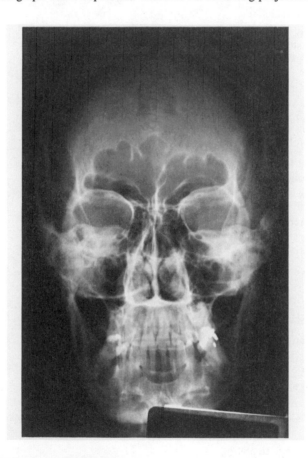

    A. PA axial projection/Caldwell method
    B. PA axial projection/Valdini method
    C. PA projection/Waters method
    D. PA axial projection/Haas method

82. Which of the following procedures involve direct instillation of contrast medium into the biliary ductal system?

       1. Percutaneous transhepatic cholangiography
       2. T-tube cholangiography
       3. Endoscopic retrograde cholangiopancreatography

A. 1 and 2
B. 1 and 3
C. 2 and 3
D. 1, 2, and 3

83. An axial plantodorsal projection of the calcaneous is performed with the

       1. ankles dorsiflexed so that the plantar aspect of the foot is perpendicular to the film
       2. central ray directed 40° cephalad to the long axis of the foot
       3. central ray directed through the bases of the metatarsals

A. 1 and 2
B. 1 and 3
C. 2 and 3
D. 1, 2, and 3

84. Which of the following eponyms describes a method that requires a 45° caudal angulation of the x-ray beam and 45° obliquity of the head?

A. Arcelin
B. Owen
C. Mayer
D. Stenvers

85. The radiograph that follows represents

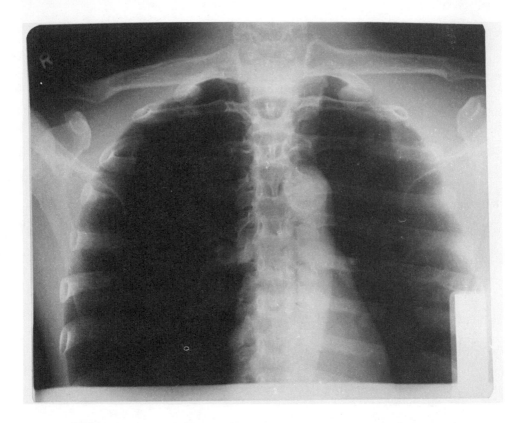

A. an AP projection with the patient supine and the central ray directed perpendicularly
B. an AP projection with the patient upright and the central ray angled cephalic
C. a PA projection with the patient prone and the central ray directed perpendicularly
D. an AP projection with the patient supine and the central ray directed caudally

86. Which of the following eponyms describes a method that is used to radiograph the zygomatic arch free of bony superimposition in patients with flat cheekbones?

A. Fuchs
B. May
C. Schüller
D. Titterington

87. Which of the following statements is FALSE concerning the radiograph below?

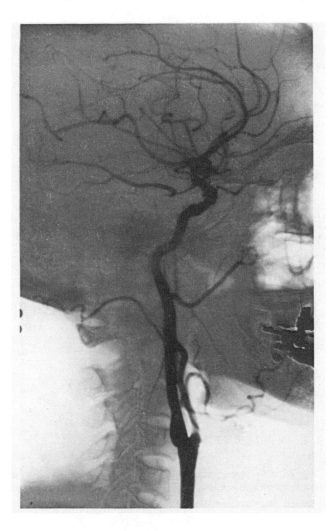

A. An opaque contrast agent has been given to the patient
B. The vertebral artery has been selectively injected
C. The angiogram has been photographically subtracted to provide a positive image
D. A lateral projection has been made

88. Surgical aseptic technique is NOT necessary for radiographic procedures involving the

A. subarachnoid space (myelography)
B. urinary bladder (cystography)
C. colon (barium enema)
D. lymphatic system (lymphangiography)

89. A balloon-tipped catheter is required in which of the following procedures?

   A. Percutaneous transhepatic cholangiography
   B. Percutaneous transluminal angioplasty
   C. Sialography
   D. Dacryocystography

90. In order to prevent the joint space from being obscured by the magnified shadow of the medial femoral condyle in the lateral projection of the knee, the

   A. central ray is angled 5° cephalad
   B. central ray is perpendicular
   C. knee is rotated so that the patella is at a 45° angle to the plane of the film
   D. knee joint is extended

91. In order to demonstrate a small amount of pleural fluid to best advantage, the patient is placed in

   A. an erect anterior oblique position
   B. a recumbent position with the affected side up and central ray horizontal
   C. a supine position
   D. a lateral decubitus position with the affected side down

92. Which of the following factors will increase the flow rate of contrast medium during angiographic injection?

   1. Multiple side holes in the catheter
   2. Increased length of the catheter
   3. Increased viscosity of the contrast medium

   A. 1 only
   B. 1 and 2
   C. 2 and 3
   D. 1, 2, and 3

Questions 93–96. For each anatomic structure listed below, choose the position that would best demonstrate it radiographically. Each lettered heading (position) may be used once, more than once, or not at all.

   A. Supine
   B. AP erect
   C. LPO
   D. RPO

93. Right intervertebral foramina of the cervical spine

94. Right articular facets of the lumbar vertebrae

95. Axillary portion of the right ribs

96. Upper posterior ribs

POSTTEST—RADIOGRAPHIC POSITIONING AND PROCEDURES
ANSWERS, EXPLANATIONS, AND REFERENCES

49. The answer is C. Medial and lateral oblique projections of the ankle are performed by turning the leg and foot of the affected side to the medial or lateral side (depending on which oblique is being performed), forming a 45° angle to the plane of the film. The foot is dorsiflexed for both projections to overcome superimposition of the calcaneous and malleoli. The central ray is directed perpendicular to the film between the medial and lateral malleoli of the ankle. Oblique projections of the ankle afford visualization of the distal tibia and fibula and malleoli and the ankle joint. *(Ballinger [Vol. 1], p 63; Bontrager and Anthony, p 147)*

50. The answer is D. Because the sigmoid is S-shaped and sometimes assumes a redundant position, it is usually necessary to perform special projections that visually "unravel" or "open up" the sigmoid radiographically. Several projections have been described for this purpose. The PA projection with a central ray angulation of 35° caudad and the reverse of this projection, AP with a 35° cephalic angulation of the central ray, are useful in demonstrating the sigmoid and rectosigmoid region. An LPO of about 35° accompanied by a 35° cephalic tube angulation is also useful in demonstrating this area of the large intestine. A Trendelenburg tilted table, with the patient in the supine or oblique position, will allow the lower bowel loops to spill upward into the abdomen and out of the pelvis, another useful method of uncoiling bowel loops, especially the sigmoid. The Chassard-Lapiné is another method of visualizing the sigmoid region using a knee-to-chest position and no angulation of the central beam. *(Ballinger [Vol. 3], p 680–682; Bontrager and Anthony, p 476–477, 479)*

51. The answer is A. The axiolateral (transaxillary) projection of the shoulder joint can be obtained by abducting the affected arm and placing the film under the axillary region for a superoinferior axial projection or by placing the film superior to the shoulder joint for an inferosuperior axial projection. For the superoinferior axial projection, the patient can be placed seated on a stool next to the examining table. With the affected arm abducted, elbow flexed, and film inferior to the shoulder and in contact with the axilla, the central ray is directed through the shoulder joint at about an angle of 10° toward the elbow. This projection demonstrates the head of the humerus, glenoid fossa, acromioclavicular joint, and other structures of the shoulder girdle. The inferosuperior axial projection is easily obtained with the patient lying down, the affected arm abducted, hand with the palm up, film positioned above the shoulder, and the central ray directed cephalad through the axilla. It demonstrates similar structures as the superoinferior axial projection. Neither of these axial projections is recommended for radiographing traumatized patients; however, the transthoracic lateral projection may be performed. *(Ballinger [Vol. 1], p 166–167; Bontrager and Anthony, p 119, 122)*

52. The answer is D. The maxillary sinuses (antra of Highmore) are best demonstrated in the parietoacanthial projection using the Waters method. In this projection, the petrous bones are demonstrated below the antral floors, thus allowing the maxillary sinuses to be projected free of superimposition. The position of the patient for this projection is PA erect, with the chin in contact with the film holder and the nose about ½ inch above the film holder. The orbitomeatal line should be adjusted so that it forms a 37° angle to the film plane. The head should be straight, without rotation, and the central ray is directed perpendicularly through the vertex of the skull, exiting the acanthion (anterior nasal spine). A projection similar to this can be performed with the patient's mouth open in order to provide additional views of the sphenoid sinuses. *(Ballinger [Vol. 2], p 514–515; Bontrager and Anthony, p 253)*

53. The answer is C. During an upper gastrointestinal series, the RAO (right PA oblique projection) will allow for separation of the duodenal cap and pyloric canal, which may be superimposed in other positions. Gastric peristalsis is also greatest in this position, allowing excellent serial projections of this important anatomic area. The patient is rotated into a 40 to 70°

oblique, larger body builds requiring the steepest obliquity. The right lateral position is important in demonstrating the duodenal cap and pylorus in patients of the hypersthenic body habitus. Supine and prone positions are not as useful in demonstrating this area but are helpful in evaluating the fundus and body portions of the stomach in most patients. *(Ballinger [Vol. 3], p 658; Meschan, p 447)*

54. The answer is C. The right sacroiliac joint is best demonstrated with patients in the RAO position with their left side elevated 25 to 30°. The RAO position will demonstrate the right sacroiliac joint, and the LAO position will demonstrate the left sacroiliac joint. Posterior obliques (RPO and LPO) can also be performed, but the side up (farthest from the film) will be best demonstrated. Both sides are usually radiographed for comparison. The central ray for these oblique projections is directed through the level of the anterior superior iliac spine, perpendicular to the film. (Cephalic angulations of 20 to 25° may also be employed.) *(Ballinger [Vol. 1], p 245–246; Meschan, p 153)*

55. The answer is C. Erect and/or decubitus positions are useful in demonstrating stratification or layering out of gallstones, as both positions require a horizontal x-ray beam. When the patient is erect or in a lateral decubitus position, the constituents of the bile will layer out according to their weight or specific gravity. Stones that may have been too small to visualize in other positions may float on the heavier constituents of bile and produce a horizontal shadow or, if heavier than the other bile constituents, may layer out on the bottommost part of the gallbladder. A horizontal beam is necessary to demonstrate this stratification effect. Anterior and posterior obliques and lateral positions do not require a horizontal beam and can be performed with the patient recumbent and a vertical x-ray beam (perpendicular to the floor). If these projections were performed in conjunction with an erect or decubitus position with the x-ray beam parallel to the floor, then stratification could be visualized. Routine studies of the opacified gallbladder employ both vertical and horizontal beam projections. *(Ballinger [Vol. 3], p 629, 631, 633; Bontrager and Anthony, p 493–494)*

56. The answer is A. Expiratory chest films are often performed in order to rule out pneumothorax (abnormal air in the pleural cavity). Chest radiographs are routinely taken at the end of inspiration to ensure maximum lung volume so that more lung area can be seen on the radiograph. The expiration chest film may, however, exaggerate the size of a small pneumothorax by decreasing lung volume and expansion. Empyema, effusions, and rib fractures do not usually require this approach. However, in the case of rib fractures, inspiration and expiration chest films may be beneficial in ruling out a pneumothorax caused by a complicated rib fracture or blunt trauma. Chest radiographs made at the end of inspiration and expiration are also useful in examining the chest for foreign bodies and diaphragm movement. *(Ballinger [Vol. 3], p 585; Armstrong and Wastie, p 16)*

57. The answer is C. In the axiolateral projections of the cranium using Lysholm's, Schüller's and Henschen's methods, a difference of 10° exists between the central ray angulation for each. In all three methods, patients are adjusted in the true lateral position, erect or recumbent, so that their interpupillary line is perpendicular to the film plane and their midsagittal plane is parallel to the film plane. For the Lysholm method, the central ray is directed at an angle of 35° caudad; for the Schüller method, 25° caudad; and for the Henschen method, 15° caudad, through the external auditory meatus of the side up. These projections may be used for radiography of the mastoid and petrous parts of the temporal bones. *(Ballinger [Vol. 2], p 435–436)*

58. The answer is C. It is desirable to obtain chest films without rotation. In order to obtain a straight PA projection of the chest, patients are positioned erect, with their weight evenly distributed on both legs; their hands are placed on their hips, with the palms up, the shoulders are rolled forward, and the chin is extended. The final radiograph should demonstrate symmetry of the sternoclavicular joints. If, however, the medial ends of the clavicles are at unequal distances from the midline or sternum, rotation of the patient can be quickly suspected. (However, in patients who have scoliosis, there usually is an asymmetric appearance of the medial end of the clavicles.) The height of the clavicles may vary between erect and supine positioning, and the scapulae may appear in the lung fields if the shoulders were not adequately rolled forward (as is usually the case in critically ill patients); however, the chest may still be straight without rotation present. Curvature of the thoracic spine may be indicative of scoliosis or degenerative disease. *(Armstrong and Wastie, p 16; Bontrager and Anthony, p 38; McInnes, p 332)*

59. The answer is A. When performing a lateral projection of the wrist, the arm is flexed approximately 90° at the elbow to bring the ulna into a lateral position. The ulnar side of the distal forearm is placed in contact with the film, and the humerus and forearm rest on the table in the same plane. The distal radius and ulna should be superimposed in this projection by lining up the styloid processes. The central ray is directed through the wrist joint, perpendicular to the film. The lateral, along with the PA and oblique projections, are usually included in the routine examination of the wrist. *(Ballinger [Vol. 1], p 132; Bontrager and Anthony, p 88)*

60. The answer is B. Intravenous urography involves the injection of aqueous iodinated contrast medium into a vein, from which it passes through the circulatory system and is filtered out of the blood by the kidneys through glomerular filtration. Kidney function, as well as visualization of the urinary collecting systems, can be assessed by excretory or intravenous urography and is the most common examination performed for evaluation of the urinary system. Retrograde or ascending urography is not a test of renal function; instead, it is primarily a urologic procedure performed after insertion of a catheter through the urethra and into the bladder. The ureters and renal pelvis can also be catheterized and opacified after injection of aqueous iodinated contrast. The anatomy of the calyces, renal pelvis, ureters, and bladder can be well seen on a retrograde urogram, and urine specimens and calculi can be removed during this procedure. Because contrast is being directly injected into the urinary system during retrograde urography and not into the bloodstream, kidney function cannot be adequately evaluated; this is the primary difference between the two types of radiographic studies. Contrast media-induced reactions are not as likely to occur in retrograde urography as in intravenous excretory urography, because the contrast is being directly injected into the urinary tract instead of intravenously. The type of contrast medium used for both examinations is of the aqueous (water-soluble) iodinated type. The number of films taken for each study is contingent on the patient situation, pathology, and physician's recommendations. *(Bontrager and Anthony, p 505–515)*

61. The answer is C. The diagram that accompanies the question is representative of the PA axial or nuchofrontal projection/Haas method. The patient with the average build is adjusted so that the head rests on the forehead and nose, and the orbitomeatal line is placed at right angles to the film plane. The central ray is directed at an angle of 25° cephalad and enters the midsagittal plane at about 1½ inches below the external occipital protruberance (inion) and exits about 1½ inches above the nasion. This projection can be taken with the patient prone or PA erect. The Haas projection is the reverse of the AP axial/Grashey or Towne method. This projection is useful in demonstrating the dorsum sellae and posterior clinoid processes within the foramen magnum shadow, as well as the occipital bone and petrous pyramids. It is also useful when the body habitus of the patient or some physical condition prevents using the AP axial projection—Towne method. *(Ballinger [Vol. 2], p 390–391)*

62. The answer is B. The position that will best "open up" the aortic arch following opacification with contrast medium is a RPO with patients rotated 30 to 45°; their right posterior aspect is in close relationship to the film, and their left side is elevated with a sponge or other radiolucent support. The central ray is directed perpendicularly to the level of the fourth thoracic vertebra and sagittal plane. Because the aorta courses upward and then descends, it is somewhat superimposed by itself when the patient is supine, in the RPO position; however, the aorta can be placed nearly parallel to the film plane. Although the RPO position will demonstrate the aortic arch and its branches, simultaneous AP and lateral projections are often performed with a single injection of contrast medium to afford visualization of the thoracic aorta. *(Ballinger [Vol. 3], p 804; Bontrager and Anthony, p 375; Snopek, p 184–185; Tortorici, p 175)*

63. The answer is C. The central ray of the x-ray beam is directed 15° cephalad through the level between the anterior superior iliac spines and symphysis pubis in order to demonstrate the sacrum. This cephalic angulation enhances visualization of the sacral foramina and sacroiliac joints, as well as an unforeshortened sacrum. The patient assumes the supine position in order to place the sacrum close to the film whenever possible. Patients who cannot lie supine may be adjusted to the prone position, with the central ray angled in the opposite direction. A 10° caudad angulation is used for demonstration of the coccyx, with the patient in the supine position. *(Ballinger [Vol. 1], p 248; Bontrager and Anthony, p 279)*

64. The answer is D. The Pfeiffer-Comberg, parallax motion, and Sweet methods are all used for radiographically localizing foreign bodies within the eye. The Pfeiffer-Comberg method incorporates a specially designed contact lens that has four lead markers spaced at intervals of 90°. This is placed over the cornea of the patient's affected eye, and a special biplane film holder unit for PA and lateral projections is placed on top of the x-ray table. The information on the location of the foreign body is recorded on a special localization graph. The Sweet method uses a special localizer device, a pedestal film tunnel, and a geometric calculator. This method requires that patients fix their eyes in one position for the duration of two exposures while in a lateral recumbent position (affected side down). Two exposures are made after positioning the patient, the localization device, and the film. The central ray should be directed perpendicular for one exposure and angled cephalad for the other. Information as to the exact position of the foreign body is charted on a localization graph. The parallax motion method does not require any special equipment; instead, two sets of PA and lateral projections are taken with the eyeball in different positions. Radiographic position of the foreign body by this parallax motion method, indicates only its general location within the eye and is not as accurate as the Pfeiffer-Comberg and Sweet methods. Preliminary projections (lateral, PA, and bone-free) of the affected eye are usually taken prior to the use of these methods to determine whether a foreign body is demonstrable radiographically. Ultrasonography can also be used for this purpose. *(Ballinger [Vol. 2], p 414–424; Meschan, p 238–240)*

65. The answer is C. Vertical fractures of the patella are best demonstrated by performing a tangential or axial projection, with the knee flexed as much as possible so that the long axis of the patella is perpendicular to the film. The central ray is directed perpendicular to the joint between the patella and condyles of the femur; the angulation of the beam depends on how much the patient can flex the knee. The patient can actually be placed in a variety of positions for this type of projection of the patella (supine, prone, sitting, or lateral). Care should be taken in flexing the affected knee so as to avoid causing increased pain to the patient, and knee flexion should only be performed after transverse fractures of the patella have been ruled out. *(Ballinger [Vol. 1], p 78–80; Bontrager and Anthony, p 165)*

66. The answer is B. The position of the patient in the radiograph that accompanies the question is left lateral recumbent (patients lie on their left side with the film in front or behind them), and the x-ray beam is directed horizontally (parallel to the horizon). This constitutes the left lateral decubitus position. (The image on the film is an AP or PA view.) The positive contrast agent seen in the intestine indicates the patient's position. Gravity will cause the positive contrast agent (heavier) to occupy the lower side of the structure it occupies, and air will tend to rise to the uppermost side. Because the positive contrast agent is heavier and tends to fall toward the left-sided walls of the intestinal lumen and air rises to the uppermost (right) side, one can assume that the patient's left side is down. The x-ray beam is horizontal, as noted by the air-fluid levels demonstrated in the intestine. A vertical beam would not allow visualization of air-fluid levels, as the beam would pass through the air and fluid, which would be superimposed over one another, and would not demonstrate a line of demarcation between them. *(Ballinger [Vol. 1], p 11; Bontrager and Anthony, p 21, 69, 480)*

67. The answer is B. For the demonstration of the greater tuberosity of the humerus in profile, the arm is positioned in external rotation so that the palm of the hand is facing forward (as in the anatomic position) and the epicondyles of the distal humerus are parallel to the plane of the film.

In external rotation, the humerus is in a true AP or anatomic position. Internal rotation of the entire arm, with the back of the hand near the side of the body and epicondyles perpendicular to the plane of the film, demonstrates the humerus in a true lateral position. Neutral position of the arm, with the palm of the hand resting on the thigh and the epicondyles forming a 45° angle to the film, may be performed when the patient cannot rotate the arm (e.g., in cases of fracture or dislocation of the humerus). This AP neutral projection is usually performed in the routine examination of the traumatized patient. For all AP projections of the shoulder, the central ray is directed to the coracoid process, perpendicular to the film. Caudal angulations of the beam may be used as additional methods for further examination of tendon and ligament attachments. *(Ballinger [Vol. 1], p 158–159; Bontrager and Anthony, p 116–118)*

68. The answer is C. Lymphography is a radiographic examination of the lymphatic system requiring injection of an opaque, iodinated (usually oil-based) contrast agent. Before the contrast can be injected into a lymphatic vessel, an indicator dye (usually blue-violet) is injected into the subcutaneous tissues of the area to be injected. This indicator dye will be picked up by the lymphatic vessels in that area so that the vessels can be more easily identified. Lymph (fluid within the lymphatic vessels) itself is colorless, and the vessels themselves are small and difficult to visualize without the use of dye. Once the indicator dye colors the lymphatics, a local anesthetic is injected subcutaneously, and a cutdown (small incision) is made over the top of the foot (for the lower extremity, abdominopelvic, and thoracic duct regions) or hand (for the upper extremity, axillary, and clavicular regions). A small lymphatic vessel is isolated and cannulated, and the contrast medium is injected with a special automatic injector that applies constant low pressure. Lymphangiography, or radiography of the lymphatic vessels, is performed within the first hour of the examination. Lymphadenography, or radiography of opacified lymph nodes, requires about 24 hours, especially when iodinated poppyseed oil, the most commonly employed contrast agent, is used. Depending on the areas of interest, 14×17-inch films may be made of the upper extremity, axilla, and thoracic region or of the femoral, groin, abdominal, pelvic, and chest regions. *(Ballinger [Vol. 3], p 812–817; Bontrager and Anthony, p 535; Meschan, p 351–354, 127; Snopek, p 221–235)*

69. The answer is C. The intervertebral foramina of the cervical spine open 45° anteriorly to the midsagittal plane and 15° inferiorly to the transverse plane. In order to visualize or "open up" the intervertebral foramina radiographically, the patient must be positioned at an angle of 45° to the plane of the film from either an AP or PA position. This will place the foramina parallel to the film. The central ray of the x-ray beam must also be angled about 15° cephalad for a RPO or LPO position or 15° caudad for a RAO or LAO position. This will allow the central part of the beam to pass through the openings in the cervical vertebrae, which open at an angle of 15° to the transverse plane. The oblique projections are most often included as a routine part of the radiographic examination of the cervical vertebrae; however, acute injuries may require alterations in patient positioning and angulation of the x-ray beam in order to protect against further injury. This can be achieved by keeping the patient's head, neck, and body straight in a supine position (no movement to head or neck) and angling the central ray 45° medially and 15° cephalic through the midcervical region. *(Ballinger [Vol. 1], p 206, 220–222, 227; Bontrager and Anthony, p 295, 299, 311)*

70. The answer is B. For an AP supraorbital projection of the internal carotid circulation, patients are placed in the supine position and their head is adjusted so that the infraorbitomeatal line and midsagittal plane are perpendicular to the film. The patient's head is secured into this position by a compression strap. The central ray is directed caudally (about 15°) so that it passes through a line about 2 cm above and parallel to the line that passes from the upper margin of the orbit to a point 2 cm above the external auditory meatus. This projection is performed in order to superimpose the supraorbital margins and petrous ridges. The final radiograph should demonstrate anterior and middle cerebral vessels above the floor of the anterior cranial fossa. This projection is most often employed in addition to a lateral projection during routine examination of the internal carotid circulation. A variety of additional projections may be used to help demonstrate aneurysms or vessel displacement. These may include the supraorbital oblique, axial, transorbital AP, and oblique projections. *(Ballinger [Vol. 3], p 784, 786–788; Bontrager and Anthony, p 374–378)*

71–73. The answers are 71-C, 72-A, 73-C. The esophagus can best be projected free of superimposition by the spine by placing the patient in the RAO position. The degree of obliquity for this routine position of the esophagus is about 40 to 45°. The patient can be positioned recumbent or erect, and the central ray is directed perpendicular to the film about the level of the sixth thoracic vertebra and left sagittal plane. The esophagus can be visualized between the spine and heart shadow after ingestion of opaque (positive) contrast medium.

Barium sulfate occupies the fundus of the stomach when the patient assumes the supine position. The stomach tends to move upward in this position, and the body and pyloric regions are demonstrated with double contrast (barium and air). The supine position is often included in routine examinations of the stomach and, with the table angled Trendelenburg, can be helpful in demonstrating hiatal hernias.

The right colic (hepatic) flexure is best seen or "opened up" in the RAO position following retrograde insertion of opaque contrast media. The patient is placed in a 45° RAO, and the central ray is directed perpendicularly to the level of the iliac crest and left sagittal plane. The LPO can also provide an opened up projection of the hepatic flexure, as it corresponds to the RAO position. The left colic (splenic) flexure is best seen in a 45° LAO or RPO position. Projections of the colic flexures are included in routine examinations of the opacified large intestine following a barium enema. *(Ballinger [Vol. 3], p 651, 654, 660–661, 682; Bontrager and Anthony, p 438, 444, 470, 473)*

74. The answer is A. The glenoid fossa of the scapula is best seen in profile by rotating the patient obliquely 45° toward the affected side (Grashey method) from an AP position (RPO or LPO). This position also demonstrates the joint space between the head of the humerus and the glenoid fossa. The central ray is directed perpendicular to the glenohumeral joint. Angling the central ray 15 to 30° cephalad with the patient positioned for an AP projection will help to demonstrate the coracoid process of the scapula. An AP projection of the shoulder with the arm internally rotated and a PA oblique projection with the scapula perpendicular to the film are useful in demonstrating parts of the shoulder joint and scapula, respectively. *(Ballinger [Vol. 1], p. 158, 162–163, 179; Bontrager and Anthony, p 120)*

75. The answer is D. The submentovertical or basilar projection, using the Schüller method, is useful in demonstrating numerous structures including the sphenoid sinuses, base of the skull, mastoid processes, mandible, nasal septum, zygomatic arches, first cervical vertebra, and portions of the temporal bones. This projection is often incorporated in many routine examinations of the skull and facial bones. It is achieved by placing patients in a supine or AP erect position, with their head extended as much as possible to rest on the vertex and their infraorbitomeatal line as parallel to the film plane as possible. The head should be straight, without any rotation, and secured in this position. The central ray is directed perpendicular to the infraorbitomeatal line through the sella turcica, entering the midsagittal plane at a point between the mandibular angles (gonia) and the central ray should pass about ¾ inch in front of the external auditory meatuses. *(Ballinger [Vol. 2], p 392–394, 435–436, 478, 520; Bontrager and Anthony, p 205, 209, 229, 256, 258)*

76. The answer is D. Proper classification of breast types and their relative density is essential in choosing the proper technical factors for exposing the breast. Though the size of the breasts of two different individuals may appear the same, the tissue composition and relative density may be quite different, warranting different sets of exposure factors. The more fat infiltration the breast has, the easier it is to penetrate compared with a more fibrous or glandular breast of the same size. Younger women tend to have more fibrous and glandular breast tissue, making it dense and requiring more exposure to penetrate it than a less dense breast with large amounts of fatty infiltration (seen especially in postmenopausal women). When radiographing a breast in the craniocaudal and mediolateral projections, it is essential to have the nipple in profile and to smooth out any wrinkles in the skin in order to obtain proper positioning. Application of breast compression evens out the breast tissues and improves definition of the breast structures. *(Ballinger [Vol. 3], p 746–747, 750–751; Bontrager and Anthony, p 333–335, 339–340)*

77. The answer is B. Inverting the feet 15° allows maximum elongation of the femoral necks and a true AP projection of the hip joints in the AP projection of the pelvis. The pelvis should not be rotated, and the patient should assume a true AP supine position. The central ray is directed perpendicular to the film at a point between the iliac crest and symphysis pubis and the midsagittal plane for this projection of the pelvis. The lesser trochanters should not be seen in profile on this projection if positioning is correct. Care should be taken *not* to invert the feet of a patient with a suspected hip fracture. For the AP projection of the hip (except in cases of suspected fracture), the feet are also inverted in order to demonstrate the femoral neck, head, and greater trochanter. *(Ballinger [Vol. 1], p 96, 102; Bontrager and Anthony, p 177–180, 183)*

78. The answer is B. The Swimmer's or Twining lateral projection is useful in demonstrating the cervicothoracic region of the spine. Requirements for this projection are that the patient be placed in a lateral erect or recumbent position with the arm nearest to the film raised above the head and the shoulders rotated in opposite directions (anterior or posterior) from each other. The shoulder remote from the film is depressed as much as possible. The central ray is directed perpendicular or a few degrees caudad (if the shoulder is not depressed) through the second thoracic vertebra. The lower cervical and upper thoracic vertebrae will be demonstrated between the shoulders. *(Ballinger [Vol. 1], p 228; Bontrager and Anthony, p 306)*

79. The answer is C. Hysterosalpingography is a radiographic examination of the uterus and fallopian tubes following instillation of opaque (positive) contrast medium into the cervix. Using aseptic technique, a vaginal speculum is introduced, followed by insertion of a cannula into the cervical canal. Backflow of the contrast medium is avoided by countertraction of the outer cervix against a rubber plug fixed to the cannula. An opaque contrast medium of the aqueous or oily iodinated type is injected through the cannula into the cervix and uterus, where it will opacify lumina of these structures as well as the fallopian tubes (a gaseous medium may be injected after opacification). If an oily iodinated contrast medium is used, ½-hour or 24-hour delayed films are often taken to check for fallopian tube patency. This can be demonstrated at the time of the initial examination if an aqueous contrast is used. Hysterosalpingography is useful in evaluating the causes of female infertility and in demonstrating uterine abnormalities as well as fallopian tube patency. AP projections are usually taken routinely; however, additional lateral, oblique, or axial projections may be required to demonstrate certain problems. Vaginography is the radiographic study of the vagina following opacification with a positive contrast medium. It may be useful in demonstrating vaginal abnormalities and fistulas. Pelvic pneumography (gynecography) is a radiographic study of the female reproductive organs following injection of a gaseous contrast agent into the peritoneal cavity. The gaseous agent provides a negative background contrast, allowing evaluation of the size, shape, and position of the ovaries, uterus, fallopian tubes, and uterine ligaments. Amniography is a radiographic study of the amniotic sac surrounding the fetus in utero following instillation of an aqueous iodinated (positive) contrast agent. Amniography and pelvic pneumography are rarely performed today because of the more efficient modalities available for evaluation of these parts, such as ultrasonography and culdoscopy. *(Ballinger [Vol. 3], p 728–732; Bontrager and Anthony, p 534; Katzen, p 105–107; Meschan, p 402–404, 411–413; Snopek, p 252–261)*

80. The answer is C. When radiographing the foot in the medial and lateral oblique projections, the sole of the foot forms a 30° angle to the plane of the film. This is best accomplished by rotating the leg medially (for the medial oblique) and laterally (for the lateral oblique) and supporting the sole on an angle sponge. The central ray is directed perpendicularly to the level of the base of the fifth metatarsal and midline of the foot. The medial oblique is very useful in demonstrating the spaces between the talus and navicular, cuboid and third cuneiform, cuboid and calcaneous, cuboid and fourth and fifth metatarsals, as well as the phalanges and metatarsals of the foot. The lateral oblique is useful in demonstrating the first and second metatarsal interspace and the first and second cuneiform interspace. *(Ballinger [Vol. 1], p 46)*

81. The answer is A. The radiograph that accompanies the question represents a PA axial projection of the skull using the Caldwell method. For this projection, patients are placed prone or erect with their forehead and nose touching the table or erect film holder, and their midsagittal plane and orbitomeatal line are adjusted so that they are perpendicular to the film. The central ray is directed 15° caudally through the glabella and midsagittal plane. This projection demonstrates the frontal bone, frontal and anterior ethmoid sinuses, the lesser and greater wings of the sphenoid within the orbital cavity, and the petrous ridges in the lower third of the orbits. *(Ballinger [Vol. 2], p 512–513; Bontrager and Anthony, p 203; Meschan, p 231)*

82. The answer is D. Percutaneous transhepatic cholangiography (PTC), T-tube cholangiography, and endoscopic retrograde cholangiopancreatography (ERCP) all require the direct injection of an opaque contrast medium into the biliary system. PTC involves the introduction of a long, thin needle through the abdominal wall and liver and into a bile duct, with subsequent injection of aqueous iodinated contrast and radiography. PTC is performed when other methods of opacifying the biliary system have failed on the jaundiced or preoperative patient. In ERCP, a fiberoptic endoscope is inserted through the mouth, esophagus, stomach, and duodenum. Then a small cannula is passed through the endoscope into the duodenal papilla, at which point aqueous iodinated contrast is injected directly into the common bile duct. This procedure is useful in diagnosing biliary and pancreatic problems and, in many cases, is used in place of PTC. Ultrasonography is usually performed before these procedures. T-tube cholangiography is a method of opacifying the biliary ducts following injection of aqueous iodinated contrast into a T tube that was placed into the common bile duct during surgery. This fluoroscopic and radiographic examination is performed in the radiology department, usually a few days after surgery, to evaluate biliary patency and to check for residual stones or strictures. *(Ballinger [Vol. 3], p 618–619, 634–635, 639; Bontrager and Anthony, p 489–491)*

83. The answer is D. The axial plantodorsal projection of the calcaneous is performed with the patient' legs extended and the affected foot placed on top of the cassette, with the sole and toes pointed vertically upward. The ankle must be dorsiflexed so that the plantar surface of the foot is perpendicular to the film; this can be accomplished by having the patient pull the upper foot toward the body with a long gauze band or folded sheet. The central ray is directed through the base of the metatarsals at an angle of 40° cephalad to the long axis of the foot and emerges just above the ankle joint. This projection demonstrates the calcaneous from its proximal to distal ends. The reverse of this position, the dorsoplantar projection, can also be performed with the central ray directed 40° caudad through the dorsal surface of the ankle, with patient prone and the plantar surface of the foot in contact with the film, ankle dorsiflexed. *(Ballinger [Vol. 1], p 54–55; Bontrager and Anthony, p 144)*

84. The answer is C. The Mayer method (axiolateral oblique projection) requires the patient's head to be oblique from the supine position so that the midsagittal plane forms a 45° angle to the plane of the film. The central ray should be directed 45° caudad through the external auditory meatus closest to the film. The infraorbitomeatal line should be almost parallel with the transverse axis of the film. The mastoid nearest to the film is being radiographed. The Mayer projection is often employed in radiography of the petrous portions of the temporal bones to demonstrate the tympanic cavity, auditory ossicles, attic, aditus, mastoid antrum, and external auditory meatus. The Owen method, a modification of the Mayer method, uses a different degree of head rotation and central ray angulation. The Stenvers and Arcelin methods, also used in radiographing the petrous portions and mastoids, employ different degrees of head rotation and beam angulations. *(Ballinger [Vol. 2], p 444–448)*

85. The answer is B. The radiograph that accompanies the question represents an AP axial projection with the patient in the upright position and the central ray directed cephalic, 15 to 20°. This projection demonstrates the pulmonary apices below the clavicular shadows because the cephalic central ray angulation tends to throw the clavicles up. A perpendicularly directed central ray would demonstrate the clavicles overlying the pulmonary apices in both PA and AP projections, recumbent or erect. An AP projection with the central ray directed caudally would place the clavicles at a lower position than normal. A similar radiograph can be obtained by positioning patients with their head and neck in contact with the film holder and having them step approximately 1 foot forward (so that they are leaning back) and directing the central ray perpendicular to the film. This is called an apical lordotic projection. *(Ballinger [Vol. 3], p 593–594; Bontrager and Anthony, p 49)*

86. The answer is B. The May method is used for the radiographic demonstration of the zygomatic arch of patients with flat cheekbones. In this tangential projection, the zygomatic arch of the side being examined is projected free of bony superimposition and is often used to demonstrate fractures of the zygoma. Patients are adjusted from the PA erect or prone position so that their head is resting on the extended chin and the midsagittal plane is rotated about 15° away from the side being radiographed. The central ray is directed caudally through the zygomatic arch of interest so that it is perpendicular to the infraorbitomeatal line. The reverse of this projection is the AP tangential, which is also helpful in demonstrating the zygoma free of superimposition in patients with depressed cheekbones. For this projection, the patient is rotated 15° from the supine or AP erect position toward the side being examined, and the central ray is directed perpendicularly to the infraorbitomeatal line, through the zygomatic arch. *(Ballinger [Vol. 2], p 480, 483; Bontrager and Anthony, p 231)*

87. The answer is B. The radiograph that accompanies the question is a lateral projection of a right carotid arteriogram. The patient's common carotid artery has been selectively catheterized and injected with an opaque water-soluble iodinated contrast agent, affording visualization of the internal and external carotid branches in the neck and head. Following angiography, the image was subtracted in order to remove unwanted bony images and provide a positive image. The final subtraction print, demonstrated in this radiograph, allows the blood vessels to be visualized clearly without much superimposition. Instead of being visualized as a negative, in which the opacified vessels appear white, the positive image projects the vessels as black. *(Ballinger [Vol. 3], p 779–782, 791–794; Bontrager and Anthony, p 376, 382)*

88. The answer is C. Surgical aseptic technique is necessary for many radiographic examinations that involve skin penetration and the introduction of catheters, needles, and contrast agents. Surgical aseptic technique is the practice of performing procedures in a sterile environment, one that is free of microorganisms and spores. It is often necessary to employ this technique so as not to introduce any pathogenic organisms into the patient's body and to prevent the spreading of organisms. The colon and most of the gastrointestinal tract are exposed to numerous organisms by way of ingestion of various foods and liquids, and indigenous bacteria inhabit the gastrointestinal system. Sterile technique is not required for radiographic procedures involving the colon and upper gastrointestinal tract—that is, barium enema examinations, intubation methods, and oral ingestion of contrast media. However, all articles used for barium enemas and other gastrointestinal examinations should be scrupulously clean (medically aseptic). Circulatory, urinary, lymphatic, subarachnoid, joint, and various other body systems and spaces require the use of surgical asepsis whenever articles and/or materials are introduced into their lumina or cavities. *(Ballinger [Vol. 3], p 685; Torres and Morrill, p 99–110)*

89. The answer is B. Percutaneous transluminal angioplasty employs a special balloon-tipped catheter and the Seldinger technique in an effort to dilate a stenotic or narrowed area of a blood vessel. This therapeutic procedure is performed on peripheral as well as coronary blood vessels in selected patients. Once the catheter is placed within the stenosed area, the balloon is inflated for a few seconds (the length of inflation time depends on the degree of stenosis and the vessel affected) and may be reinflated many times if the physician believes it necessary. A successful (dilatation) angioplasty can be demonstrated by an angiogram of the treated vessel. Percutaneous transhepatic cholangiography is a diagnostic radiographic procedure using a specially designed needle that is directed through the abdomen into a bile duct. Contrast medium is directly injected into the biliary ducts for opacification. Sialography is the radiographic study of the salivary glands and ductal system, and dacryocystography is the radiographic study of the tear ducts and lacrimal apparatus. Both procedures require the use of an opaque contrast agent and small catheters. Elective embolization is another therapeutic procedure, but it does not usually require the use of a balloon catheter; instead, it employs various substances, chemicals, or devices (such as Gelfoam, ethanol [absolute alcohol], Gianturco coils, and spring embolus), which can be used to embolize (occlude) a vessel that may be affected by malformation, tumor, or hemorrhage. *(Ballinger [Vol. 3], p 811; Katzen, p 97–98, 124–131)*

90. The answer is A. In order to prevent the joint space from being obscured by the magnified shadow of the medial femoral condyle in the lateral projection of the knee, the central ray is angled 5° cephalad through the knee joint. The distal femoral condyles will be superimposed, thus affording an obstructed view of the joint space. The affected leg is positioned with the lateral aspect in contact with the film, knee flexed to the angle desired, and long axis of the leg horizontal. A true lateral position of the knee will show the patella-femoral interspace, knee joint, proximal tibia and fibula, and the distal structures of the femur. *(Ballinger [Vol. 1], p 69; Bontrager and Anthony, p 162)*

91. The answer is D. A small amount of pleural fluid (effusion) is best demonstrated with the patient in a lateral decubitus position with the affected side down, so that the fluid will not be superimposed by mediastinal shadows. The affected side should be elevated (with pads or sponges), with the patient's arms above the head and the body in a true lateral position. The central ray is directed horizontally to the midsagittal plane at a level between the fourth and seventh thoracic vertebrae, depending on the area of interest. The supine and erect anterior oblique positions, although not suited for demonstration of small pleural effusions, may be useful in evaluating other processes. When a small pneumothorax is to be demonstrated, the patient may be positioned in a recumbent or lateral decubitus position with the affected side up and central ray directed horizontally. Air will rise to the uppermost region of the side up, avoiding superimposition by mediastinal structures. *(Ballinger [Vol. 3], p 596; Bontrager and Anthony, p 48)*

92. The answer is A. By increasing the number of side holes in a catheter, more contrast can be delivered per unit of time because there are more points of exit (holes) from which the contrast agent flows into vessels. There is a 10 to 20% increase in delivery rate for catheters with side holes over those without. Side holes also help reduce the "whiplash effect" that may be caused by the pressure of injection of the contrast medium. Increased catheter length would decrease flow rate, as the contrast medium would have to travel farther before filling the desired vessel, and increased resistance to flow would occur. Increased viscosity of the contrast medium increases the resistance of this fluid to movement, making it difficult to inject. Warming the contrast will decrease its viscosity and make injection easier. *(Tortorici, p 157–158; Snopek, p 53, 76)*

93–96. The answers are 93-C, 94-D, 95-D, 96-B. The right-sided intervertebral foramina of the cervical spine are best demonstrated with the patient in the LPO position. When performing posterior obliques (RPO and LPO) of the cervical spine, the intervertebral foramina and pedicles farthest from the film (closest to the x-ray tube) are best seen. For these posterior oblique positions, the patient is rotated 45° from the supine or erect position and the central ray is angled 15 to 20° cephalad through the fourth cervical vertebra and sagittal plane of the neck side that is up. RAO and LAO positions can also be employed; however, the intervertebral foramina closest to the film will be best demonstrated. That is, the RAO will demonstrate the right-sided intervertebral foramina, and the LAO will demonstrate the left-sided intervertebral foramina. The central ray must be angled in the opposite direction—that is, 15 to 20° caudally.

The articular facets on the right side of the lumbar spine are best seen with the patient in the RPO position. When performing posterior oblique positions (RPO and LPO), the facets and apophyseal joints closest to the film will be demonstrated. For these positions, the patient is rotated 45° from the supine position and the central ray is directed perpendicularly to the third lumbar vertebra. RAO and LAO positions can also be performed. However, the articular facets and apophyseal joints farthest from the film will be demonstrated—that is, the RAO will demonstrate left-sided articular facets and the LAO will demonstrate the right-sided articular facets and apophyseal joints.

The axillary portion of the ribs on the right side can be demonstrated with the patient in a 45° RPO position. The axillary portion of the ribs is located laterally and curves around and is not well seen on straight AP or PA projections; therefore, rotation of the patient so that the affected side is closest to the film is required.

The upper posterior ribs are examined with the patient in the AP erect position whenever possible. By positioning the patient in the AP erect position and taking the exposure at the end of inspiration, the diaphragm is able to fall to its lowest level, allowing more of the upper posterior ribs to be visualized. If the patient cannot stand or be seated, then the AP supine position may be used. The lower ribs should be radiographed with the patient supine, and the exposure should be taken at the end of expiration. *(Ballinger [Vol. 1], p 194–199, 220–222, 242–243; Bontrager and Anthony, p 283, 311, 327–330)*

RADIOGRAPHIC EXPOSURE AND PROCESSING

Questions 97–100 consist of four lettered headings followed by a list of numbered words or phrases. For each numbered word or phrase, select the one heading with which it is most closely related. Each heading may be used once, more than once, or not at all.

A. Radiographic grid
B. Transducer
C. Vidicon tube
D. Primary-beam restriction

97. Grid cutoff

98. Aperture diaphragm

99. Dose reduction

100. Grid radius

101. Determining the correct level of radiographic density for each examination is a triumph of art and science when one considers the number of factors to be manipulated each time. Which of the following variables does NOT affect radiographic density?

A. The focus-film distance (FFD) or source-image distance (SID)
B. The size of the focal spot
C. Whether the equipment is single phase or three phase
D. The speed of the intensifying screen

102. The quality, or penetrability, of the x-ray beam is measured by reference to its half-value layer (HVL) and is affected by exposure factors such as

    1. kVp of tube operation
    2. FFD/SID and mAs selected
    3. total aluminum filtration in the primary beam

A. 1 and 2
B. 1 and 3
C. 2 and 3
D. 1, 2, and 3

103. Which of the following formulas are used to calculate heat units that will be generated in the anode when x-rays are produced (where s stands for seconds)?

    1. $kVp \times mA \times s$
    2. $kVp \times mA \times s \times 1.35$
    3. $kVp \times mA \times s \times 1.41$

A. 1 and 2
B. 1 and 3
C. 2 and 3
D. 1, 2, and 3

Questions 104–107 consist of four lettered headings followed by a list of numbered words or phrases. For each numbered word or phrase, select the heading with which it is most closely related. Each heading may be used once, more than once, or not at all.

    A. Density
    B. Contrast
    C. Sharpness
    D. Distortion

104. Intensifying screen contact

105. Voltage waveform

106. Filament heating

107. Inverse square law

108. Of the following groups of exposure factors, which would provide the LEAST optical density in a processed radiograph?

    A. 150 mA, 1.0 second, 53 kVp, 36 inches FFD/SID
    B. 200 mA, 0.4 second, 40 kVp, 32 inches FFD/SID
    C. 300 mA, 0.6 second, 73 kVp, 72 inches FFD/SID
    D. 400 mA, 0.3 second, 46 kVp, 42 inches FFD/SID

109. On single-phase generators, the technnologist can test the accuracy of the exposure timer with a simple gadget—a metal top with one small hole near its edge. When the top is spun manually while resting on a cassette, the processed image will show a series of dots indicating the number of pulses of current that occurred during the elapsed exposure period. How many dots would appear for a correctly functioning timer set at 0.3 second on a full-wave rectified generator?

    A. 6
    B. 12
    C. 36
    D. 48

110. The tomographic method isolates one plane or slice of the anatomy, which is imaged clearly, while blurring out the anatomy above and below that selected plane. The thickness of the in-focus plane is decreased by

    A. increasing the tomographic (exposure) angle
    B. increasing focus-object distance (FOD) and keeping tube travel distance the same
    C. changing the level of the objective plane
    D. keeping FOD constant and decreasing tube travel distance

111. In the following diagram of an image-intensifier, or amplifier, tube, the component labeled with the number 6 is the

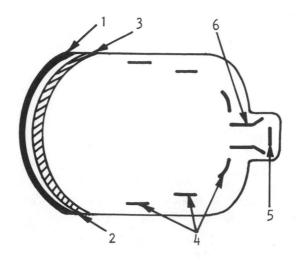

A. output phosphor
B. photocathode
C. focusing electrode
D. anode

112. Image-intensified fluoroscopy not only improves the quality of the fluoroscopic image but also increases the scope of viewing and imaging methods available with it, as compared with direct fluoroscopy. Which of the following imaging methods produces the best-quality image in a still format?

A. Video disk
B. Cassette spot films
C. Strip spots (70 mm, 90 mm, 105 mm)
D. Videotape

113. A number of elements must be considered in order to produce stereoradiographic images that will "stereo" properly. All of the following promote the production of a stereo pair of images EXCEPT

A. a tube shift:focus-image distance (FID) of 1:10
B. the first image made with the central ray centered to the cassette
C. the cassettes in an identical location for each exposure
D. tube shift direction perpendicular to the dominant anatomic lines

114. An automatic exposure control, or "phototimer," is a very useful piece of equipment. Acceptable fluoroscopic spot films would be impossible to obtain without it, and patients with unsuspected pathology might require more than one exposure. Certain parameters, however, must be observed when it is being used. In the production of an accurate phototimed radiograph, it is essential that

    A. backup time be set at 0.1 second
    B. all pickup chambers or detectors be selected, regardless of the anatomy being radiographed
    C. x-ray field size be as large as or larger than pickup chamber size
    D. lead shields be avoided near the pickup chamber, because the scatter they generate can affect radiographic density

115. The anode heel effect, which results in a variation in the output from the anode to the cathode side of the tube, can be annoying when it cannot be used to advantage. The anode heel effect might be visible when radiographing uniformly thick anatomic parts on

    A. a 14 × 14-inch chest examination at 72 inches
    B. a 14 × 17-inch abdomen examination supine at 40 inches
    C. a 10 × 12-inch hip joint examination at 40 inches
    D. a 8 × 10-inch right upper quadrant abdomen examination erect at 40 inches

116. The radiographic image of any object is always larger than the object because of the divergence of the x-ray beam and the distance between the object and the imaging plane. When a series of radiographs have been made on different x-ray units, the amount of magnification is an important factor in comparing object sizes (organ or lesion sizes) over time. What is the object size if the magnification factor (MF) is 1.25 and the image size is measured as 3.5 mm?

    A. 2.5 mm
    B. 2.8 mm
    C. 3.0 mm
    D. 3.2 mm

117. The radiologist who is comparing many examinations of the same part finds it helpful to have all radiographs exhibit comparable density, regardless of the circumstances under which they were exposed. A portable chest radiograph is initially made at 40 inches with 3 mAs. As the patient improves and is able to sit up, a 6-foot radiograph is obtained. What mAs will show comparable density at this new FFD?

    A. 5.4
    B. 7.0
    C. 9.7
    D. 92.5

118. Of the x-ray interactions with matter that occur in the diagnostic energy range, the greatest positive contribution to radiographic contrast is made by

    A. Compton interaction
    B. photoelectric interaction
    C. pair production
    D. Thompson scatter

119. Restriction of the primary beam to the smallest area of clinical interest contributes to both reduced patient dose and increased radiographic quality. When a variable-shutter light-beam collimator is not available, other beam restrictors may be used and, if selected specifically for the situation at hand, can be quite effective. Which of the following would best restrict the beam?

   A. Lead mask on the cassette
   B. Flare cone
   C. Aperture diaphragm
   D. Extension cylinder cone

120. As tubes begin to age, whether normally or at an accelerated rate, changes occur in their operation that make achieving correctly exposed radiographs very difficult unless an automatic exposure system is used. Impending failure in the x-ray tube may be evidenced by

   A. absence of tube current
   B. increased tube ouput
   C. complete lack of exposure
   D. decreased and variable tube output

121. Radiographic contrast is so very important in the perception of image detail that special attention must be given to ensure an adequate level when a contrast medium is not being used. All of the following will alter radiographic contrast EXCEPT

   A. increasing screen speed
   B. increasing FFD or SID
   C. decreasing the size of the x-ray field
   D. decreasing kV and increasing mAs proportionally

122. Using exposure factors that supply a longer gray or contrast scale in the image gives the technologist room to make a small error and still have an acceptable radiograph. Which of the following offers the greatest amount of exposure latitude for the same density?

   A.   63 kVp, 160 mAs
   B.   74 kVp, 80 mAs
   C. 102 kVp, 20 mAs
   D. 138 kVp,   5 mAs

123. The same computer technology that produced the CT image has been applied to some fluoroscopy and radiographic examinations and has been termed digital imaging. Digitization has proved to be tremendously advantageous in

   A. angiography
   B. contrast studies of the gastrointestinal tract
   C. tomography
   D. pediatric radiography

124. Which of the following sets of exposure factors will contribute to a radiograph with the sharpest image details, or the least penumbra (where OFD stands for object-film distance)?

   A. 1.0-mm focal spot, 48-inch FFD, 2-inch OFD
   B. 1.5-mm focal spot, 40-inch FFD, 2-inch OFD
   C. 2.0-mm focal spot, 40-inch FFD, 4-inch OFD
   D. 2.0-mm focal spot, 36-inch FFD, 3-inch OFD

125. Detail sharpness and resolution are very closely related characteristics of the radiographic image. Detail sharpness can be measured by line-spread function and the definition of penumbra. Resolution is measured by means of a

A. spinning top test
B. pinhole camera
C. wire mesh screen test
D. bar test pattern

126. To be able to use a radiographic grid correctly and to best advantage, the technologist must be in command of much information about its structure and function. To avoid grid cutoff, particular attention must be paid to the grid's

A. ratio
B. radius
C. frequency
D. total lead content

127. Imaging a soft-tissue anatomic part such as the breast presents difficulties in the trade-off of dose and image quality, but certain modifications of the x-ray tube have more recently made mammography an essential component in breast cancer diagnosis. Which of the following would NOT be part of a dedicated mammographic unit?

A. Tungsten target
B. 2.5-mm aluminum primary-beam filter
C. Molybdenum target
D. Beryllium tube window

128. Radiographic contrast is often described as having either a long scale (low contrast), or short scale (high contrast). In which of the following examinations is a relatively short scale of contrast required for best diagnostic results?

A. PA and lateral projections of the chest
B. Intravenous pyelogram (urogram)
C. Barium enema
D. Upper gastrointestinal series

129. If the characteristic curve of a given film shows that 10 mR is needed to produce a density of 1.0 on that film, then the film speed is

A. 1.0
B. 10
C. 100
D. 1,000

130. An abdominal examination using high-speed intensifying screens is taken at 80 kVp, 50 mAs, and results in a patient exposure of 120 mR. If the same examination is repeated without using screens, resulting in an exposure to the patient of 5,760 mR, what is the intensification factor of the film-screen combination?

A. 0.02
B. 4
C. 48
D. 57

131. One of the most important image characteristics is the sharpness with which details of anatomy are recorded in the radiograph. Radiographic detail sharpness is not at all affected by

A. the mA station
B. primary-beam filtration
C. the intensifying screen speed
D. focal spot size

132. The established technique chart for any radiographic unit serves the technologist only as a detailed guide for "normal" tissue volumes and densities in "average" situations. Radiographic contrast can be increased for any specific examination if the

    1. kVp is decreased by 15%
    2. mAs is doubled
    3. screen imaging system is changed to rare earth

A. 1 and 2
B. 1 and 3
C. 2 and 3
D. 1, 2, and 3

133. Which of the following components is located in the gantry assembly of the CT unit?

A. Computer
B. Detector array
C. Autotransformer
D. Microprocessor

134. Radiographic contrast in skeletal imaging of trauma victims is not usually a problem, but when an elderly patient has primary or metastatic disease in the facial bones, special precautions must be taken to minimize the loss of contrast. Which of the following strategies would be appropriate in such a situation?

    1. Extending the FID as much as possible
    2. Using low-latitude film
    3. Using a high-speed intensifying screen

A. 1 and 2
B. 1 and 3
C. 2 and 3
D. 1, 2, and 3

135. For an intravenous pyelogram examination on a 1-year-old child measuring 9 cm at the abdomen it would be appropriate to use a

    1. radiographic grid
    2. low to medium kVp range
    3. high-speed (200) screen system

A. 1 and 2
B. 1 and 3
C. 2 and 3
D. 1, 2, and 3

136. The sharper an anatomic detail is imaged in the radiograph, the more diagnostic that radiograph will be. Radiographic sharpness is the sum of a number of geometric factors, some of which can be controlled by the technologist and some of which cannot. Which of the following factors is directly proportional to radiographic sharpness and can almost always be controlled by the technologist?

A. OFD
B. Effective focal spot size
C. Intensifying screen speed
D. Patient motion

137. To prevent damage to tubes that have no circuitry to prevent unsafe exposures, a chart is given indicating maximum values for single exposures on a relatively cold anode. Which of the following statements correctly describe the tube-rating chart below?

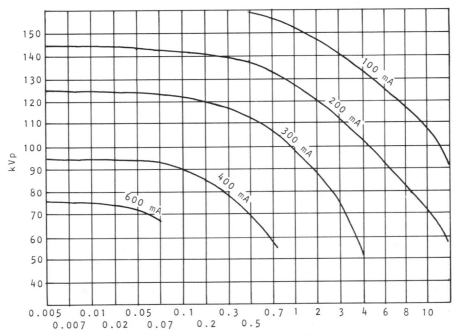

Maximum exposure time in seconds

1. 125 kVp, 300 mA, 0.3 second can be made
2. 85 kVp, 400 mA, 0.05 second can be made
3. 140 kVp, 200 mA, 0.5 second cannot be made

A. 1 and 2
B. 1 and 3
C. 2 and 3
D. 1, 2, and 3

138. With the purchase of a new, higher-powered generator, one x-ray department found that film quality could be improved (by reducing penumbra) in some upright examinations of joints by using an 8-foot FFD. At the original 40-inch FFD, 12 mAs produced the desired radiographic density. What mAs was required when the FFD was increased to 8 feet?

A. 21 mAs
B. 29 mAs
C. 50 mAs
D. 69 mAs

139. Edge enhancement is an advantageous characteristic of which of the following imaging systems?

A. Rare earth screens
B. Xeroradiography
C. Digital subtraction
D. Magnetic resonance imaging

140. The kVp selected for each examination is probably the most significant exposure factor because it affects so many aspects of the finished radiograph. Which of the following remains unaffected by variations in kVp?

A. Exposure latitude
B. Radiographic density
C. Scattered radiation at the image plane
D. Image magnification

141. If the following four sets of exposure factors were used to make four radiographs, which of the four radiographs would exhibit the LEAST optical density?

A.   75 mA, 0.5   second, 67 kVp, 34 inches FFD/SID
B.   250 mA, 0.75 second, 58 kVp, 36 inches FFD/SID
C.   400 mA, 0.2   second, 79 kVp, 60 inches FFD/SID
D.   800 mA, 0.03 second, 93 kVp, 72 inches FFD/SID

142. Which of the following statements is (are) true concerning the fixing solution used in the chemical processing of exposed film?

1. Unexposed silver halide crystals are removed from the film emulsion
2. The emulsion shrinks and hardens as a result of fixation
3. Fixation takes place in an alkaline pH solution

A. 1 only
B. 1 and 2
C. 2 and 3
D. 1, 2, and 3

143. An intensifying screen's ability to intensify the action of x-rays on radiographic film is a function of its active ingredient, phosphors. Phosphors should possess

    1. high atomic number
    2. phosphorescence
    3. conversion efficiency

A. 1 and 2
B. 1 and 3
C. 2 and 3
D. 1, 2, and 3

144. Which of the following statements are true concerning automatic rapid processing?

    1. Replenishment occurs as each film passes through the processor
    2. The rinse, or stop bath, is eliminated between the developer and fixer tanks
    3. Better image quality is obtained in automatic processing than in manual processing

A. 1 and 2
B. 1 and 3
C. 2 and 3
D. 1, 2, and 3

POSTTEST—RADIOGRAPHIC EXPOSURE AND PROCESSING
ANSWERS, EXPLANATIONS, AND REFERENCES

97–100. The answers are 97-A, 98-D, 99-B, 100-A. Grid cutoff is the undesirable absorption of primary-beam x-rays by the radiographic grid. A grid is made up of very thin strips of lead spaced with wood, plastic, or aluminum to permit passage of the transmitted radiation while absorbing the scattered photons. If the primary beam is not centered and perpendicular to the grid center, the transmitted photons will not pass through the spaces between the lead strips but will be absorbed, or cut off, along with the scattered radiation. The radiograph will show decreased density in the area where both scattered and remnant beams have been absorbed by the grid.

An aperture diaphragm is the simplest type of beam restrictor, usually just a cutout lead sheet attached to the tube itself to confine the beam to a specific area at a set focus-film distance (FFD). These are still found on head stand units with a fixed FFD, where only two cassette sizes are used. The aperture diaphragm should restrict the beam to an area slightly smaller than the film size.

The primary beam is restricted to the area of clinical interest only, to prevent unnecessary exposure. Patient dose increases as tissue area irradiated increases. Evidence of collimation should be visible on every radiograph (an unexposed border should be visible). Correct collimation also increases the quality of the image by reducing scatter production.

Radius refers to the convergence line or point, an imaginary point above the grid at which the lead strips of a focused grid would meet if they were extended. The significance of radius is that it indicates the correct FFD at which the grid should be employed for maximum transmission of primary beam photons. Cutoff results when a focused grid is used at less or greater distance than 25% of its stated radius. *(Bushong, p 187–188, 201–202, 204, 206–209, 547)*

101. The answer is B. The size of the focal spot (or actually, the width of the focal track) selected has no effect on the quantity or quality of the beam produced, nor does it attenuate the beam in any way and so has no effect on radiographic density. Focal spot size is related to the geometry of beam formation, whereas radiographic density is a photographic property. Radiographic density is inversely proportional to the square of the focus-film distance (FFD)/source-image distance (SID). Three-phase generation produces a higher effective kV than does single-phase generation for the same control panel factors, resulting in increased radiographic density. Intensifying screens give off light proportional to the x-ray exposure received by them. Higher-speed screens are those that emit more light for any given x-ray exposure received, thus amplifying the resultant exposure to the film. Varying intensifying screen speed changes radiographic density dramatically. *(Bushong, p 278–288; Selman, p 263–264, 286, 327, 340)*

102. The answer is B. The quality of the useful x-ray beam is primarily determined by the kVp of tube operation and is modified by the amount of aluminum filtration in the beam's path. The kVp controls the energy, or penetrating power, of the beam: As kVp increases, penetrability, or beam quality, increases. The purpose of the aluminum filtration in the primary beam is to totally absorb the lower-energy photons, but it also slightly reduces energy, or quality, of every photon that it does not absorb completely. The SID and mAs affect only the numbers of photons in the beam, or the beam quantity, at any point. *(Bushong, p 177, 210; Selman, p 176, 200)*

103. The answer is D. When electrons from the cathode filament interact with atoms of the target, both x-ray photons and heat are produced. Roughly 99% of the kinetic energy of the electrons produces heat, leaving about 1% for x-ray production. Anode heat is directly proportional to tube current and kVp. For single-phase machines, heat units are calculated by multiplying kVp × mAs. When three-phase generation is used, slightly more heat is generated, so heat units are calculated by multiplying kVp × 1.35 for 6-pulse generation and kVp × mAs x 1.41 for 12-pulse generation. *(Selman, p 224)*

104–107. The answers are 104-C, 105-A, 106-A, 107-A. Radiographic sharpness is dependent on very close contact between the film and the two intensifying screens used. Each burst of light from the screen should be immediately incident on the film so that the light photons do not spread out and enlarge the detail they represent and make the image less sharp. Inadequate contact between the screens and the film is almost always the result of rough handling or dropping the cassette.

X-ray generators produce a variety of voltage waveforms, including half-wave and full-wave rectification (single-phase generation) and 6-pulse and 12-pulse (three-phase generation). The number of x-rays being produced at the target (and the resulting radiographic density) increases when peak voltages are reached. Peak voltage is reached twice as frequently with full-wave generation as with half-wave, so radiographic density will be doubled. Three-phase generation maintains the voltage at a high level, very close to peak, resulting in the production of more photons and higher-energy photons. Radiographic density is increased (with exactly the same kVp and mAs used) when three-phase generation is used compared with single-phase generation.

Heating the x-ray tube filament produces thermionic emission. Those emitted electrons drawn across the x-ray tube by the applied high voltage constitute tube current, or mA. The mA times the length of time of exposure (mAs) is directly proportional to radiographic density.

The inverse square law describes the reduction in intensity or exposure rate of an x-ray beam as it spreads out over distance from the focus, or source. At 4 feet from the source, the original intensity is covering four times the area that it covered at 1 foot from the source, so area-for-area, the beam is one-quarter its original intensity. X-ray intensity, or exposure, causes film blackening, or radiographic density. Radiographic density varies inversely with the square of the distance from the source. *(Bushong, p 154; Selman, p 336, 340–344)*

108. The answer is B. Of the choices listed in the question, 200 mA, 0.4 second, 40 kVp, 32 inches FFD/SID will produce the least optical density in a processed radiograph. This can be shown in the following steps: *Step 1:* Multiply mA × seconds; mAs is directly proportional to optical density, or in choice **A**, 150 mAs; choice **B**, 80 mAs; choice **C**, 180 mAs, and choice **D**, 120 mAs. *Step 2:* kVp is related to optical density in that increasing kVp by 15% doubles optical density; reducing kVp by 15% halves optical density. Increasing kVp by 15% *and* halving mAs or decreasing kVp by 15% *and* doubling mAs will keep optical density constant. For **B**, increase the original kVp of 40 by 15%, to 46, and halve the original mAs of 80, to 40. Again, increase kVp by 15%, to 53, and halve mAs, to 20. Optical density has not changed. For **C**, decrease the original kVp of 73 by 15%, to 62, and double the original mAs of 180, to 360. Again, decrease kVp by 15%, to 53, and double mAs, to 720. Optical density remains constant. For **D**, increase the original kVp of 46 by 15%, to 53, and halve the original mAs of 120, to 60. Optical density remains constant. To summarize, **A:** 150 mAs, 53 kVp; **B:** 20 mAs, 53 kVp; **C:** 720 mAs, 53 kVp; and **D:** 60 mAs, 53 kVp. *Step 3:* Optical density varies inversely as the square of the FFD/SID. Halving FFD/SID will quadruple optical density, and doubling FFD/SID will reduce optical density to one-quarter of its original level. Use the mAs/distance equation to keep optical density proportional as FFD/SID is changed:

For **B**, $\dfrac{mAs_1}{mAs_2} = \left(\dfrac{D_1}{D_2}\right)^2 \rightarrow \dfrac{20}{X} = \left(\dfrac{32}{36}\right)^2 \rightarrow \dfrac{20}{X} = \dfrac{1{,}024}{1{,}296} \rightarrow 1{,}024X = 25{,}920 \rightarrow$

$X = 25.3$ mAs.

For **C**, $\dfrac{mAs_1}{mAs_2} = \left(\dfrac{D_1}{D_2}\right)^2 \rightarrow \dfrac{720}{X} = \left(\dfrac{72}{36}\right)^2 \rightarrow \dfrac{720}{X} = \dfrac{5{,}184}{1{,}296} \rightarrow 5{,}184X = 933{,}120 \rightarrow$

$X = 180$ mAs.

For **D**, $\dfrac{mAs_1}{mAs_2} = \left(\dfrac{D_1}{D_2}\right)^2 \rightarrow \dfrac{60}{X} = \left(\dfrac{42}{36}\right)^2 \rightarrow \dfrac{60}{X} = \dfrac{1{,}764}{1{,}296} \rightarrow 1{,}764X = 77{,}760 \rightarrow$

$X = 44.08$ mAs.

Final summary:
A. 150 mAs, 53 kVp, 36 inches FFD/SID
B. 25 mAs, 53 kVp, 36 inches FFD/SID
C. 180 mAs, 53 kVp, 36 inches FFD/SID
D. 44 mAs, 53 kVp, 36 inches FFD/SID
Now that all factors have been brought to the same terms, it can be seen that radiograph **B** would have the least optical density.

109. The answer is C. Full-wave rectified units using all the alternating current pulses of 60-cycle current will emit 120 bursts of x-ray photons per second. This would result in 120 dots of density visible on the processed radiograph of a spinning top (if this were possible in a practical situation). If the x-ray exposure timer were set for 0.3 second and were operating accurately, then 36 dots would be visible (120 dots per second divided by 0.03 second). *(Bushong, p 125–127; Selman, p 242–243)*

110. The answer is A. The tomographic (exposure) angle, or the number of degrees that the central ray moves through, is the controller of "cut," or in-focus plane thickness: The larger that angle, the greater the blurring of details above and below the in-focus plane and the thinner that in-focus slice will be. Amplitude, or linear distance of tube travel, and focus-object distance (FOD) can affect cut thickness in that they can change the exposure or tomographic angle. Either increasing FOD without changing linear amplitude or decreasing linear amplitude without changing FOD will decrease tomographic or exposure angle, increasing the thickness of the in-focus plane. The level of the objective plane selected is unrelated to the thickness of the slice. *(Bushong, p 305; Selman, p 425–427)*

111. The answer is D. In the figure that accompanies the question, the number 6 identifies the positive terminal of the image intensifier, the point at which the electrons cross over the anode. The component labeled 2 is the input phosphor, where the remnant x-ray beam is made visible as a light image. The number 3 labels the photocathode, or negative terminal, in which the light photons cause emission of electrons in the same pattern. The focusing lenses (4) force the electron beam to converge at the anode, and 5 represents the output phosphor, in which the received electron image is emitted as a light image. A glass envelope (1) encloses the vacuum and components of the image-intensifier tube. *(Bushong, p 294–296; Selman, p 405–409)*

112. The answer is B. Cassette spot films, in which the image is formed by a relatively high mAs radiographic beam and is recorded on a film-screen system, provide the best image quality of those methods listed in the question. Cassette spot films are actually radiographs taken during fluoroscopy. Their disadvantages include interruption of fluoroscopic viewing and a time lapse for chemical development before the image can be viewed. Strip spot films, which record the image on film from the output phosphor, have good image quality (especially the larger format), but not equal to that of cassette spot films. Video disk is a magnetic recording system mainly used for "still" images. The recording medium itself offers reduced resolution, and the image is taken from the output phosphor of the image intensifier, with inherently less resolution than a primary-beam-generated image. *(Bushong, p 302; Chesney and Chesney [1984], p 398–402)*

113. The answer is B. To produce a stereoscopic pair of radiographs, the central ray must initially be directed through the appropriate part of the anatomy and to the center of the cassette. Then move the central ray one-half of the total tube-shift distance, perpendicular in direction to the dominant lines of the anatomy (if grid direction is not a problem) and make the first exposure. The central ray is then moved the whole distance of tube shift, back through the original centering position to a location one-half the distance of tube shift on the other side of the original central ray location, and the second exposure is made. If one exposure is made with the central ray centered to the cassette, the stereoscopic effect will be greatly diminished. The cassettes must be in the same location for each exposure, plus the tube shift:focus-image distance (FID) ratio must be 1:10. *(Bushong, p 307–310; Selman, p 411–415)*

114. The answer is C. An automatic exposure control, or phototimer, is a timing device that terminates the exposure when correct film density is achieved. Pickup chambers or detectors (which monitor the radiation exiting the patient or the dose at the film, depending on the type of device used) are centered over areas of the anatomy considered to be representative of the entire anatomy. If the x-ray field size is smaller than the detector or pickup chamber, so little radiation will be monitored that the time of exposure will be extended, resulting in an overexposed anatomic part. Backup time is a safety control set by the technologist; it will vary with the size of the part to be radiographed. Pickup chamber or detector selection depends on the number of density or thickness variations in the anatomy to be radiographed. Lead shields must never cover the pickup chambers or detectors, but they can be used for regular shielding. *(Bushong, p 124–125; Chesney and Chesney [1984], p 177–185)*

115. The answer is B. The anode heel effect produces a beam with greater intensity at the cathode side of the beam than at the anode side. The x-ray beam diverges from its source, so the entire beam, with its edge intensity variations, is not always used in its entirety for every radiograph. The greater the distance from the source or focal spot at which the image plane is placed, the smaller is the area of the beam used. In a 72-inch chest film that uses a small central portion of the beam, the variations caused by the anode heel effect would not be visible. Similarly, a small film size, such as 8×10 inches or 10×12 inches, even at 40 inches would use the central part of the beam, which is uniform in intensity. Depending on anode angle, the entire beam is generally needed at 40 inches to cover a 17-inch length corresponding to the anode-cathode axis, and if the patient is positioned with the thicker part of the anatomy toward the cathode end of the tube, uniform radiographic density would result. If the patient were uniformly thick, however, greater radiographic density would be visible at the cathode end of the radiograph. *(Bushong, p 118; Chesney and Chesney [1984], p 221)*

116. The answer is B. The magnification factor (MF) is equal to the ratio of image size to object size, or MF = image size/object size. The following calculations determine the object size for the example given in the question *(Bushong, p 272–273; Selman, p 356):*

$$1.25 = \frac{3.5 \text{ mm}}{X} \rightarrow 1.25X = 3.5 \text{ mm} \rightarrow \frac{1.25X}{1.25} = \frac{3.5 \text{ mm}}{1.25} \rightarrow X = .28 \text{ mm.}$$

117. The answer is C. The mAs-distance formula is derived form the inverse square law, which quantifies the reduction in beam intensity over distance. The mAs must be multiplied by a factor of 4 if the FFD is doubled. The following calculations yield the answer to the example given in the question *(Bushong, p 63–65; Selman, p 341–344):*

$$\frac{mAs_1}{mAs_2} = \left(\frac{D_1}{D_2}\right) \rightarrow \frac{3}{X} = \left(\frac{40}{72}\right)^2 \rightarrow \frac{3}{X} = \frac{1,600}{5,184} \rightarrow 1,600X = 15,552 \rightarrow$$

$$X = 9.72 \rightarrow X = 9.7 \text{ mAs.}$$

118. The answer is B. In the photoelectric interaction, the x-ray photon is completely absorbed in the tissue when the tissue atomic number is high and the photon energy is not sufficient to penetrate to the film. This results in a relatively unexposed area of film, which provides high contrast when compared with adjacent film areas receiving exposure from photons that were transmitted through tissues of lower atomic number. Compton scattered photons reduce image contrast without supplying information. Thompson scatter has very little effect on the image, and pair production does not occur in the diagnostic energy range. *(Bushong, p 161–162, 283; Selman, p 347–348)*

119. The answer is D. An extension cylinder cone can be almost as effective as a variable-shutter collimator in restricting the primary beam, because it restricts the beam both at the top, where it attaches to the x-ray tube, and at the bottom, closest to the image receptor. Although the image receptor is almost always rectangular, the circular extension cylinder cone can be adjusted in length until it shows an unexposed border on the radiograph, at the usual FFD. Flare cones and aperture diagrams restrict the beam only at the x-ray tube, and, although an aperture diaphragm can be designed to show an unexposed border on the film, a flare cone exposes an area larger than the film size. A cassette mask does not restrict the beam until it reaches the image plane. *(Bushong, p 187–191; Selman, 394–399)*

120. The answer is D. Gas molecules are liberated and accumulate during tube use, interfering with the passage of electrons from cathode to anode. Cathode electrons are deviated from their path and lose energy by interacting with the gas, therefore having less kinetic energy left when they reach the anode. Tube output is reduced from what would be anticipated from the control console setting. Tube output is also variable because the presence of gas is variable, as is the amount of interference it will cause. A lack of tube current would signal a severed filament or a failure in delivery of the current to the tube. Increased tube output is unrelated to aging but might be caused by variations in incoming line voltage. Complete lack of exposure (if tube current were indicated on the meter) would indicate a problem with the anode, unless the collimator were closed. *(Bushong, p 133–137; Chesney and Chesney [1984], p 268, 626–627)*

121. The answer is B. Increasing FFD or SID does not affect radiographic contrast. Those factors that increase or decrease contrast are related to the photographic aspects of image formation, not the geometry of the beam. Contrast is increased or enhanced by increasing intensifying screen speed, mainly because of the characteristics of the screen-type film that is used in combination with the intensifying screens. Scatter production is limited when x-ray field size is limited, and any decrease in scatter results in an increase in contrast. Decreasing kVp and increasing mAs proportionally (in accordance with the 15% rule) will increase contrast while maintaining a constant density. *(Bushong, p 282–284, 288; Selman, p 345–351)*

122. The answer is D. Radiographic contrast is controlled by kVp and is inversely proportional to exposure latitude. As kVp increases, more of the beam is transmitted through tissues of all densities, and a longer image gray scale results. A 9-kVp error at 63 kVp (a 15% increase in kVp) will result in an unacceptable doubling (100% increase) of density, but a 9-kVp error at 138 kVp (a 6.5% increase in kVp) will result in less than a 50% density increase, which allows the radiograph to be acceptable from a diagnostic standpoint. Therefore, 138 kVp offers the greatest amount of exposure latitude in comparison with the other factors presented in the question. *(Selman, p 345–351; Thompson, p 122–125)*

123. The answer is A. The digitization of the angiographic examination has permitted multiple subtracted images to be made electronically during the examination. Subtracted images in angiography aid in a more accurate and rapid diagnosis by eliminating bony or soft-tissue structures that may be superimposed on the image of the vascular dye column. What was previously done using a time-consuming photographic process can now be achieved instantaneously through electronic manipulation of images. The other examinations listed in the question do not require the use of subtraction. *(Bushong, p 345–362; Curry et al., p 420–424)*

124. The answer is A. The geometric factors governing sharpness can be solved or evaluated using the penumbra (P) formula:

$$P = \frac{\text{width of focus} \times \text{object-film distance (OFD)}}{\text{FOD}}$$

The following calculations show how to find P for the examples listed in the question (OFD is calculated by subtracting FOD from FFD):

A.$P = \dfrac{1.0 \text{ mm} \times 2 \text{ inches}}{46 \text{ inches}}$ $P = 0.0434 \text{ mm}$

B. $P = \dfrac{1.5 \text{ mm} \times 2 \text{ inches}}{38 \text{ inches}}$ $P = 0.0789$ mm

C. $P = \dfrac{2.0 \text{ mm} \times 4 \text{ inches}}{36 \text{ inches}}$ $P = 0.2222$ mm

D. $P = \dfrac{2.0 \text{ mm} \times 3 \text{ inches}}{33 \text{ inches}}$ $P = 0.18181$ mm

The least penumbra is 0.0434 mm, from the combination of factors used in **A.** *(Bushong, p 278–281; Selman, p 329)*

125. The answer is D. Resolution is defined as the ability of an imaging system to produce separate images of two closely spaced objects. A bar test pattern of equal-sized lead lines and spaces is generally used to define resolution in line pairs/mm or cm. The spinning top test is primarily used to test an x-ray exposure timer for accuracy when the generator is single phase. A pinhole camera is used to image the focal spot; this image is then measured, and focal spot size can be determined from it. A wire mesh screen test involves radiographing a piece of ordinary wire mesh embedded in lucite and placed directly on a cassette to evaluate film-screen contact. *(Bushong, p 247–248, 258; Selman, p 333–334)*

126. The answer is B. All focused grids have a "radius" designation: that distance from the target at which the grid should be used to have the maximum amount of primary beam coincident with the angle of the grid spaces. If the grid is used at a shorter or longer FFD/SID, the angle of the diverging primary rays will not permit their passage through the grid and the rays will strike the lead strips and be absorbed. This uneven absorption of primary beam radiation is called *cutoff.* Ratio (the height of the lead strip to the width of the space) and frequency (the number of lead strips per centimeter or inch of grid) can be combined to express total lead content of the grid, a measure of its efficiency in absorbing scattered photons. *(Bushong, p 206–207; Selman, p 380–385)*

127. The answer is B. The breast is a very low-contrast part, made up of fat, glandular, and connective tissues that exhibit very little radiographic difference one from another. Using low kVp (between 30 and 50) maximizes the small tissue differences that do exist, but a 2.5-mm aluminum filter (the filter in the usual radiographic beam) would eliminate many of those very low-energy photons that would be useful. Dedicated mammographic units may have a tungsten target with a small amount of added filter to absorb those photons with too little energy to contribute to the image or may employ a molybdenum target with a molybdenum filter and a beryllium or a thinner glass tube window. *(Bushong, p 313–316; Chesney and Chesney [1984], p 283–285)*

128. The answer is B. Radiographic contrast is primarily the result of beam characteristics, subject characteristics, and film characteristics. In a body part that has low inherent contrast or little atomic density differences between adjacent tissues, relatively low kVp will amplify these small differences and increase detail visibility by increasing radiographic contrast. The intravenous pyelogram is an attempt to visualize part of a low-contrast area by using a contrast medium (injected intravenously). However, that medium loses contrast through the biologic processes that bring it to the urinary system. The kVp should be kept below 85, preferably below 75 kVp, for optimum contrast in this examination. Chest examinations benefit from relatively low contrast; high kVp permits visualization of both the lungs and the mediastinum. Barium studies also exhibit greater diagnostic information when the barium is penetrated by quite high kVp, permitting simultaneous visualization of the outer dimensions of the gastrointestinal tube, details of the mucosal pattern inside the lumen, and adequate presentation of the surrounding anatomy. *(Bushong, p 164–170; Selman, p 348–349)*

129. The answer is C. In sensitometry, the density specified for determining the speed of a radiographic film is 1.0. Speed can be measured in reciprocal roentgens using the following formula:

$$\text{Speed} = \frac{1}{\text{number of roentgens needed to produce a density of 1.0.}}$$

If 10 mR are needed to produce a density of 1.0 using a given type of film, one must first convert mR to R (1 R = 1,000 mR). Then compute the speed factor:

$$\frac{1.0}{10 \text{ mR}} = \frac{1.0}{0.01 \text{ R}} = 100.$$

The speed of this film is 100. Speed is an important factor to consider when choosing a film, as slower films require more exposure than faster films in order to produce the same radiographic film density. The more exposure required, the greater the dose to the patient. Faster films may exhibit poorer image quality, however, due to increased radiographic noise. *(Bushong, p 268–269; Chesney and Chesney [1981], p 63–68)*

130. The answer is C. The intensification factor (IF) is the ratio of exposure required with screens to those without screens in order to produce the same density on film, or IF = Exposure required without screens/Exposure required with screens. For the example given in the questions, IF = 5,760 mR/120mR, or 48. The high-speed screen described in the example intensified the action of x-rays 48 times that of the system that did not use a screen, resulting in less exposure to the patient. Screens are most often used for abdominal radiography today because of the intensification factor. *(Bushong, p 245–246; Selman, p 287)*

131. The answer is B. The aluminum filtration placed in the primary beam to absorb the lower-energy photons can decrease both radiographic density and radiographic contrast, but it does not affect beam geometry or image resolution and so has no effect on radiographic detail sharpness. The size of the focal spot selected is most imporant: When its size doubles, unsharpness doubles. The selection of mA station also affects the size of the focal spot: The higher the mA station, the greater the number of electrons striking the focal spot. As electron numbers increase, it becomes more difficult for the focusing cup to confine the beam. Thus it spreads out, striking a larger area of the focal track and creating a larger source of x-ray photons. As intensifying screen speed increases, resulting image sharpness decreases proportionally as the light image diffuses, producing slightly overlapping images in the film emulsion. *(Bushong, p 178, 272–276; Selman, p 327–338)*

132. The answer is A. Radiographic contrast is increased (in the well-calibrated x-ray machine) by using the "15%" rule, or the relationship between kVp, mAs, and radiographic density. The kVp controls image contrast, and reducing kVp will increase image contrast but will reduce image density. Reducing kVp by 15% will halve radiography density; doubling mAs will double radiographic density. When both changes are made simultaneously, image density remains constant but image contrast will have been reduced. For example, 80 kVp with 40 mAs has the same radiographic density as 68 kVp with 80 mAs, but the latter has greater contrast. Rare earth screens are not uniform in their density response across a wide range of kVp values and so are not generally used to control contrast. *(Bushong, p 174–175; Thompson, p 111, 116–117)*

133. The answer is B. The CT unit is organized into three main components—the operating console, the computer, and the gantry. The gantry consists of the x-ray tube, the detectors, and usually the high-voltage transformer as well. The computer (and there may be a separate computer for each additional viewing console) has a primary memory and a microprocessor or an array processor. The operating console houses the controls for exposure factors and the monitoring meters, plus the autotransformer, but it may be separate from the console that communicates with the computer. *(Bushong, p 370–372; Chesney and Chesney [1984], p 480)*

134. The answer is C. X-ray film that has low latitude is normally called high-contrast film, and its use in an elderly patient with primary or metastatic disease in the facial bones would greatly improve radiographic contrast. High-contrast film is manufactured to amplify small differences in beam absorption, thereby increasing total radiographic contrast. A high-speed intensifying screen rather than a detail or fine screen will expand film contrast, again adding to an increase in radiographic contrast. Extending the FID does not affect the pattern of differential absorption of the beam and so will not change contrast in any way. *(Bushong, p 265–272; Selman, 345–351)*

135. The answer is C. An intravenous pyelogram examination of a 1-year-old child measuring 9 cm at the abdomen is aimed at imaging a low-contrast system with the use of an iodinated contrast agent. Radiographic contrast must be maintained by the use of low to medium kVp ranges, as some effectiveness of the contrast agent is lost through dilution in body fluids. If a variable kVp technique were used, 58 kVp would transmit enough photons for suitable part penetration when coupled with the correct mAs to provide acceptable film density. A high-speed system will maintain contrast while keeping dose low, without generating distracting mottle. A radiographic grid is not required on a body part of this size, because the amount of scatter generated would not interfere with image contrast if tight collimation were used. Of course, mAs (dose) would have to be doubled, tripled, or quadrupled to accommodate a radiographic grid. *(Selman, p 348–349; Thompson, p 98, 122)*

136. The answer is B. Geometric unsharpness, or penumbra, is defined as being directly proportional to both effective focal spot size and OFD and inversely proportional to FOD. Therefore, the smaller the effective focus, the sharper the image. OFD is also crucial to radiographic sharpness but cannot always be selected by the technologist, as effective focal spot size can. OFD depends on patient size, location of the anatomy of interest within the patient, and also the distance that has been designed between the tabletop and the image plane. Increasing intensifying screen speed and patient motion increase unsharpness but are not directly proportional. *(Bushong, p 278–281; Selman, p 329)*

137. The answer is C. To determine if the exposure can be safely made, find the point on the vertical axis between 80 and 90 that represents 85 kVp. Follow that point or draw a line to the right until the 400-mA curve is met. Now move straight down to the horizontal axis and read the maximum time permissible with 85 kVp and 400 mA: 0.2 second. The time selected is only 0.05, much shorter than the maximum, so this exposure is safe and can be made. For 3, find the point on the vertical axis for 140 kVp; follow that line to the right until it intersects the 200-mA curve. Continue straight down to the horizontal axis and read the maximum safe time: 0.3 second. A longer time than 0.3 second (0.5 second) cannot be safely made. For 1, find the point on the vertical axis for 125 kVp, follow along to the last point at which the 125-kVp line is superimposed on the 300-mA line, move straight down to the horizontal axis, and read the maximum permissible time: 0.07 second, much shorter than 0.3 second. Exposure 1 cannot be safely made. *(Selman, p 222–223)*

138. The answer is D. The mAs distance formula can be applied when a constant film density is required even though the FFD must be changed. The following calculations demonstrate the formula's use in this problem *(Bushong, p 63–65; Selman, p 341–344):*

$$\frac{mAs_1}{mAs_2} = \left(\frac{D_1}{D_2}\right) \rightarrow \frac{12}{X} = \left(\frac{40}{96}\right)^2 \rightarrow \frac{12}{X} = \frac{1,600}{9,216} \rightarrow 1,600X = 110,592 \rightarrow$$

$$X = 69.12 \rightarrow X = 69 \text{ mAs.}$$

139. The answer is B. Edge enhancement is a characteristic of the xeroradiographic imaging system that accentuates contrast at tissue interfaces that normally have low inherent contrast. Edge enhancement is a desirable effect, as abrupt edges can be seen between one tissue and another, enhancing detail visibility because of the distribution of the blue toner in the image. For instance, a body part composed of two different tissues that differ in density only slightly will show noticeable enhancement of the edge or interface between the two tissues. This is because of the difference in the number of residual charges on the plate following exposure; the tissue of slightly lower density will have fewer charges remaining on the xeroradiographic plate beneath, whereas the tissue of slightly higher density will have more charges left on the plate beneath. When the xeroradiographic plate is processed, charged blue toner particles will be blown over the plate. More toner will be attracted to and will adhere to areas on the plate with a greater amount of residual charge, and less will adhere to areas with little residual charge. At the interface of these two slightly different regions of charge, there will be a robbing of toner on the side with greater charge, creating a defined edge with an adjacent halo (area of no toner due to robbing), thus creating edge enhancement. This characteristic is especially useful in mammography. *(Bushong, p 322–324; Curry et al., p 312, Selman, p 439–440)*

140. The answer is D. Film latitude refers to the range of exposures through which the film responds with useful densities, a property that is inversely proportional to contrast. The kVp is the variable used to change radiographic contrast from a short scale at low kVp through to a long scale at high kVp, increasing exposure latitude with decreasing contrast. The kVp increases in increments of 15%, each constituting a doubling of radiographic density. As kVp increases through the diagnostic energy range, Compton scattering occurs more and photoelectric absorption occurs less, increasing the proportion of scattered radiation reaching the image plane. Magnification in the image is the result of x-ray beam divergence plus the location of the part being radiographed, with magnification increasing as the part is moved away from the image plane, or toward the tube focus or source. Magnification is unrelated to variations in kVp. *(Bushong, p 269–273, 284–287; Selman, p 340)*

141. The answer is D. Of the choices given in the question, 800 mA, 0.03 second, 93 kVp, 72 inches FFD/SID will produce the least optical density. This can be shown in the following steps: *Step 1:* Multiply mA × seconds; mAs is directly proportional to optical density, or in choice **A,** 37.5 mAs; choice **B,** 187.5 mAs; choice **C,** 80 mAs; and choice **D,** 24 mAs. *Step 2:* kVp is to optical density in that increasing kVp by 15% doubles optical density; decreasing kVp by 15% halves optical density. Decreasing kVp by 15% *and* doubling mAs or increasing kVp by 15% *and* halving mAs will keep optical density constant. For **B,** increase the original kVp of 58 by 15%, to 67, and halve the original mAs of 187.5, to 93.75. Optical density has not changed. For **C,** decrease the original kVp of 79 by 15%, to 67, and double the original mAs of 80, to 160. Optical density has remained the same. For **D,** decrease the original kVp of 93 by 15%, to 79, and double the original mAs of 24, to 48. Again decrease the kVp by 15%, to 67, and double the mAs, to 96. Optical density has not varied. To summarize, **A:** 37.5 mAs, 67 kVp; **B:** 93.75 mAs, 67 kVp; **C:** 160 mAs, 67 kVp; **D:** 96 mAs, 67 kVp. *Step 3:* Optical density varies inversely as the square of the FFD/SID. Doubling FFD/SID will reduce optical density to one-quarter of its original level. Use the mAs/distance equation to keep optical density proportional as FFD/SID is changed:

$$\text{For A, } \frac{mAs_1}{mAs_2} = \left(\frac{D_1}{D_2}\right)^2 \rightarrow \frac{37.5}{X} = \left(\frac{34}{36}\right)^2 \rightarrow \frac{37.5}{X} = \frac{1,156}{1,296} \rightarrow 1,156X = 48,600 \rightarrow$$

$$X = 42.04 \text{ mAs.}$$

$$\text{For C, } \frac{mAs_1}{mAs_2} = \left(\frac{D_1}{D_2}\right)^2 \rightarrow \frac{160}{X} = \left(\frac{60}{30}\right)^2 \rightarrow \frac{160}{X} = \frac{3,600}{1,296} \rightarrow 3,600X = 207,360 \rightarrow$$

$$X = 57.6 \text{ mAs.}$$

$$\text{For } \mathbf{D}, \frac{mAs_1}{mAs_2} = \left(\frac{D_1}{D_2}\right)^2 \rightarrow \frac{96}{X} = \left(\frac{72}{36}\right)^2 \rightarrow \frac{96}{X} = \frac{5,184}{1,296} \rightarrow 5,184X = 124, 416 \rightarrow$$

$$X = 24 \text{ mAs.}$$

Final summary:
A. 42 mAs, 67 kVp, 36 inches FFD/SID
B. 94 mAs, 67 kVp, 36 inches FFD/SID
C. 58 mAs, 67 kVp, 36 inches FFD/SID
D. 24 mAs, 67 kVp, 36 inches FFD/SID
It is now apparent that the radiograph exhibiting the least optical density is **D**, as its mAs is the least.

142. The answer is B. Fixation is the chemical process that follows the development of an exposed film. One function of the fixing solution is to neutralize and stop development; therefore, acetic acid is used as an acidifier to neutralize development, which took place in an alkaline solution. The clearing agent (hypo), usually ammonium thiosulfate, removes or "clears" the unexposed, undeveloped silver halide crystals from the film emulsion, constituting another important function of the fixer solution. The hardener, also a major component of the fixer, shrinks and hardens the emulsion before the film is washed and dried. Potassium alum, chromium alum, and aluminum chloride are commonly employed hardening agents. A chemical such as sodium sulfite is also added to the fixing solution to help preserve chemical balance. Water is used as a solvent for the chemicals contained in the fixer as well as in the developer. Development takes place before fixation and changes exposed silver halide crystals to visible black metallic silver. Washing occurs after fixation, followed by drying of the film. *(Bushong, p 230–231; Chesney and Chesney [1981], p 149–156; Selman, p 314–315; Thompson, p 261–262)*

143. The answer is B. The phosphors in an intensifying screen should have a high atomic number so that the probability of x-ray photon interaction is high (quantum detection efficiency). Conversion efficiency is another important characteristic of the phosphor, as each phosphor should emit a large amount of light per interaction with x-ray photons. One of the primary advantages of intensifying screens is their ability to convert x-ray energy into visible light, which is much more efficient in exposing film emulsion than is direct x-ray action. Therefore, fewer x-rays are needed to expose a film when intensifying screens are used, resulting in reduced exposure (dose) to the patient. The color or wavelength of light emitted by phosphors (spectral emission) should match that to which the x-ray film emulsion is sensitive (spectral sensitivity). Spectral matching is essential in order to derive the maximum efficiency or speed in an imaging system. Phosphorescence is not a necessary characteristic of intensifying screens. It may be undesirable, because if the phosphors continue to emit light after x-ray exposure (stimulation) has been removed, this "afterglow" or "lag" may cause unwanted darkening of the film, resulting in an overexposed and possibly unacceptable radiographic image. Fluorescence is a necessary characteristic of the phosphors in an intensifying screen, as it means that they give off light only during x-ray exposure (stimulation). *(Bushong, p 245–255; Chesney and Chesney [1981], p 91–96; Selman, p 281–294; Thomspon, p 66–72)*

144. The answer is D. Automatic processors have not only reduced the time it takes to completely develop, fix, wash, and dry a radiographic film but have also ensured better image quality because of the consistency in processing. The element of human error has almost been eliminated, as the automatic processor develops, fixes, washes, and dries all films exactly the same way. As chemicals are used up during the processing cycle, new chemical (developer and fixer) is automatically pumped into the processor tanks as each film passes through the feed tray, activating a microswitch that turns on the replenishment for as long as the film travels through the microswitch. There is no need for a rinse or stop bath between the developer and fixer tanks of an automatic processor, because special rollers situated between the tanks squeegee excess chemical off the surface of the film. *(Bushong, p 231-235; Chesney and Chesney [1981], p 176, 204–218; Selman, 318–322; Thompson, p 258–270)*

PHYSICS AND EQUIPMENT

145. Of the following types of electromagnetic radiation, which sequence is arranged in order from the longest to the shortest wavelength of the spectrum?

    A. Infrared light—radio waves—visible light—ultraviolet light—x-rays—gamma rays
    B. Cosmic rays—radio waves—infrared light—visible light—ultraviolet light—x-rays—gamma rays
    C. Radio waves—infrared light—visible light—x-rays—gamma rays—cosmic rays
    D. Radio waves—visible—ultraviolet light—infrared light—x-rays—gamma rays

146. What is $68\,°F$ equal to on the Celsius scale?

    A. $12\,°C$
    B. $20\,°C$
    C. $65\,°C$
    D. $341\,°C$

147. Atoms that have the same mass number but different atomic numbers are called

    A. isotones
    B. isobars
    C. isomers
    D. isotopes

148. A material that is strongly attracted by a magnet is described as

    A. ferromagnetic
    B. paramagnetic
    C. nonmagnetic
    D. diamagnetic

149. Between 1895 and 1936, the target of an x-ray tube was a stationary tungsten disk surrounded by a larger copper block. When the rotating anode became available, its use revolutionized radiography by increasing

    1. actual target area 2 or 3 times
    2. tube heating capacity dramatically
    3. penumbra

    A. 1 only
    B. 2 only
    C. 3 only
    D. 1, 2, and 3

150. Certain factors are essential to the production of a reliable beam of x-ray photons suitable for diagnostic radiography. Which of the following are required for the generation of a diagnostic x-ray beam?

     1. An oil-immersed glass vacuum tube

     2. A wire filament heated by 3 to 5 A of current

     3. A high-voltage circuit (thousands of volts) between the filament and a suitable target

A. 1 and 2

B. 1 and 3

C. 2 and 3

D. 1, 2, and 3

151. What is the total resistance in the circuit diagramed below if $R_1 = 10$ ohms (Ω), $R_2 = 25\,\Omega$, and $R_3 = 40\,\Omega$.

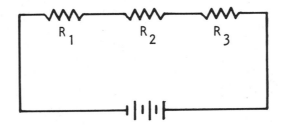

A. $6\,\Omega$

B. $33\,\Omega$

C. $75\,\Omega$

D. $10{,}000\,\Omega$

152. How much power would be consumed by a mobile x-ray unit that had a total resistance of $30\,\Omega$ and was plugged into a power outlet supplied with 220 V?

A. 1.613 kW

B. 6.60 kW

C. 7.33 kW

D. 30 kW

153. In the following radiograph, blurriness of part of the image is probably caused by

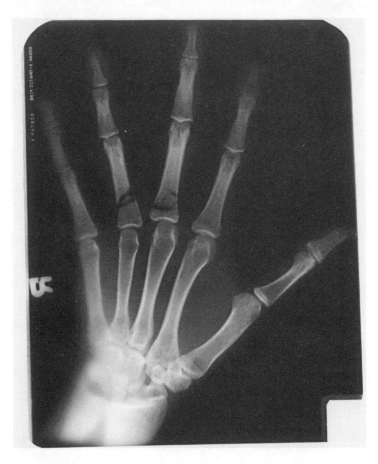

  A. movement of the x-ray tube and film
  B. patient movement
  C. poor film-screen contact
  D. noise due to increased system speed

154. In a Compton scatter interaction between x-rays and matter, the scattered photon retains most of its energy, but some energy is transferred to the electron that is removed from the atom. The amount of energy transferred to the secondary or recoil electron is affected by the

  A. mAs or tube current
  B. density of the material irradiated
  C. angle at which the photon is deflected
  D. atomic number of the material irradiated

155. A variety of materials are used in the construction of the x-ray tube and housing because of the different functions of the individual components. In most modern tubes, a tungsten-rhenium alloy is used in the

- A. filament
- B. rotor assembly
- C. focusing cup
- D. anode target

156. In an x-ray tube, x-ray photons are produced by more than one process. Which of the following occurs in the generation of bremsstrahlung radiation?

- A. An electron approaching a positively charged nuclear field changes direction and loses energy
- B. An electron moves from an outer shell to an inner shell of an atom
- C. A metal is heated to incandescence by a high-amperage current
- D. A high-speed electron interacts with an inner-shell electron of a tungsten atom

157. The image-intensifier tube makes the fluoroscopic image brighter electronically. The output phosphor differs from the input phosphor in that it

- A. is much larger but made of the same crystals
- B. emits electrons where the input phosphor emits light
- C. is considerably smaller than the input phosphor
- D. receives x-rays and the input phosphor receives electrons

158. If the primary side of a step-up transformer consists of 110 turns and the secondary side consists of 13,200 turns, what is the voltage induced in the secondary coil if 220 V of alternating current is supplied to the primary coil?

- A. 1.83 V
- B. 2,640 V
- C. 18.3 kV
- D. 26.4 kV

159. Many modern x-ray units, especially those designed for angiographic procedures, use three-phase generation of x-rays even though this increases the cost of the unit. Three-phase generation is an improvement over single-phase because

1. angiographic contrast is enhanced
2. the quantity and quality of x-rays produced are greater
3. this voltage waveform does not require rectification

- A. 1 only
- B. 2 only
- C. 3 only
- D. 1, 2, and 3

160. In which of the following x-ray interactions with matter does the photon lose some energy and also change direction?

    A. Photoelectric absorption
    B. Compton scattering
    C. Thompson or unmodified scattering
    D. Characteristic secondary

161. The composition of the primary beam is the main factor that dictates the photographic quality of the resulting radiograph, although variation in tissue thickness and condition must also be acknowledged. Which of the following factors *decreases* the total number of photons in the primary beam?

    A. Increasing added filtration in excess of minimum
    B. Three-phase rather than single-phase generation
    C. Increasing the kinetic energy of the cathode electrons
    D. Increasing tube current

162. To convert alternating current to half-wave rectified current requires

    1. no rectifiers
    2. one rectifier
    3. two rectifiers

    A. 1 and 2
    B. 1 and 3
    C. 2 and 3
    D. 1, 2, and 3

163. X-ray technologists adjust the quality or penetrability of the x-ray primary beam by altering the kVp. Increasing kVp increases the percentage of photons that are transmitted through the patient to make up the image. X-ray quality is also specified by HVL. What is the HVL of an x-ray beam, with an initial exposure rate of 120 mR/minute, on which the following measurements were made?

Thickness of added aluminum	Exposure rate
A. 1 mm	82 mR/minute
B. 2 mm	60 mR/minute
C. 3 mm	40 mR/minute
D. 4 mm	30 mR/minute

Questions 164–165 consist of four lettered headings followed by a list of numbered words or phrases. For each crystal listed below, select the imaging method in which it is used. Each lettered method may be used once, more than once, or not at all.

    A. Film-screen radiography
    B. Magnetic resonance imaging
    C. Ultrasonography
    D. Xeroradiography

164. Gadolinium oxysulfide

165. Piezoelectric

166. A technique used to enhance image characteristics by removing unwanted or superimposing anatomic images from a finished radiograph is called

    A. magnetic resonance imaging

    B. xeroradiography

    C. tomography

    D. subtraction

Questions 167–168 consist of four lettered headings followed by a list of numbered phrases. For each cause of radiographic artifacts listed below, select the artifact with which it is usually associated.

    A. Guide shoe marks

    B. Pi lines

    C. Black branch-like marks

    D. Reticulation marks

167. Chemical and dirt buildup on a roller in an automatic processor

168. Improper position of an automatic processor part

POSTTEST—PHYSICS AND EQUIPMENT
ANSWERS, EXPLANATIONS, AND REFERENCES

145. The answer is C. The electromagnetic spectrum comprises various forms of electromagnetic radiation, which travel at the speed of light (186,000 miles/second in air) but have different wavelengths and frequencies. Since velocity is equal to the product of wavelength times frequency, and the velocity of electromagnetic radiation is constant, then as wavelength increases, frequency decreases proportionally. In the electromagnetic spectrum, the longest wavelength and low-frequency radiation are at one end and the shortest wavelengths and higher-frequency radiations are at the other. From longest to shortest wavelength, the range of the electromagnetic spectrum is as follows: radio waves—microwaves—infrared light—visible light—ultraviolet rays—x-rays—gamma rays—cosmic rays. There is some overlap between various forms of electromagnetic radiation on this spectrum. Radiologic technologists should be familiar with the range of useful x-ray wavelengths, 0.1 to 1.0 nm. Because these wavelengths are extremely short, their frequency is proportionally higher (increased) in order to produce the constant velocity (that of the speed of light). Radio waves, important in magnetic resonance imaging, have a longer wavelength and proportionally lower (decreased) frequency. The differing wavelengths and frequencies of various forms of electromagnetic radiation result in different interactions between their photons and matter. *(Bushong, p 53–63; Selman, p 155–157)*

146. The answer is B. The three scales developed for measuring temperature are Fahrenheit (F), Celsius (C), and Kelvin (K). In order to convert °F to °C, the following formula is used: $°C = 5/9(°F-32)$. For the example given in the question, $°C = 5/9(68-32) \rightarrow °C = 5/9(36) \rightarrow °C = 20°$. Therefore, 68°F is equal to 20°C. The following formula is used to convert °C to °F: $°F = 9/5 \ °C + 32$. To convert °C to °K, the following formula is used: $°K = °C + 273$. *(Bushong, p 28–29; Selman, p 30–31)*

147. The answer is B. *Isobars* are atoms that have the same atomic mass but different atomic numbers. They have the same total number of particles in their nucleus, but the number of protons and the number of neutrons is not the same (atomic mass equals the combined number of protons and neutrons in the nucleus; atomic number [Z] equals the number of protons only). If two atoms both have a mass number of 48 but their ratio of protons to neutrons is different (e.g., one has 12 neutrons and 36 protons and the other has 20 neutrons and 28 protons), then they are isobars. *Isotones* are atoms that have the same number of neutrons but different numbers of protons in their nuclei. Their atomic mass numbers and atomic numbers would be different. *Isomers* are atoms that have the same atomic mass number and the same atomic number but differ in their arrangement of nucleons. *Isotopes* are atoms that have the same atomic number but different atomic mass; the nuclei of these atoms contain the same number of protons but different numbers of neutrons. Knowledge of atomic arrangement, structure, and terminology is essential to understanding the fundamentals of chemistry and physics. *(Bushong, p 43–44; Selman, p 43–45)*

148. The answer is A. Ferromagnetic materials are strongly attracted by a magnet. They are very susceptible to becoming magnets themselves because of their high permeability. Examples of ferromagnetic materials are iron, steel, aluminum, and nickel. Paramagnetic materials are only slightly attracted, nonmagnetic materials are not attracted, and diamagnetic materials are actually weakly repelled by magnets. *(Bushong, p 85; Selman, p 94–95)*

149. The answer is B. Heat production at the target, the limiting factor to x-ray tube use, can quickly lead to tube failure. The stationary target was very limited in the amount of heat it could tolerate at one time; consequently, exposures were very long and motion was frequently a problem. By increasing the actual target area 20 to 50 times, the rotating anode increased tube heating capacity 100 to 200 times, thereby permitting larger exposures in very short times. As rotating anode technology improved, effective focal spot sizes were reduced, giving a sharper image with reduced penumbra. *(Bushong, p 114–116; Selman, p 215)*

150. The answer is D. Three basic requirements must be satisfied to produce a diagnostic x-ray beam. The insert must be made of a material that will not greatly attenuate the beam but will permit the massive amounts of heat generated to escape rapidly. Efficient thermionic emission requires a filament-heating circuit of 3 to 6 A. In order to propel the electrons released from the filament to the high-atomic-number target with sufficient speed to produce a primary beam with enough energy to penetrate a typical large body part, between 40,000 and 150,000 V are required. *(Bushong, p 106–114; Selman, p 208–215)*

151. The answer is C. The circuit diagramed in the question is a series type, in which all component elements are placed in a row along the conductor of the circuit. In a series-type circuit, the total resistance in ohms (Ω) is equal to the sum of each of the resistances. In this example, $R_T = R_1 + R_2 + R_3 \rightarrow R_T = 10\Omega + 25\Omega + 40\Omega \rightarrow R_T = 75\Omega$. ($R_T$ = total resistance. R_1, R_2, and R_3 are individual resistors.) *(Bushong, p 78–80; Selman, p 75–78)*

152. The answer is A. In order to determine the power used in the example given in the question, the voltage must be multiplied by the current: power (P) = voltage (V) $\times$ current (I). Since the amount of current in the example is unknown, Ohm's law must first be applied (R stands for resistance):

$$I = \frac{V}{R} \rightarrow I = \frac{220\ V}{30\Omega} \rightarrow I = 7.33 \text{ A.}$$

Now that the current is known, the formula for power is used as follows: $P = IV \rightarrow P = 7.33\text{ A} \times 220\ V \rightarrow P = 1{,}612.6$ W (round off to 1,613), or 1.613 kW would be consumed (1 kW = 1,000 W). *(Bushong, p 78, 82; Selman, p 71–72, 84)*

153. The answer is C. Poor film-screen contact will result in blurred areas in a radiographic image. If an intensifying screen does not have direct, close contact with the film being exposed, then light spreads from the distant screen phosphors before reaching the film, resulting in blurred areas. The causes of this problem are many, including warped cassettes or screens, broken cassette locks (hinges, latches, etc.), worn contact felt, and unwanted particles of matter under or between screens. Poor film-screen contact can be further determined by performing a wire mesh test. This test is done by placing a wire mesh on top of a cassette loaded with film, exposing it to x-rays, and then processing the exposed film from the cassette. On examination, any blurred areas of the wire mesh image signify poor film-screen contact. Movement of the x-ray tube and film, as in tomography, would provide a more uniform and expected blurring across the film with good detail of the anatomy at the fulcrum level. In the radiograph that accompanies the question, patient movement would not likely cause a single blurred area with sharp images surrounding it, as it would be difficult to move only that small isolated area of the hand shown. This is a radiograph of a "phantom" hand (a part of a skeleton has been imbedded in plastic in order to be tissue-equivalent to a human hand), which was completely still on top of the cassette during radiographic examination. (Note: The phantom hand has fractured third and fourth fingers.) Noise or mottle due to fast film-screen combinations would not normally produce an isolated area of blurring as in this radiograph; instead, graininess or mottle related to film or screen construction (inherent in the image receptor) would be observed throughout the image. *(Bushong, p 255–256, 258–259; Chesney and Chesney [1981], p 350–353; Selman, p 290–293, 335–337)*

154. The answer is C. Although a scattered photon retains the greater portion of its original energy, as the angle at which the photon is deflected from its original path increases, more energy is transferred to the secondary, or recoil, electron. Variations of density (quantity per unit volume) or atomic number (number of protons in the nucleus) of the irradiated material are unrelated to energy transfer in a Compton interaction. The mAs, or tube current, is proportional to the number of photons produced but does not affect how energy is transferred in a Compton interaction. *(Bushong, p 158; Selman, p 187)*

155. The answer is D. Originally, the anode target was a simple tungsten button embedded in a copper block—the stationary anode, which limited use of the tube to the thermal load that the tungsten could withstand before it melted. This was followed by the rotating tungsten disk, which improved the heat-loading capability of the tube enormously and left target abrasion as the limiting factor. A molybdenum disk is now in general use with an alloy coating that lasts longer and affords higher-efficiency x-ray production by combining tungsten (atomic number 74) and rhenium (atomic number 75). The filament is constructed of thoriated tungsten; the rotor assembly is copper, steel, plus a metal lubricant; and the focusing cup is molybdenum. *(Bushong, p 110–116; Chesney and Chesney [1984], p 275)*

156. The answer is A. In the generation of bremsstrahlung radiation, a high-speed electron from the cathode is deviated from its original path by the very strong positive nuclear field of a target atom. The cathode electron loses some of its energy as it is slowed down, and that lost energy is emitted as an x-ray photon. An interaction between a high-speed electron and an inner-shell electron of a tungsten atom generates characteristic x-rays. A metal heated to incandescence causes thermionic emission, the method used to produce free electrons in the x-ray tube. Movement by an electron from an outer to an inner shell in an atom also produces a characteristic photon. *(Bushong, p 141–144; Selman, p 161–163)*

157. The answer is C. The output phosphor has a diameter of 1 or 2 inches, whereas the input phosphor may have a diameter of 4, 6, 9, or 14 inches. The output phosphor receives electrons and emits light photons; the input phosphor receives x-rays and emits light photons. The output phosphor crystals are usually zinc cadmium sulfide, and the input phosphor crystals are cesium iodide. *(Bushong, p 294–295; Selman, p 407–408)*

158. The answer is D. In order to solve the problem presented in the question, the transformer law must be applied. This law states that the ratio of voltage induced in the secondary coil to the voltage induced in the primary coil is directly related to the ratio of turns in the secondary coil to the ratio of turns in the primary coil. This may be expressed as $V_s/V_p = N_s/N_p$, where $V_s =$ voltage in the secondary coil (unknown), $V_p =$ voltage in the primary coil (220 V), $N_s =$ the number of turns in the secondary coil (13,200 turns), and $N_p =$ the number of turns in the primary coil (110 turns). In order to determine the unknown voltage induced in the secondary coil (V_s), manipulate the equation as follows:

$$V_s = V_p \left(\frac{N_s}{N_p} \right) \rightarrow V_s = (220 \ V) \left(\frac{13,200}{110} \right) \rightarrow V_s = 220 \times 120 \rightarrow$$

$$V_s = 26,400 \ V \ (1,000 \ V = kV) \rightarrow V_s = 26.4 \ kV.$$

The type of transformer described here is a step-up transformer because it steps up the voltage from the primary coil to the secondary coil. If 110 turns are on the primary side of the transformer and 13,200 turns are on the secondary side, then there are 120 times more turns on the secondary side than on the primary, so voltage induced in the secondary will be increased, or "stepped-up," by a factor of 120 times that of the primary side. *(Bushong, p 97–100; Selman, p 124–127)*

159. The answer is B. A three-phase generator requires three single-phase currents out of step by 120°, or one-third of a cyle. The number of photons produced and the average energy of photons produced are significantly increased because the voltage never drops to zero, the voltage waveform exhibiting less than 5% ripple. This alternating current still requires rectification, usually with 6 or 12 rectifiers. Contrast is actually decreased slightly for any selected kVp, because the average energy of the beam is greater. *(Bushong, p 132–133; Selman, p 263–267)*

160. The answer is B. In the Compton interaction, the incoming x-ray photon removes an outer-shell electron, ionizing the atom and losing some energy in the process. The photon then continues in an altered direction, with an energy loss equal to the energy gained by the removed electron. In photoelectric absorption, all the photon's energy is lost, and it disappears. In Thompson scattering, there is no energy lost although there is a change in direction of the photon. A charactersitic secondary interaction is a process by which x-ray photons are generated. *(Bushong, p 157–160; Selman, p 187)*

161. The answer is A. The purpose of added filtration is to remove nonuseful photons from the primary beam. More total filtration in the primary beam than is required to provide adequate patient protection will require greater electric energy to produce a radiograph of suitable density, as the filter will decrease the number of photons in the beam. Three-phase generation, increasing kinetic energy of electrons (kVp), and increasing tube current (mA) will all *increase* the quantity of photons in the primary beam. *(Bushong, p 149–154; Selman, p 169)*

162. The answer is D. If no rectifiers are used to convert alternating current to half-wave rectified current, the high voltage is applied to the x-ray tube itself, which acts as its own rectifier, passing current from cathode to anode only during the positive half-cycle. When one rectifier (valve tube, vacuum tube diode) is used, current flows through it and then through the x-ray tube from cathode to anode during the positive half-cycle and is suppressed by the rectifier during the negative half-cycle. When two valve tube rectifiers are used, current again is passed only during the positive half-cycle, but the inverse voltage is divided between the two valve tubes, permitting heavier loading of the x-ray tube. A half-wave rectified voltage waveform results from each system. *(Bushong, p 130–131; Selman, p 143–146)*

163. The answer is A. Half-value layer (HVL) is defined as that thickness of an absorber that will reduce x-ray intensity to one-half its original value. In the example given in the question, the original beam intensity was 120 mR/minute, and that value of absorber (aluminum filter) that reduced the beam to 60 mR/minute (one-half the original exposure rate) was 2 mm of aluminum. *(Bushong, p 175; Selman, p 176–178)*

164–165. The answers are 164-A, 165-C. Gadolinium oxysulfide crystals are used in some of the newer intensifying screens available for radiography. Gadolinium oxysulfide is a rare earth type of phosphor that is usually activated with other compounds, causing it to emit light mainly in the green region of the visible-light spectrum, in response to x-ray exposure. Rare earth elements are classified as such because they are not as abundant as other natural minerals, and they are found in the periodic table of elements in group III. The advantage of gadolinium oxysulfide and other rare earth phosphors is their efficiency or speed in converting x-ray energy into visible (fluorescent) light. Rare earth phosphors are faster than most conventional phosphors such as calcium tungstate; their use in imaging allows for decreased exposure times, longer tube life, and a significant reduction in patient dose. Because gadolinium oxysulfide emits mainly green light, special green-sensitive or orthochromatic film must be used with the screens that employ it as a phosphor.

A piezoelectric crystal is the active element of the transducer of an ultrasound unit that is responsible for transmitting and receiving high-frequency sound waves. As the crystal is stimulated by electric energy, it is set into mechanical motion, which produces sound of the same frequency as the electric stimulation it received. When applied to a patient, sound waves are generated and passed through the tissues of the body, some being reflected back to the transducer from tissue interfaces. The piezoelectric crystal can then convert the returning sound waves back into an electric signal that can be viewed and imaged on a television monitor or cathode ray tube. Ultrasonography, a very useful imaging modality, uses ultrasound instead of x-rays in the production of diagnostic images. *(Bushong, p 250–255, 554–588; Chesney and Chesney [1981], p 93–96; Curry et al., p 351–399)*

166. The answer is D. Subtraction is a technique used to remove unwanted images from a finished radiograph by superimposing a positive mask image over a selected negative image. This technique is useful in angiography, especially of cerebral circulation, where many bony structures lie over contrast-filled vessels. The first step in subtraction is to obtain two radiographs, one with contrast media and one "scout" film without contrast media. Ideally, there should not be any patient movement between these two films in order to make the subtraction process as precise and as easy as possible. A positive subtraction mask film is made of the scout film; this mask will be the exact reversal of images from the scout film, and blacks will be white and vice versa. Once the mask is obtained, it is superimposed over the angiogram with contrast until soft tissues and bones are "subtracted," or only faintly seen. The dark images of the mask will cancel out the same light images on the angiogram and vice versa; this is called registration. The contrast-filled vessels that were not on the scout film (therefore not on the mask) will not be cancelled out of the image; instead, they will be enhanced without obscuring bone and soft-tissue structures. A final subtraction print is made following registration of the mask and angiogram. This print will demonstrate the vessels without the superimposition of other structures, in contrast to the original angiogram film. This procedure requires the use of special single-emulsion subtraction film and can be performed using a printer containing a white light source. Some of the principles of subtraction have been applied to digital subtraction angiography, in which a computer-processed image is formed without the use of radiographic film as an image receptor. Magnetic resonance imaging is a newly developed imaging process using magnetic fields and applied radio frequency. Tomography is a commonly employed technique used to take section radiographic images that blur out superimposing anatomic structures above and below the desired body level or fulcrum point, as the x-ray tube and film move in opposing directions during exposure. Xeroradiography is an electrostatic imaging technique that produces blue-toned images following exposure of a part to x-rays, using a special selenium-coated image receptor that is then processed in a special Xerox "dry" processor. *(Chesney and Chesney [1981], p 491–500, 508–518; Curry et al., p 243–261, 290–319, 461–503)*

167–168. The answers are 167-B, 168-A. Pi lines are produced on a film when dirt, gelatin, or chemicals build up on a roller of the automatic processor, marking or staining the radiograph during processing. These lines appear at intervals of approximately 3.14 inches, or one revolution of a 1-inch diameter roller. Guide shoe marks are produced by displaced guide shoes, curved metal plates with grooves that guide the film around a turn. The guide shoes are usually located in the lower portion of a roller rack and constitute the turnaround assembly. If these plates are out of the normal position, they press against the film being processed and produce marks on the film in the direction of film travel. Black branch-like marks on a film are due to static electricity induced during the handling of radiographic film. A lack of humidity increases the possiblity of static artifacts. Reticulation marks can occur when a film is processed in chemical solutions that vary greatly in their temperatures. They appear as a network of weblike grooves, usually across the entire film; these are not generally produced in automatic processors but can occur in manual processing. *(Bushong, p 236–239; Chesney and Chesney [1981], p 232–238; Thompson, p 272–273)*

RADIATION PROTECTION
AND RADIOBIOLOGY

169. The overall response of a cell to ionizing radiation exposure depends mainly on how cell DNA responds. Observable effects following DNA irradiation include

    1. malignant disease
    2. genetic damage
    3. cell death

  A. 1 and 2
  B. 1 and 3
  C. 2 and 3
  D. 1, 2, and 3

170. In order to reduce radiation levels in the diagnostic x-ray room, the federal government has instituted certain performance standards. One standard defines the diagnostic-type protective tube housing as a tube housing constructed so that leakage radiation measured at 1 meter from the source, when the tube is operated at its maximum continuous current for maximum-rated potential, does not exceed

  A. 10 mR/minute
  B. 100 mR/hour
  C. 50 R/hour
  D. 2 R/minute

171. A pregnant x-ray technologist is subject to a maximum permissible dose (MPD) that is different from that of other technologists in order to avoid unnecessary exposure to a member of the general public (the fetus). What is this MPD?

  A. 0.5 mrem
  B. 5 mrem
  C. 50 mrem
  D. 500 mrem

172. Human death from doses of radiation to the whole body comes as a result of damage to three major systems—hematopoietic (hematologic), gastrointestinal, and central nervous systems. Which of the following dose ranges would be anticipated to cause death from damage to the gastrointestinal system?

  A. 75 to 100 rem
  B. 200 to 1,000 rem
  C. 1,000 to 5,000 rem
  D. 4,000 rem or more

173. The National Council on Radiation Protection (NCRP) recommends that the lead equivalent of the fluoroscopic primary barrier meet certain requirements depending on the energy potential of the x-ray unit itself. The recommendation for units capable of operating at 125 kVp or higher is

A. 1.0 mm of lead
B. 1.5 mm of lead
C. 1.8 mm of lead
D. 2.0 mm of lead

174. To reduce the possibility of genetic mutations, patients should be provided with gonadal shielding if

1. necessary clinical information is not obscured
2. the gonads are a few centimeters outside the edge of the x-ray field
3. they have reproductive potential

A. 1 and 2
B. 1 and 3
C. 2 and 3
D. 1, 2, and 3

175. During any fluoroscopic examination, everyone (except the patient) should be wearing a lead apron that covers the trunk and that contains a minimum of 0.25 mm of lead. This recommendation assumes that these people could be exposed to at least

A. 2 mR/hour
B. 5 mR/hour
C. 10 mR/hour
D. 100 mR/hour

176. Therapeutic radiation doses in the thousands of rad are frequently used to kill or control the growth of malignant cells, and yet the $LD_{50/30}$ for humans is in the range of 400 to 500 R. What factors account for this?

1. The amount of body area exposed
2. The methods of measuring radiation dose
3. The treatment schedule

A. 1 and 2
B. 1 and 3
C. 2 and 3
D. 1, 2, and 3

177. Biologic factors have a great effect on the quality of a cell's response to radiation. Which of the following cell types is the least sensitive to radiation?

A. Lymphocytes
B. Erythroblasts
C. Muscle cells
D. Osteoblasts

178. The wall of an x-ray room is designed as a secondary radiation barrier and is expected to shield against

      1. radiation of the useful beam
      2. scattered radiation
      3. leakage radiation

  A. 1 and 2
  B. 1 and 3
  C. 2 and 3
  D. 1, 2, and 3

179. The biologic state of the tissue irradiated affects the total biologic effect resulting from any dose of radiation. Which of the following decreases the radiosensitivity of any tissue?

  A. Youthfulness of the tissue
  B. High metabolic activity of cells
  C. Low proliferation rate of cells
  D. Aerobic tissues

180. After an x-ray interaction with an atom in which an inner-shell electron is removed, another series of events will occur to fill the initial vacancy. The x-ray photons that are emitted when electrons move from one energy level to another to fill that vacancy are called

  A. bremsstrahlung radiation
  B. Compton scattering
  C. pair production
  D. characteristic radiation

181. The principle "patient dose is linearly related to mAs" is helpful to the technologist in choosing exposure factors and imaging systems that provide adequate radiographic density and lowest achievable dose. Which of the following combinations of exposure factors and imaging systems would deliver the lowest patient dose?

  A. Detail, 50-speed system, 200 mAs, 80 kVp
  B. High speed, 200-speed system, 25 mAs, 92 kVp
  C. Par speed, 100-speed system, 100 mAs, 80 kVp
  D. Rare earth, 200-speed system, 50 mAs, 80 kVp

182. The unit used to describe absorbed dose, or the quantity transferred from ionizing radiation to the material through which it passes, is the

  A. roentgen
  B. rad (or gray)
  C. rem
  D. sievert

183. Much information on the effects of ionizing radiation has come from human populations. Which of the following groups have contributed to knowledge of radiocarcinogenesis?

    1. Infants treated for thymus enlargement
    2. Patients who received Thorotrast as a contrast agent
    3. Early cyclotron physicists

A. 1 and 2
B. 1 and 3
C. 2 and 3
D. 1, 2, and 3

184. Of the gas-filled detectors listed below, which can also be used as a personnel monitor?

A. Geiger counter
B. Ionization chamber
C. Proportional counter
D. Scintillation detector

185. There are several types of ionizing radiations, all of which cause the same general kinds of response in tissue but to different degrees. Which of the following compares the response of a specific absorbed dose of any type of radiation to a standard absorbed dose?

A. Protraction
B. Relative biologic effect (RBE)
C. Oxygen enhancement ratio (OER)
D. Linear energy transfer (LET)

186. Our environment is the source of several types of ionizing radiations, both photon and particulate. The source of x-rays is

A. emissions from radioactive decay
B. nuclear reactors
C. interaction of high-speed electrons with metals
D. helium nuclei

187. Individuals who have incurred immediate or short-term effects from exposure to ionizing radiation may have a number of other effects to anticipate. Sequelae to whole-body or local large exposures may include

    1. leukemia
    2. acute radiation syndrome
    3. skin cancer

A. 1 and 2
B. 1 and 3
C. 2 and 3
D. 1, 2, and 3

188. Film badges have been used for personnel monitoring for many years despite some drawbacks associated with their use. Diagnostic technologists are aware of other devices used to monitor personnel exposure (e.g., the pocket ionization chamber and the thermoluminescent dosimeter). Since none is perfect, useful comparisons can be made between them. Which of the following is a disadvantage of film badges?

    A. Low-level exposure (below about 20 mR) cannot be accurately quantified
    B. Daily tabulation of the exposure received is too time-consuming
    C. Exposure in excess of the stated range cannot be measured
    D. They are extremely expensive to read

189. Not all patients who come to the radiology department are capable of the physical cooperation necessary for the completion of the examination. When assistance is required, the best person to restrain the patient during the exposure is the

    A. nurse who is caring for the patient on the unit
    B. technologist responsible for the examination
    C. friend or relative who accompanies the patient
    D. transportation aide who brings the patient to the department

190. In assessing radiation damage to any cell, it becomes important to know at what stage of the cell cycle the irradiation occurred. The stage of the somatic cell cycle that occurs between G_1 and G_2 is called

    A. mitosis
    B. interphase
    C. synthesis
    D. telophase

191. The magnitude of the area of the human body exposed to a large dose of radiation is directly related to the amount of damage received. At what dose range would erythema be anticipated following irradiation of a limited skin area?

    A. 100 to 500 mrad
    B. 0.5 to 100 rad
    C. 100 to 250 rad
    D. 250 to 600 rad

192. The MPD for a radiation worker is the maximum dose of radiation that, if received annually, would not be expected to produce significant radiation effects. The current numeric value for the MPD is

    A. 5 rem/year
    B. 10 to 12 rem/year
    C. 15 rem/year
    D. 100 rem/year

193. Which of the following methods will tend to reduce patient dose?

      1. Using a slow-speed imaging system
      2. Collimating to a specific area of clinical interest
      3. Using relatively low-contrast exposure factors

  A. 1 and 2
  B. 1 and 3
  C. 2 and 3
  D. 1, 2, and 3

194. When a patient with an internal source of radiation requires a diagnostic examination, the technologist might use (in addition to the regular dosimeter) a dosimeter that will show total exposure received as soon as the examination is completed. This second dosimeter will be a

  A. self-reading pocket chamber
  B. film badge
  C. sensitometer
  D. proportional counter

195. In circumstances in which structural shielding or another barrier is not available, technologists can use distance from the source to minimize their exposure. If technologists' exposure at 2 feet from a source is 16 mR/hour, what would their exposure be if they retreated to a position 6 feet from the source of radiation?

  A. 0.56 mR/hour
  B. 1.77 mR/hour
  C. 2.40 mR/hour
  D. 4.00 mR/hour

196. During mobile radiography, technologists will probably receive some exposure. Besides wearing a protective shield, they should also keep exposure low by

  A. using only the small focal spot
  B. making use of the anode heel effect
  C. staying as far from the tube and patient as possible
  D. using a grid imaging system when possible

Questions 197–200 consist of four lettered headings followed by a list of numbered words or phrases. For each numbered word or phrase, select the one heading that is most closely related to it. Each heading may be used once, more than once, or not at all.

  A. Hematopoietic syndrome
  B. Nonthreshold dose-response relationship
  C. Relative risk
  D. Skin cancer

197. Leukemia

198. Long-term response

199. Short-term response

200. Genetic response

POSTTEST—RADIATION PROTECTION AND RADIOBIOLOGY
ANSWERS, EXPLANATIONS, AND REFERENCES

169. The answer is D.   The DNA molecule contains the genetic information necessary for all cell functions, including growth, reproduction, and daily cell activities. Severe damage to cell DNA can cause abnormally rapid mitosis, which, if not repaired, can result in a malignancy. Point mutations can occur, resulting in the transfer of incorrect genetic information to one daughter cell when the cell divides. The most serious damage to the DNA can prevent any normal cell functions from being carried out, and, when the damage cannot be repaired, the cell will die. *(Bushong, p 450-451; National Council on Radiation Protection [NCRP, No. 39], p 33-38)*

170. The answer is B.   The federal government has set certain standards regarding the permissible level of leakage radiation from an operating x-ray tube, primarily to reduce exposure to the patient but also to anyone else who may be in the room during the exposure. All x-ray tubes (radiographic and fluorographic, fixed or portable) are required to comply with the recommendation to ensure that leakage does not exceed 100 mR/hour under any circumstances. *(NCRP [No. 33], p 37; Bushong, p 512)*

171. The answer is D.   The MPD for a pregnant radiation worker to receive throughout the duration of the pregnancy is 500 mrem. This dose limit does not exceed the fetus' own dose-limiting recommendation of 500 mrem/year as a nonoccupationally exposed person. In many institutions, few technologists actually receive more than 500 mrem/year because of care and caution exercised in the workplace, and so it may not be necessary for a pregnant technologist to make any changes in her work habits. A separate radiation monitor may be desirable, however, to record any exposure at the surface of the abdomen. *(Bushong, p 511; NCRP [No. 39], p 92-93)*

172. The answer is C.   At a dose below 100 rem, the acute radiation syndrome would not be expected to occur, although sufficient damage could cause deleterious effects at a later date. A range of 200 to 1,000 rem is usually associated with the hematologic syndrome. The hematologic system is the least radioresistant system and is composed of the bone marrow, circulating blood, and lymphoid tissue. A range of 1,000 to 5,000 rem would involve the intestinal crypt cells and bring about the gastrointestinal syndrome, although there is considerable overlap of syndromes as these dose ranges do not indicate the dose rate or the sensitivity of individuals exposed. A dose of 4,000 rem or more would result in the central nervous system syndrome and ensuing death within hours. *(Bushong, p 467-468; NCRP [No. 39], p 45-47)*

173. The answer is D.   The primary barrier of the fluoroscopic tube is the conventional fluoroscopic screen and carriage or image-intensifier side of the C-arm assembly. In most modern fluoroscopic units, unless the primary barrier is in place, the unit will not generate x-rays. For fluoroscopic units with potential capability greater than 125 kVp, the primary barrier must be equivalent to at least 2.0 mm of lead, and the image-intensifier tube itself must also be adequately shielded. This recommendation is for the safety of both the operator and the patient. *(Bushong, p 513; NCRP [No. 33], p 8)*

174. The answer is D.   The prime objective of every diagnostic x-ray examination is the acquisition of essential information, and gonadal shielding may be used if it does not reduce the amount of information gathered. Females requiring abdominal or pelvic radiographs cannot have their gonads shielded. The gonads should be shielded if there is a possibility of their being exposed to the primary beam, and because x-ray field/light field congruence is rarely exact, shielding should be used if the gonads lie a few centimeters outside of the edge of the light field. All individuals with procreative potential should be shielded, generally up to the age of 40 years for females and 50 years for males. *(Bushong, p 547-549; Frankel, p 106)*

175. The answer is B.   The requirement for wearing protective clothing in fluoroscopy is based on the MPD recommendations. It is believed that exposure above the level of 5 mR/hour in fluoroscopy for a reasonable number of hours each week, plus other routine exposures, could easily add up to an annual exposure of one-quarter of the MPD. The possibility that an individual could receive one-fourth of the MPD defines that person as a radiation worker who should be monitored for radiation exposure. *(NCRP [No. 33], p 12)*

176. The answer is D.   Radiation effects are far more significant as larger areas of the body are exposed. The $LD_{50/30}$ refers to whole-body exposure measured in air at the skin surface. Radiation therapy is directed at the site of disease only, and adjacent healthy tissue is protected from exposure as much as possible. Therapeutic doses are frequently calculated at the target site and are expressed in rads. The $LD_{50/30}$ dose is assumed to be delivered at one time, whereas radiation therapy is delivered as a course of treatment made up of fractions of the total dose. *(Bushong, p 465-466; NCRP [No. 39], p 44-47)*

177. The answer is C.   Of those cell types listed in the question, muscle cells or fibers are least sensitive to radiation exposure, primarily because they do not divide. Lymphocytes, formed in either the lymphoid tissue or in bone marrow, are one of the most radiosensitive types of cells in the body. Erythroblasts, which are immature nucleated RBCs, are less sensitive than lymphocytes but more sensitive than muscle cells. Osteoblasts, which are bone-forming cells, are less sensitive than the blood cells but more sensitive than muscle cells. *(Bushong, p 437; Frankel, p 20)*

178. The answer is C.   Both leakage and scatter are considered secondary radiation, always lower in energy than primary-beam, or useful, radiation. Leakage radiation is that radiation that is emitted from the tube housing in other directions than through the tube port. Scatter occurs when the primary beam strikes any object, and the patient is the most important scatter source in all diagnostic examinations. A secondary barrier requires less shielding material than a primary barrier because it shields against a lower-energy radiation. *(Bushong, p 515; Noz and Maguire, p 150-154)*

179. The answer is C.   When the cells that compose any tissue have a low mitotic or proliferation rate, the radiosensitivity of that tissue is decreased. Generally, the more youthful a tissue is, the more rapidly it is growing and the more radiosensitive it is. The higher the level of metabolic activity and the more oxygenated or aerobic the cells are, the more radiosensitive they are. These concepts were first presented by Bergonié and Tribondeau in 1906. *(Bushong, p 438; Frankel, p 20)*

180. The answer is D.   In the photoelectric process, the x-ray photon loses all its energy in ejecting an inner-shell electron from the target atom, leaving the atom in an ionized state. An electron from an outer shell will move down to fill the inner-shell vacancy, with the emission of a characteristic photon — "characteristic" of the difference in binding energy of each shell involved in the transition. Bremsstrahlung is an x-ray generating process between a cathode electron and the target. Compton scattering and pair production are x-ray interactions with matter. *(Selman, p 185)*

181. The answer is B.   All of the combinations listed in the question would result in equal radiographic density, but the high-speed 200 system only requires 25 mAs, because the system is one of the fastest and the kVp is 92. Increasing either the mAs or kVp will increase radiographic density (doubling mAs doubles density; increasing kVp by 15% doubles density), but increasing mAs increases patient dose linearly and increasing kVp does not. The dose-reducing advantage of a high-speed imaging system can be negated by the choice of high mAs/low kVp exposure factors. *(Bushong, p 245, 547; Frankel, p 108)*

182. The answer is B.   The unit of absorbed dose is the rad (or gray), the rad being the older term. The rad or gray quantifies the amount of energy transferred from any ionizing radiation to any material per unit mass of that material. Biologic effects are related to the absorbed dose. The roentgen is the unit of x-ray intensity or quantity. The rem or sievert are units of dose equivalent. *(Noz and Maguire, p 59, 182; Bushong, p 13)*

183. The answer is A.   Thirty to 40 years ago, radiotherapy was used to shrink a large thymus gland in very young infants. Between 15 and 20 years later, many of those so treated discovered thyroid gland nodules, some of which were malignant. During the 1930s, Thorotrast was a commonly used angiographic contrast agent that contained radioactive isotopes and decay products of thorium. Many cases of liver and spleen cancer became evident 15 to 20 years later. The early cyclotron physicists experienced cataract formation resulting from lens exposure to high-energy particles. *(Bushong, p 489-497; NCRP [No. 39], p 36, 39)*

184. The answer is B.   When personnel are exposed to continuous sources (patients with internal radiation sources), the ionization chamber can be used as a personnel monitor to measure either the amount of radiation per unit of time or the total of all radiation received by the chamber for the measurement period. Unlike the film badge, this method provides immediate dose information. The proportional counter is mainly a laboratory instrument, the Geiger counter is used for field survey, and the scintillation detector is used in the laboratory and in many imaging devices. *(Noz and Maguire, p 22; Bushong, p 517)*

185. The answer is B.   Relative biologic effect (RBE) is defined by the following ratio:

$$\frac{\text{Dose of standard radiation that produces a given effect}}{\text{Dose of test radiation that produces the same effect}}$$

RBE is determined by experiment and depends on many factors relative to the tissue or cell irradiated and to the radiation used. Linear energy transfer (LET) is a measure of the energy transfer rate from the radiation beam to the tissue or cell. LET affects RBE in that RBE increases as the LET of the radiation increases. Oxygen enhancement ratio (OER) refers to the increased radiosensitivity of tissues when they are well oxygenated. Protraction is a means of delivering a dose of radiation at a low dose rate over a long period of time. *(Bushong, p 439, 462-463; NCRP [No. 39], p 29)*

186. The answer is C.   X-ray photons are generated by two processes of energy transfer after the collision of high-speed electrons with a metal target. A helium nucleus (two protons and two neutrons) is also known as an alpha particle, a highly ionizing particle. Ionizing radiations emitted by radioactive materials could be either alpha or beta particles or gamma rays. Nuclear reactors can be used to generate radionuclides or to release energy from an atomic nucleus. *(Bushong, p 140; Selman, p 157)*

187. The answer is B.   Both skin cancer and leukemia have developed in individuals who initially experienced immediate or short-term effects after large doses of radiation. Skin cancer has been documented after a latent period of 5 to 10 years in patients who received radiation therapy. Radiation-induced leukemia was experienced by Japanese people surviving the atomic bombs. The acute radiation syndrome is an immediate or short-term effect of radiation exposure. *(Bushong, p 484, 490-492, 495)*

188. The answer is A.   Each method of monitoring personnel exposure to radiation has its inherent disadvantages. Film badges report exposures below about 20 mR as "M," or minimum exposure, as they are not sufficiently sensitive to assess accurately that small a dose. Daily tabulation of exposure and inability to measure exposures in excess of the stated range are disadvantages of the pocket ionization chamber. The thermoluminescent dosimeter is expensive to read; it requires a costly piece of equipment to determine exposure received by the chip. *(Bushong, p 539-541; Frankel, p 60-69)*

189. The answer is C.   The relative or friend who accompanies a patient to the radiology department is the best person to assist during a radiological procedure. This person is not normally exposed to radiation and, when providing assistance, will be provided with protective clothing and will not be exposed to the primary beam. Other hospital employees could be used for this task, but they are likely to accrue some exposure from portable radiography or from patients with internal radiation sources, and so they should only be called on if there are no other alternatives. The technologist should perform this task only in emergency situations when mechanical restraining devices are not appropriate and no other person is available to assist. *(Bushong, p 545-546; NCRP [No. 33], p 16)*

190. The answer is C.   The synthesis phase, that period in which DNA is synthesized, comes between G_1 and G_2 of the cell cycle. It is during the synthesis phase that the DNA molecule replicates itself, becoming two identical daughter molecules. Interphase is that period of the cell cycle between mitoses (or cell division), including G_1, G_2, and synthesis. Telophase is the last subphase of mitosis. *(Bushong, p 434-435)*

191. The answer is D.   Skin erythema, a reddening of the skin similar in appearance to a sunburn, would be expected at radiation doses greater than 250 rad. As the dose increases above this level, more of the basal skin cells will become damaged or killed, with the initial reaction still being erythema. With higher doses, however, erythema will be followed by ulceration of the outer skin layer (the epidermis), and ulceration could progress to necrosis if the dose were high enough so that no functioning stem cells were left. *(Bushong, p 470-472; NCRP [No. 39], p 49)*

192. The answer is A.   For radiation workers, the current MPD for whole-body exposure, including the gonads and the lens of the eye, is 5 rem/year. In general, the diagnostic technologist receives much less than this maximum, because shielding is always used in fluoroscopy and on portable units. Because shielding is used, exposure levels recorded on personnel monitors indicate a level received only by those parts of the body outside the shielded (trunk) area. *(Bushong, p 508, 510)*

193. The answer is C.   Collimating every radiograph to the specific area of clinical interest requires skill and technical knowledge, but it eliminates unnecessary or unproductive exposure of the patient. Using high-kVp (lower-contrast) exposure factors results in reduced patient dose. The use of 25 mAs and 85 kVp will result in the same radiographic density as 50 mAs and 72 kVp, but with about half the dose. A slow-speed imaging system requires greater exposure to reach the required optical density than does a high-speed system. Use of a slow-speed system would increase patient dose. *(Bushong, p 546-547; Frankel, p 102)*

194. The answer is A.   The self-reading pocket dosimeter (chamber) is a very small ionization chamber with a built-in electrometer to measure the charge received by the device. The device must be charged to a predetermined voltage before use so that the indicator of the reading scale is at zero. Then, as the air becomes ionized, the indicator moves, showing to what extent the device has been discharged. The amount of discharge is proportional to the amount of radiation received and is expressed in milliroentgens. *(Noz and Maguire, p 51; Frankel, p 62)*

195. The answer is B.   Radiation intensity varies inversely with the square of the distance from the source. To solve the problem given in the question, the following formula is used:

$$\left(\frac{\text{Intensity}_1}{\text{Intensity}_2}\right) = \left(\frac{\text{Distance}_2}{\text{Distance}_1}\right)^2.$$

Intensity$_1$ is 16 mR/hour, the original exposure rate. Intensity$_2$ is the unknown new exposure rate. Distance$_2$ is 6 feet, the new distance from the source. Distance$_1$ is 2 feet, the original distance from the source. The following calculations yield the new exposure rate *(Selman, p 343):*

$$\frac{16}{X} = \frac{6}{2}^2 \qquad \frac{16}{X} = \frac{36}{4} \quad 36X = 64 \qquad X = 1.77 \text{ mR/hour.}$$

196. The answer is D.   Because radiation reduces in intensity over distance, simply moving away from a radiation source will reduce one's exposure. Usually, the exposure switch cord of a mobile unit is about 6 feet long, permitting the technologist to make the exposure from a considerable distance. Using the small focal spot or anode heel effect to advantage will not vary dose at all. Using a grid imaging system rather than a nongrid system will increase patient and technologist dose slightly. *(NCRP [No. 33], p 17)*

197–200. The answers are 197-B, 198-D, 199-A, 200-B.   Leukemia is a somatic effect of radiation, but a nonthreshold dose-effect relationship is suggested. This response has been studied extensively in laboratory animals, and much other information has been gained from human populations exposed to radiation from various sources. Radiation-induced leukemia appears to have a short latent period, between 5 and 10 years, but a long at-risk period, thought to be as long as 20 years.

A long-term response to radiation exposure is one that occurs from many months after the irradiation to many years or even a generation afterward. The long-term or delayed effects can be the result of both high-dose acute exposures and chronic low-level exposures spread over a period of time. The very early radiologists who frequently checked the penetrating power of the fluoroscopic beam by examining their own hands are known to have developed skin cancer over a latent period of up to 10 years. Another human population with documentation of radiation-induced skin cancer are therapy patients treated with x-rays up to about 350 kVp.

A major short-term or immediate effect of radiation exposure of the whole body simultaneously is the hematopoietic aspect of the acute radiation syndrome. In this syndrome, after a latent period of several weeks, the numbers of cells circulating in the peripheral blood will have markedly declined. This leads to clinical symptoms of hemorrhage, infection, and weakness. Recovery, if it occurs, may take as long as 6 months to be complete.

There are no direct human data relating to genetic effects of ionizing radiation exposure, although the Japanese survivors of atomic bombing in the 1940s and their progeny have been observed extensively since that time. Information gained from laboratory experiments of animals has shown that a nonthreshold dose-response relationship seems to exist. It was also observed that exposure to radiation affected only the frequency of mutations, not the type or quality of the mutation. *(Bushong, p 466-467, 484, 490-495, 502-503)*

BIBLIOGRAPHY

Armstrong, P., and M. L. Wastie. X-ray diagnosis. Blackwell Scientific Publications, Inc., Boston. 1981.

Austin, M. Young's Learning Medical Terminology Step by Step. C. V. Mosby Co., St. Louis. 1983.

Ballinger, P. W. Merrill's Atlas of Roentgenographic Positions and Radiologic Procedures. C. V. Mosby Co., St. Louis. 1982. Fifth edition.

Bontrager, K., and B. T. Anthony. Textbook of Radiographic Positioning and Related Anatomy. Multimedia Publishing Corp., Denver. 1982.

Boyd, W., and H. Sheldon. An Introduction to the Study of Disease. Lea & Febiger, Philadelphia. 1977. Seventh edition.

Bushong, Stuart C. The Development of Radiation Protection in Diagnostic Radiology. Chemical Rubber Company Press, Cleveland. 1973.

Bushong, S. C. Radiologic Science for Technologists. C. V. Mosby Co., St. Louis. 1984. Third edition.

Cawson, R. A., A. W. McCracken, and P. B. Marcus. Pathologic Mechanisms and Human Disease. C. V. Mosby Co., St. Louis. 1982.

Chaffee, E. E., and I. M. Lytle. Basic Physiology and Anatomy. J. B. Lippincott Co., Philadelphia. 1980. Fourth edition.

Chesney, D. N., and M. O. Chesney. Care of the Patient in Diagnostic Radiography. Blackwell Scientific Publications, Inc., Boston. 1978. Fifth edition.

Chesney, D. N., and M. O. Chesney. Radiographic Imaging. Blackwell Scientific Publications, Inc., Boston. 1981. Fourth edition.

Chesney, D. N., and M. O. Chesney. X-ray Equipment for Student Radiographers. Blackwell Scientific Publication, Inc., Boston. 1984. Third edition.

Chiu, L. C., and R. L. Schapiro. Atlas of Computed Body Tomography: Normal and Abnormal Anatomy. University Park Press, Baltimore. 1980.

Curry, T. S., J. E. Dowdey, and R. C. Murry. Christensen's Introduction to the Physics of Diagnostic Radiology. Lea & Febiger, Philadelphia. 1984. Third edition.

Frankel, R. Radiation Protection for Radiologic Technologists. McGraw-Hill Book Co., New York. 1976.

Frenay, A. C., and R. M. Mahoney. Understanding Medical Terminology. The Catholic Hospital Association, St. Louis. 1984. Seventh edition.

Gray, J. E., N. T. Winkler, J. Stears, E. D. Frank. Quality Control in Diagnostic Imaging. University Park Press, Baltimore. 1983.

Gylys, B. A., and M. E. Wedding. Medical Terminology: A Systems Approach. F. A. Davis Co., Philadelphia. 1983.

Hole, J. Jr. Human Anatomy and Physiology. William C. Brown Co., Publishers, Dubuque, Iowa. 1984. Third edition.

Katzen, B. T. Interventional Diagnostic and Therapeutic Procedures. Springer-Verlag New York, Inc., New York. 1980.

McInnes, J. Clark's Positioning in Radiography. Year Book Medical Publishers, Inc., Chicago. 1974. Ninth edition.

Meschan, I. Radiographic Positioning and Related Anatomy. W. B. Saunders Co., Philadelphia. 1978. Second edition.

Montgomery, W. H., and T. J. Herrin. Student Manual for Basic Life Support. American Heart Association, Dallas. 1981.

National Council on Radiation Protection (NCRP). Medical X-ray and Gamma-Ray Protection for Energies up to 10 meV — Equipment Design and Use. (Report No. 33.) National Council on Radiation Protection, Bethesda. 1973.

National Council on Radiation Protection (NCRP). Basic Radiation Protection Criteria. (Report No. 39.) National Council on Radiation Protection, Bethesda. 1982.

Noz, M. E., and G. Q. Maguire. Radiation Protection in the Radiologic and Health Sciences. Lea & Febiger, Philadelphia. 1979.

Rose, J. S. Invasive Radiology: Risks and Patient Care. Year Book Medical Publishers, Inc., Chicago. 1983.

Selman, J. The Fundamentals of X-ray and Radium Physics. Charles C. Thomas, Publisher, Springfield, Ill. 1978. Sixth edition.

Snopek, A. Fundamentals of Special Radiographic Procedures. McGraw-Hill Book Co., New York. 1975.

Thompson, T. Cahoon's Formulating X-Ray Techniques. Duke University Press, Durham, N.C. 1979. Ninth edition.

Torres, L., and C. Morrill. Basic Medical Techniques and Patient Care for Radiologic Technologists. J. B. Lippincott Co., Philadelphia. 1983. Second edition.

Tortora, G., and N. P. Anagnostakos. Principles of Anatomy and Physiology. Harper & Row, Publishers, Inc., New York. 1984. Fourth edition.

Tortorici, M. Fundamentals of Angiography. C. V. Mosby Co., St. Louis. 1982.

Wroble, E. Terminology for the Health Professions. J. B. Lippincott Co., Philadelphia. 1982.